COVID Chaos Dedications

To those who lost the battle with COVID, you will be remembered.

To all those who fought the battle to save lives through caring for those sick with COVID, who implemented public health measures to decrease the impact of COVID, and who created drugs and vaccines to treat and prevent COVID.

COVID Chaos

What Happened and Why

COVID Chaos

What Happened and Why

Robert J Sherertz
Wake Forest School of Medicine, USA

Jon S Abramson
Wake Forest School of Medicine, USA

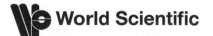

NEW JERSEY · LONDON · SINGAPORE · BEIJING · SHANGHAI · HONG KONG · TAIPEI · CHENNAI · TOKYO

Published by

World Scientific Publishing Co. Pte. Ltd.

5 Toh Tuck Link, Singapore 596224

USA office: 27 Warren Street, Suite 401-402, Hackensack, NJ 07601

UK office: 57 Shelton Street, Covent Garden, London WC2H 9HE

British Library Cataloguing-in-Publication Data
A catalogue record for this book is available from the British Library.

COVID CHAOS
What Happened and Why

ISBN 978-981-126-457-3 (hardcover)
ISBN 978-981-126-560-0 (paperback)
ISBN 978-981-126-458-0 (ebook for institutions)
ISBN 978-981-126-459-7 (ebook for individuals)

For any available supplementary material, please visit
https://www.worldscientific.com/worldscibooks/10.1142/13093#t=suppl

Contents

List of Abbreviations   xv

Foreword   xix

Sherertz – Abramson Collaboration   xxi

Prologue: Overwhelmed Hospitals   xxiii

1. Making of a Pandemic   1

  1. Introduction   1

  2. Coronaviruses — Structure and Replication   3

  3. Evolution of Human Coronaviruses   5

  4. Differences Between Outbreaks, Epidemics and Pandemics   7

  5. Factors Affecting the Severity of a Pandemic   8

  6. Impact of Genetic Mutations on Viral Transmission and
Mortality   12

  7. Containment, Mitigation and Flattening
the Curve   15

  8. Pandemic Waves   16

  References   16

2. Path of Destruction   23

  1. The SARS-CoV-2 Outbreak Begins and Spreads Across the
Globe (December 2019–March 11, 2020)   24

    a. Spread through all regions   30

    b. Initial attempts to contain and mitigate the spread of
SARS-Cov-2 vary across regions and countries   32

    c. WHO Director General declares the COVID-19 pandemic   32

  2. The COVID-19 Pandemic Intensifies (March 12,
2020–December 31, 2020)   35

    a. WHO develops the Solidarity Call to Action and the
Access to COVID-19 Tools Accelerator programs to help
create equity in supplies, drugs and vaccine availability   37

b. Formation of the WHO Task Force to investigate the
origins of SARS-CoV-2   40
3. Success of Containment and Mitigation Policies Vary
Across Regions and Countries   41
a. Asian region with spotlight comparing China and India   43
b. European region with spotlight comparing Sweden
and Norway   45
c. Americas regions with spotlight comparing the United
States and Canada   45
d. African region with spotlight comparing South Africa and
the rest of the region   48
e. Eastern Mediterranean region with spotlight
comparing Iran and Jordan   51
f. Antarctica   54
References   54

3. Disorganized Global Response   **61**

1. Overview   62
a. WHO issues technical reports on how countries can contain
and mitigate the spread of SARS-CoV-2   62
b. Effectiveness of various containment and mitigating steps   64
i. Government policies   64
2. Lessons Learned from How Various Regions/Countries
Responded to the Pandemic   70
a. Asia   70
i. China vs. India   71
b. Europe   76
i. Sweden vs. Norway   78
c. Americas   86
i. US vs. Canada   86
d. Africa   97
i. South Africa vs. the African Region   98
e. Eastern Mediterranean Region   100
i. Iran vs. Jordan   101
3. Conclusions   105
References   109

4. Airborne Assassin   **119**

  1. Clinical Presentations   120
    a. Case #1 — Risk of transmission   121
      i. No symptoms vs. symptoms   121
      ii. Superspreaders   123
      iii. Risk of transmission to healthcare workers   123
      iv. How well do personal protective equipment work?   124
      v. SARS-CoV-2 survival on surfaces   125
    b. Case #2 — Mild COVID-19 pneumonia   126
      i. COVID-19 presentations at Emergency Departments   126
      ii. Laboratory abnormalities   126
      iii. Imaging: Chest computerized tomography
        vs. chest X-rays   129
      iv. Diagnostic testing: PCR vs. antigen vs. antibodies   130
      v. Risk factors for COVID-19 admissions   133
    c. Case #3 — COVID-19 with embolic and thrombotic events   134
      i. Deep venous thrombosis   136
      ii. Pulmonary emboli   138
      iii. Myocardial infarctions and strokes   138
    d. Case #4 — COVID-19 reinfection with fatal outcome   139
      i. Reinfection vs. persistent infection   140
      ii. Treatment effectiveness   142
      iii. Overall impact of treatment on mortality   147
      iv. Ethics   147
    e. Case #5 — MIS-C in children   148
    f. Case #6 — Pregnant females with COVID-19   152
    g. Case #7 — Immunocompromised patients   153
    h. Case #8 — Central nervous system manifestations   154
    i. Case #9 — "Long Haulers" or "Long COVID"   156
  2. Pathogenesis of COVID-19   159
    a. ACE2 receptor   159
      i. Role of binding to ACE2 receptor
        (angiotensin-converting enzyme 2 receptor)   159
    b. Lung disease   161
    c. Heart disease   162

   d. Immune response 165
     i. Are asymptomatic COVID-19 infections due to
      persistent immunity from prior nonSARS-CoV-2
      coronavirus infections? 165
     ii. Are the most severe COVID-19 pneumonias
      a consequence of cytokine storm? 166
   e. Coagulopathy 166
   f. SARS-CoV-2 mutation 167
  References 173

5. Vaccine Salvation? 195

  1. Development of COVID-19 Vaccines 196
   a. Two recent technologies used to make the SARS-CoV-2
    spike protein antigen 201
     i. Viral-vector vaccines 201
     ii. mRNA vaccines 204
  2. SARS-CoV-2 Variants 209
   a. Potential impact of SARS-CoV-2 variants alpha (B.1.1.7)
    and beta (B.1.351) on transmission, Case Fatality
    Rate (CFR) and vaccine efficacy 210
   b. Potential need for repeated vaccination with new
    variant strains 211
  3. COVID-19 Vaccine — Challenges in Delivery and Distribution 212
   a. WHO develops programs to create equitable vaccine
    distribution 212
     i. Solidarity program and access to COVID-19 tools
      (ACT)-Accelerator programs 213
     ii. COVAX — COVID-19 vaccine access program
      and facility 214
   b. Prioritizing groups for vaccination 219
     i. High risk including elderly and healthcare workers 221
     ii. Do people known to have been infected with
      SARS-CoV-2 need vaccination or can they wait? 223
   c. Delivery of vaccines to vaccinations sites 223
     i. How well did various countries do in rolling
      out vaccines? 224

4. Vaccine Hesitancy 228
   a. Overview of issues impacting vaccine hesitancy 228
   b. COVID-19 and vaccine hesitancy 229
      i. Examples of vaccine hesitancy across regions
         and countries 231
      ii. How vaccine hesitancy in one region can affect
         another region 233
   c. Overcoming vaccine hesitancy 235
5. Conclusion 237
References 238

6. **Collateral Damage** **249**

1. Introduction 250
2. Impact on Birth Rate 250
3. Impact on Other Diseases 251
   a. Drug shortages 251
   b. Declining outpatient visits and elective surgeries 251
   c. Increasing TB, malaria, HIV, and sexually
      transmitted infections 252
   d. Decrease in vaccination rate for routine
      preventable diseases 252
   e. Decreased in incidence of influenza and RSV
      infections 253
   f. Psychological impact: Community and healthcare workers 254
   g. Excess deaths due to COVID-19 versus other causes 255
4. Misinformation, Countering Misinformation 257
5. Ethical Issues 258
   a. Drug trials 258
   b. Equipment shortages 258
   c. Racial disparities 259
   d. Prisoners 260
   e. Immigrants 261
   f. Vaccines 261
      i. Exclusion of pregnant women 262
      ii. Vaccine passports 264
      iii. Jumping the line for vaccines 266

iv. Should vaccines be mandated?   267
v. Countries using vaccines to advance their
    foreign policy agenda   268
g. School closure — Impact on children, families
    and teachers   270
6. Conclusion   272
References   273

7. Origin Story   287

1. What is an Infectious Disease?   288
2. What is an Emerging Infectious Disease (EID)?   288
3. When and Where did COVID-19 Become an EID?   288
4. What was the Source of SARS-CoV-2?   288
5. Why are Bats the Likely Animal Long-term Host for
   SARS-CoV-2?   290
6. Is there an Intermediate Host for SARS-CoV-2?   291
7. How does COVID-19 Compare with Other
   Coronavirus-caused Infections?   293
8. Does the Recent Appearance of More Lethal
   Coronaviruses Globally Suggest that these Viruses have
   the Ability to Evolve Rapidly?   294
9. Is there any Possible Explanation for How a Coronavirus
   can Suddenly Appear in the Human Population and
   Cause Disease?   295
10. Are these Three New Coronavirus-caused EID (COVID-19,
    MERS, SARS) Isolated Events, or Are they Part of a Larger
    Global Phenomenon?   296
11. What Risk Factors can Play a Role Increasing the
    Likelihood of an EID Event?   299
    a. Transition to an agricultural society   299
    b. City size   300
    c. War   300
    d. Famine   301
    e. Slavery   301
    f. Colonization   302

  g. Ignorance = Undiscovered 302
  h. Climate change 303
 12. Summary 303
 References 304

8. **Pantheon of Plagues** **317**

 1. Epidemiology Definitions 317
  a. What defines an outbreak, an epidemic or a pandemic? 317
 2. Outbreaks 321
 3. Epidemics 324
 4. Pandemics 335
 5. Superspreaders 354
 6. Global trends 357
 7. Summary of Factors Leading to Pandemics 361
 References 364

9. **Are There Geopolitical Solutions?** **403**

 Introduction 403
 1. Improve WHO and member countries pandemic
  capabilities 404
 2. Determine the impact of mitigation strategies on
  global economies 409
 3. Study the relationship between longCOVID and
  persistent SARS-CoV-2 infection 411
 4. Evaluate the relationship between the immune system
  and 2nd SARS-CoV-2 infections 412
 5. Find ways to decrease global vaccine inequity 413
 6. Improve education for all ages during a pandemic 416
 7. Understand the importance of bat reservoirs related
  to SARS-CoV-2 evolution and human adaptation 416
 8. Investigate the reasons for the asymptotic increase
  in global epidemic/pandemic infectious diseases 420
 9. Learn from all countries how best to handle future
  pandemics (investigation, early mitigation, global
  treatment trials, vaccine development and deployment) 422
 References 424

10. Epilogue   **431**

  1. COVID-19 Pandemic Continues   432
    a. Endemic disease is likely   434
    b. Excess mortality   435
  2. COVID-19 Vaccines   435
    a. Global availability   435
    b. Impact of SARS-CoV-2 variants   436
  3. Collateral Damage   438
    a. Economic impact   438
    b. Other (non-COVID vaccines) vaccination programs   439
    c. Tuberculosis, HIV, and malaria control and mortality   439
  4. COVID-19 Clinical Updates   440
    a. Immunocompetent adults   440
    b. Long-COVID = Persistent infection   441
    c. Immunocompromised patients   442
    d. Treatment effectiveness   443
  5. SARS-CoV-2 Mutations   445
  6. SARS-CoV-2 Origin: Revisited   446
  References   447

11. The Human Side   **459**

Acknowledgments   479
Index   481
Figures and Tables   505

List of Abbreviations

ACE 2 receptors:	angiotensin 2 receptors
ACT-Accelerator:	(Access to COVID-19 Tools)-Accelerator
AIDS:	Acquired Immunodeficiency Syndrome
ARDS:	Adult Respiratory Distress Syndrome
ASTM:	American Society of Testing and Materials
BARDA:	Biomedical Advanced Research Development Authority
BMGF:	Bill and Melinda Gates Foundations
CAC:	coronary artery calcium
CDC:	Centers for Disease Control and Prevention (United States)
CD4:	type of lymphocyte defined by surface glycoprotein 4
CD8:	type of lymphocyte defined by surface glycoprotein 8
CEPI:	Coalition for Epidemic Preparedness Innovation
CFR:	case fatality rate
CK:	creatinine kinase
CNS:	central nervous system
COVAX:	COVID-19 Vaccine Access Program and Facility
COVAX AMC:	COVAX Advanced Market Commitment
COVID-19:	coronavirus disease of 2019, the pandemic caused by SARS-CoV-2 virus
CRP:	C-reactive protein
CT:	Computerized Tomography
CTA:	Computerized Tomography Angiogram
DDT:	dichlorodiphenyltrichloroethane, a pesticide
DNA:	deoxyribonucleic acid
DTP:	diphtheria tetanus pertussis
DVT:	deep venous thrombosis
ED:	emergency department
EEG:	electroencephalogram

EID:	Emerging Infectious Disease
EMA:	European Medicines Agency
EN:	European standard for surgical masks
ESR:	erythrocyte sedimentation rate
EU:	European Union
EUA:	Emergency Use Authorization (United States)
FDA:	Food and Drug Administration (United States)
GAP:	Global Alliance Partners
GDP:	gross domestic product
Gavi:	Global Alliance for Vaccines and Immunizations
H:	Hemagglutinin protein
HCW:	healthcare workers
HIV:	human immunodeficiency virus
HR:	hazard ratio, statistical measure of risk
ICU:	intensive care unit
IFR:	infection fatality rate
IgA:	immunoglobulin type A, type of antibody
IgG:	immunoglobulin type G, type of antibody
IgM:	immunoglobulin type M, type of antibody
IOAC:	Independent Oversight and Advisory Committee
IHR:	International Health Regulations
IMF:	International Money Fund
LDH:	lactate dehydrogenase
MERS-CoV	the coronavirus causing the Middle East Respiratory Syndrome outbreak
MHRA	Medicines and Healthcare Regulatory Agency (United Kingdom)
MIS-C:	Multisystem Inflammatory Syndrome in Children
MRI:	magnetic resonance imaging
mRNA:	messenger RNA vaccines
MRSA:	methicillin resistant *Staphylococcus aureus*
N:	Neuraminidase protein
N95:	filters 95% of airborne particles (NIOSH)
NIH:	National Institutes of Health (United States)
NIOSH	National Institute for Occupational Safety and Health
O_2	oxygen

OR:	odds ratio, statistical measure of risk
OxCGRT:	Oxford Coronavirus Government Response Tracker
PCR:	polymerase chain reaction
PE:	pulmonary embolus
PFR:	population fatality rate
PMN:	polymorphonuclear, type of white blood cell
PPE:	personal protective equipment
PHEIC:	Public Health Emergency of International Concern
PMH:	past medical history
PREDICT:	Pandemic Preparedness for Global Health Security (USAID iniative)
PREVENT:	Pregnant Women & Vaccines against Emerging Epidemic Threats
R_0:	basic reproductive number, a measure of contagiousness
RCT:	randomized controlled trial
RNA:	ribonucleic acid
RRT:	renal replacement therapy
RSV:	respiratory syncytial virus
SAGE	Strategic Advisory Group of Experts on Immunization
SARS:	Severe Acute Respiratory Syndrome
SARS-CoV-1:	also known as SARS-CoV, the coronavirus strain that caused the 2002–2003 Severe Acute Respiratory Syndrome outbreak
SARS-CoV-2:	coronavirus strain causing the COVID-19 pandemic
STI:	sexually transmitted infection
TB:	tuberculosis
UK:	United Kingdom
UN:	United Nations
UNICEF:	United Nations Children's Fund
US:	United States of America
USAID:	United States Agency for International Development
VDRL:	Venereal Disease Research Laboratory, test for syphilis
VoC:	variants of concern
WHA:	World Health Assembly
WBC:	white blood cell
WHO:	World Health Organization

Foreword

This book focuses on events that occurred in 2020–2021, during the COVID-19 pandemic.

The Prologue provides a first-person account from three physicians working in hospitals during the first six months of the pandemic when healthcare systems were overwhelmed with those seeking care and there was inadequate manpower, equipment and supplies to provide care for all the patients.

Chapter 1 provides background information about the SARS-CoV-2 virus causing the COVID-19 pandemic and various basic concepts that are useful for describing the transmission, morbidity and mortality caused by the virus.

Chapters 2 and 3 detail what happened in various regions and countries during the first year of the pandemic and why some countries were able to contain/mitigate the spread of the virus reasonably well while others were unable to do so. The figures in these chapters show timelines of various aspects of the pandemic through the end of December 2020.

Chapter 4 details clinical aspects of COVID-19 disease, testing, treatment and long-term symptoms that have persisted in some patients.

Chapter 5 describes the development and use of COVID-19 vaccines and problems related to distribution, delivery and vaccine hesitancy. The timetable of some of the figures extends into 2021, since these vaccines first became available for use in countries beginning in December 2020.

Chapter 6 examines the indirect impact the COVID19 pandemic had on other infectious and non-infectious diseases.

Chapters 7 and 8 look at historically important infectious diseases that cause epidemics and pandemics that help frame our understanding of the current pandemic.

Chapter 9 examines some possible solutions to problems that arose during this pandemic that could allow us to better deal with the ongoing and future pandemics.

Chapter 10, The Epilogue, contains important updates during the time frame January 2022 through mid 2022, including figures that contain global maps of the COVID-19 cases and deaths per capita and distribution of COVID-19 vaccines in each country.

Chapter 11 includes various pictures that visually show aspects of the pandemic and the physical and emotional impact it had on people across the world.

Sherertz – Abramson Collaboration

Drs. Sherertz and Abramson have a common heritage at Wake Forest University School of Medicine (WFUSM) that goes back 30 years, culminating in this effort to write about the COVID-19 pandemic in real time. During their many years of friendship, Drs. Sherertz and Abramson worked together on outbreak investigations, educational initiatives, and in 2009, when the influenza pandemic occurred, they collaborated to make WFUSM one of the first medical schools in the US to require mandatory flu vaccines. Both Drs. Sherertz and Abramson are Emeritus Professors of WFUSM.

In 1968, Dr. Sherertz went to Wake Forest University, in 1972, attended the University of Virginia for medical school and his Internal Medicine Residency (1972–1979), and from 1979–1982, attended the University of North Carolina School of Medicine for his adult Infectious Disease Fellowship. In 1982, Dr. Sherertz joined the Division of Infectious Diseases in the Department of Internal Medicine at the University of Florida School of Medicine, where he was the Hospital Epidemiologist, in charge of all outbreak investigations, and became the National President of the American Society of Microbiology Division of Nosocomial Infections. In 1988, he joined the faculty in the Section of Infectious Diseases, Department of Medicine at WFUSM, initially as the Hospital Epidemiologist, and later in his career, he became the Chief of Adult Infectious Diseases (1997–2006). Pertinent to this book, Dr. Sherertz did 30 years of research focused on the pathogenesis of hospital acquired infections and the mechanism of transmission of many microorganisms, but mainly *S.aureus*. Between 1983 and 2007 he published a series of papers about how *S.aureus* is transmitted in the hospital setting, particularly through the air, culminating in NIH funding to investigate "Cloud Adults", airborne superspreaders of *S.aureus* in the setting of nasal rhinovirus infection. Dr. Sherertz has taught 3 university courses in Microbial Pathogenesis, and in the last two years, been involved with the care of more than 100 hospitalized COVID-19 patients, as part of his role in teaching Internal Medicine and Family Practice Residents.

Dr. Abramson graduated from Boston University in 1972, attended WFUSM for medical school and a pediatrics residency (1972–1979), and did his pediatric Infectious Diseases Fellowship at the University of Minnesota (1979–81). Dr. Abramson joined the faculty at WFUSM in the Department of Pediatrics Section of Pediatric Infectious Diseases. He served as Chair of the Department of Pediatrics from 1996–2014. His research interests included studies on how influenza virus affects neutrophil function and how to optimize vaccine use in children. He was elected President of the US Society for Pediatric Research in 1995. Dr. Abramson's mid and late career has increasingly focused on first national, and then international pediatric vaccine issues. From 1995–2003 he was a member and later Chair of the American Academy of Pediatrics Committee on Infectious Diseases that writes the Red Book that serves as an important reference for pediatricians on the prevention, diagnosis and treatment of pediatric infectious diseases. From 2003–2007 he was appointed as a member and later Chair of the US CDC Advisory Committee on Immunization Practices (ACIP). Internationally, he has worked on various WHO-related committees, including as a member and later Chair of the Strategic Advisory Group of Experts on Immunization (SAGE) from 2009–2016, Chair of the Gavi 2021–2025 Vaccine Investment Strategy Steering Committee (2017–2018), Chair of the Global Alliance (WHO, Gavi, UNICEF, Bill and Melinda Gates Foundation and PATH) Vaccine Innovation Prioritization Strategy Committee (2018–2020) and a member of the WHO COVID-19 Vaccine Target Product Profile working group (2020–2021). Pertinent to the current "COVID Chaos: What Happened and Why", he previously wrote the book, "Inside the 2009 Influenza Pandemic."

Prologue: Overwhelmed Hospitals

"I felt totally helpless, because more and more people with respiratory symptoms were coming... It was like a tsunami movie where you see the wave coming and no one is doing anything."

Victor Pedrera, a doctor from a healthcare centre in the Spanish port city of Alicante

COVID-19: Three Physician First-Person Accounts

The COVID-19 Pandemic has been very difficult for the general public to understand. Politicians were overwhelmed, so they often blamed others, including other countries, other politicians, scientists, doctors, and even their predecessors. Public Health authorities were overwhelmed and made many mistakes early on because they never had to deal with anything like this before. Many hospitals were overwhelmed as they found themselves having to cancel admissions for surgeries or non-COVID problems, forbidding families from being with their dying loved ones and dealing with situations involving mass casualties, with no end in sight. Doctors, nurses and other healthcare workers quickly found themselves overwhelmed due to exhaustion, short staffing, and an unimaginable number of patient deaths. The media tried to cover what was going on but found themselves shut out or being given sanitized versions of what was actually happening, and even worse, they sometimes misreported or politicized the information they had. In actual fact, what was going on in hospitals was much more akin to a war zone disaster than hospital medicine.

We asked three physicians who worked in these COVID hospital war zones to give their perspective on what it was like. The first was a fellow at a midwestern hospital in the United States (US) until she was told to cease her fellowship activities and report to an inpatient medical ward to

begin caring for COVID-19 patients. The second was an internal medicine physician when he decided to volunteer for two weeks in a New York City hospital during the time that they were overwhelmed. The third was a physician at a small hospital in India. All physicians and hospital names are withheld due to retaliations that have already occurred. These are their accounts. Code blue = cardiac arrest.

COVID Wards, Midwestern Hospital, US

Since my childhood I wanted to be a doctor. I never considered any other path. I moved to the US to pursue the American Dream and made it happen. The United States is where medical miracles happen. Where evidenced based medicine is above all. Where we save people. Where there is no diagnosis that is a mystery, and there is always a "Dr. House" with all the answers at every institution. Where I take pride to practice medicine.

How can COVID-19 be so devastating in this powerful country? Why do we not know what to do? Why are we so vulnerable? Why do I feel like I've been punched in the gut every day?

COVID made me feel so angry!

Angry at the virus.

Angry for impacting my subspecialty training.

Angry at feeling isolated, at having to stay at a hotel alone.

Angry I cannot go home to my two toddlers and hug them because I might infect them. Angry that if my husband and I get sick or die, who will care for our children?

Angry I have to stay away from co-workers for fear of getting or sharing the disease.

Angry that my patients are isolated, so alone. Angry because I cannot be with them all the time. Angry that families cannot visit.

Angry that it takes an extra minute to don PPE (personal protective equipment) before I can rush into a "code blue". What if that extra minute causes their death?

It made me bargain!

If I make it through the shift without a "code blue", I will not be angry for being isolated.

If my family stays healthy, I will not be angry for spending time away from my family and losing out on my subspecialty training.

If my patient makes it through the night, I will try not to wake up angry. Yet...

Still, so many code blues.

Still so much anger.

In denial again: ...but Mrs. Smith was just fine 2 minutes ago. If she makes it without intubation, I will not be angry that she is so alone. I will not be angry that I cannot stay in her room. I will stand outside her room and she will know I am there. I am sure she knows... I AM HERE.

It made me feel depressed!

Face shields and goggles hide tears that can also be blamed on the disinfectant.

Wearing two masks hides your voice cracking while breaking bad news to families.

Talking to patients and families is important, but sometimes I only manage being there without talking.

Isolation is depression, for me, for the patient.

Debriefing is important, if I can go through it. Having a purpose helps.

Opening windows while driving helps, but just for a moment.

On rare days I can accept!

We are strong and resilient

Our patients depend on us.

Isolation is temporary.

People survive code blues.

I was put in this place to do what I am doing now. It is a privilege to do what we do.

The human body is resilient. We will unite and win.

COVID-19 made us stronger. We have learned more, we have become more appreciative of what we have.

In the end, I wondered: Is this a dream?

If patients worsened on a general medical ward, they were upgraded to either a stepdown unit or ultimately an intensive care unit (ICU) where the highest intensity of care Is provided.

COVID ICUs, New York City Hospital, US

In April 2020, while practicing in my hospital in the US, I began contacting colleagues in New York City. They described horrific numbers of deaths due to COVID-19. We had not seen our first case at my hospital, and this made me feel like I should be working right alongside these pandemic doctors.

Two events triggered me to action. The first event was the governor of New York urgently calling for physicians from other states to come help without the need for a medical license. The second event was when a physician risked her career by recording a video that showed refrigerator trucks containing piles of dead bodies in body bags (due to the hospital morgue being full) and an emergency room full of patients on ventilators because there was no room in their ICUs. She said they were downplaying the severity of the pandemic and that it was only going to get worse. It was a cry for help!

I felt I could no longer sit idly by and called a friend at a large hospital in New York City to help me get emergency credentialing. They told me I was their first volunteer physician. When I spoke on the phone to the medical officer aiding in my credentialing, a nephrologist, I could hear the desperation in her voice. She explained that in spite of FEMA (Federal Emergency Management Agency), there simply weren't enough ventilators or dialysis machines. They had reached the point of rationing life support.

I arrived at my airplane check-in to go to New York City and there were only seven people waiting for the flight, all wearing masks. Everyone's eyes showed concern and fear. The whole trip, I heard no laughter, no conversations, just unnerving silence. After landing in NYC, I walked through an empty airport and was picked up by my friend, a critical care physician. She had just gotten off her shift and looked exhausted, both in her stance and tone of voice. A once energetic and upbeat soul, my friend explained that she had been working for at least two weeks straight in the ICUs due to several colleagues contracting the virus.

My friend drove me to my hotel, which the hospital system I would be volunteering in, had reserved in its entirety for staff who chose to live apart from their families during the pandemic. On the way there, the streets were eerily empty, rather than the usual bumper-to-bumper traffic and a sea of people talking on their cellphones. Upon checking in, the hotel clerk informed me that I was only their third guest in spite of their 100-room capacity. By the time I left, the number of guests had increased to 20; none of us ever spoke to each other or got any closer than 25 feet.

The next morning, I drove to the hospital and obtained my identification badge with the label "Voluntary Physician". The person handing me the badge told me I must be either a saint or the craziest person she had ever met. I was then thermally scanned and directed inside to collect scrubs from a vending machine. Next, I was given a bag with my daily PPE, one N95 mask, and a surgical mask to be worn over the N95 mask; neither could be removed all day except when eating. There followed a crash course in their EMR (electronic medical record), which I had never used before, and it was quite complex. Finally, I was assigned to shadow my friend for a day in the critical care unit so that I could learn the routine.

Walking into the ICU, I felt as though I was in a dystopian novel. Every member of the team, including myself, was wearing an N95 mask with a surgical mask over it, a bouffant cap, a face shield, a plastic gown, as well as gloves and shoe covers. The only part of us visible was our eyes, and those eyes spoke volumes about exhaustion. Before this trip, I had never seen healthcare providers working together with such intense determination toward a common goal. I felt immediate respect, but also intimidation, wondering whether I would measure up.

For every patient, we rounded as a team, nurse, resident, fellow, and attending. Every single patient was intubated because of COVID. Most were also receiving dialysis. Almost all were on vasopressors (medications to raise blood pressure). One patient, in particular, caught my eye, a 24-year-old Hispanic male who was maxed out on three vasopressors and receiving ECMO (where blood is run through a machine outside the body to provide oxygenation because the lungs can't do it). I was shocked to see such a young person so sick; by the end of that day, the patient had died, along with several other patients. I also learned over the course of that day that at that point in the pandemic, no one really knew how to treat this infection. All they could do was just treat the complications as they developed. At the end of my shadowing day, I was given my long-term assignment of helping out an ICU in another one of the health system's hospitals in the Bronx.

I arrived the next morning at the ICU to which I had been assigned. This particular ICU had previously been a telemetry unit for patients requiring heart monitoring and was not equipped to be an ICU. The nurses worked in a 4:1 patients-to-nurse ratio (usually 2:1), and there was only one ICU-trained nurse on this unit that housed over 65 intensive care unit patients. Each room was only intended for one person, yet housed two patients on ventilators provided by the FEMA (Federal Emergency Management Agency). The physician call rooms on that floor had been modified to hold patients and had become patient rooms as well. We continued to add more rooms during my stay, but more patients did not mean more providers. Instead, it simply meant that we had more people to take care of without any additional support.

I was introduced to the physician team, which consisted of one pulmonary-critical care attending, one fellow, and three residents. This team was caring for far more patients than under normal circumstances, but they didn't seem to notice. While their exhaustion was physically evident, their motivation and determination to help others allowed them to push through.

This particular ICU had been struggling harder than other nearby ICUs in the previous few weeks of the surge due to inadequate staffing, and the sight of me created brief euphoria. Upon my arrival, I shared with the team that the world had been watching and respected their work and that I would provide any help I could. They were so happy to see extra support that the critical care fellow took my picture and sent it out to a large group of physicians to announce that help had arrived. It seemed my presence alone had already done something positive.

My assignment was to act as a supporting physician by managing up to ten patients in collaboration with the critical care attending and aiding the other physician members in any way possible. This included performing bedside procedures, such as central line placements and other standard ICU procedures. My first procedure was placing a dialysis catheter in a woman who needed emergent dialysis. The patient's skin felt as though she was on fire — her temperature was almost 109°F despite antipyretics and ice packs being all over her. Her fiery skin was to foreshadow the myriad ways this virus could bring about death.

Rounding on patients was a continuous circuit. We moved to our first patient and drew the necessary blood for laboratory studies, titrated the vasopressors, the analgesia (pain medications) and sedation, adjusted the ventilator settings, and then moved on to the next, and so on until it was time to start over. We had to run our blood samples down to the laboratory ourselves due to short staffing. With so many patients and so few providers, we all had to work together and accept that all providers must play all roles, else the team would fail. We rapidly ran out of certain medications such as fentanyl and versed, and we had to find alternatives. We did not have enough pumps to provide artificial nutrition through feeding tubes in the normal continuous way, so every patient received bolus feeding. If the patients stooled in bed, we all pitched in to clean them.

Between these encounters were orders for medicines and tests, EMR notes to be written, and routine code blues. A code blue is when someone's heart stops beating, and providers have to initiate CPR in an attempt to restart the heart. Under normal circumstances, attempts at resuscitation are unlikely to be successful, and this seemed even more true with COVID. If the heart did restart, it usually stopped again soon, and the patient would finally die. We had so little time that we could not continue CPR for very long, or we would neglect other patients. Sometimes there were more codes than personnel to run them, and so some patients just died without resuscitation attempts. Each CPR event exposed us to more COVID aerosolization, with many providers becoming ill or dying while I was there.

If the code blue was unsuccessful, the patient was pronounced deceased, and the staff would call down to the morgue and ask if it was still at capacity. I had never heard anyone ask that question — one more sign of how different this was from normal ICU medicine. If the morgue was still at capacity, then the deceased patient needed to be taken to the refrigerator trucks, where bodies in dark body bags were stacked one on top of another. When full, these trucks would take the bodies to Hart Island, where they would be either cremated or buried in a mass grave. Each family was allowed only two family members present for the state-run funeral. Then, instead of debriefing as a team or taking a moment to reflect, we would simply fill that empty bed with yet another COVID patient that was intubated and seemingly waiting to die.

The entire hospital was closed to the public, and thus, it was our responsibility to contact the families of each patient daily by phone, typically 5 to 15 minutes per patient per day. Some of the families were understanding, but most were fearful and blameful. We had taken away their ability to see for themselves what was happening, and as a consequence, there was an intense amount of distrust. As a specialist in Palliative Medicine, I normally felt comfortable with end-of-life discussions, but I had never encountered such a high level of distrust. Every family demanded to know if their loved one had received all the experimental drugs that they had heard about on the news. Some of the family discussions were truly difficult, up to and including conspiracy theories.

The first few days, I didn't pay attention to the number of code blues we performed except to note that it was high. On day five, I decided to make a tally every time we performed CPR, and I subsequently recorded an average of just over one code per hour on our unit. Almost all of these eventually resulted in death, a body bag thrown into a truck on top of other bodies, with the bed immediately filled by another sedated, unresponsive COVID patient on life support. It was on this day that one of the nurses broke down and cried on my shoulder. She proclaimed that she had been working 12-hour shifts for 14 straight days and had no idea why she kept doing this when everyone died anyway.

Moving on from a death without any pause was difficult, but it was even more difficult when one of those deaths had been your colleague who had been working by your side only days earlier. For me, the hardest death was seeing a resident physician die. As an attending who regularly taught resident physicians and students, I can only compare that feeling to the scenario of watching an innocent child die, a child who has not yet had the opportunity to live a real and full life. To witness someone in the beginning of their career taken so quickly and unfairly makes you realize that this virus truly does not discriminate.

After the nurse cried on my shoulder, the endless stream of deaths suddenly seemed more apparent. I went to the emergency department only to see a patient heading toward my ICU and found that I had to push carts full of dead bodies out of my way just to get to my patient. It was horrific. It became clear that a significant number of patients never reached the ICU; they just died alone in the emergency room and were left there until they could be moved into a refrigerator truck. It felt more like a war zone than a hospital; COVID had taken the thing most precious to us, our humanity. Sometimes it felt as if God himself had left us entirely.

After each 12-hour shift, I went back to my hotel and allowed the emotions to hit me. I cried for the deceased who had to suffer so needlessly. I cried for the exhausted providers because there was no end in sight. I cried for the families who suffered from a distance while their loved ones died alone and isolated. I especially cried for the nurses, physicians and other staff who lost their lives trying to fight this virus. One unfortunate nurse who succumbed to the virus was so dedicated that her last words prior to intubation were: "You forgot to set up the suction."

I spent only a short time in New York City compared to the amazing hero clinicians that had already worked weeks in the non-stop chaos I experienced, but a part of me was lost forever in that city. We spent every day trying to save lives only to find that the vast majority of our ICU patients never left that unit alive. Every day we made decisions about who got the ventilators and dialysis, and those that didn't get them died almost immediately. No person can be the same after that. There were even more horrific things that I intentionally chose not to include in this recount simply because they were and are too painful.

After I returned home, I was asked to give talks to different groups. In every talk I was asked if COVID was really as bad as the media was saying, or was it simply overhyped as a fear tactic. Each time I gave the same reply, COVID was not like the media portrayed it — it was much worse.

Late in the pandemic, India had an explosion of cases that overwhelmed many of their hospitals. A physician working with COVID-19 patients provided the following account.

Small Community Hospital, Rural India

I am a physician who works in a hospital in rural India. In March 2020, we went into coronavirus lockdown, and the fear of the virus came and has not left. It permeates all our activities. If you went to a market to buy some food, people would stare at you, like they were waiting to see you cough so that they could tell you to leave. If a person developed a fever after such a trip, they were quick to blame it on something else, something other than coronavirus, such as "cold foods" like certain fruits or vegetables. I remember looking for apartments during the summer of 2020, and since I was a doctor, people were scared of me, and I was refused places to live in. People were so fearful, but still, they didn't wear masks. I have not been able to figure that one out.

Later in the Pandemic, many people in our charitable organization developed COVID after trying to help others. A woman in her 30s developed a cough and had trouble breathing. She was admitted to our hospital and steadily declined, such that she was going to need ICU-level care. Our hospital does not have ICU capabilities so we had to find her a hospital. We desperately tried to find her a hospital in Delhi, the city where we send our sickest patients. All hospitals in Delhi, a city of 19 million people, were full. After continued searching, we finally found one hospital in Delhi that accepted her, if she could be there within 30 minutes, but we were hours away...

We eventually found a local hospital that had ventilators! But, it was not enough to find a hospital with ventilators; the hospital had to have staff who knew how to use them. As an internal medicine physician, I never had trouble using a ventilator because a respiratory therapist usually did the actual work. However, in this time of COVID, we were short-staffed in all areas. Many nurse assistants found themselves becoming nurses, and other untrained staff became medicine specialists, such as respiratory therapists. There was one more problem: hospitals had ventilators but no available patient rooms unless you were a family member of a politician. So when we sent the above woman to this local hospital, she was kept in the emergency department. Her temperature was not checked. Food was not provided, so we sent her food from our organization. Then we found out they were only giving her oxygen sporadically. Humanity had left, and they were clearly just checking a box, whether the patient was alive or not. In desperation, we brought her back to our hospital.

Fortunately, we were able to get her admitted to a hospital in Delhi. Later we found out that only when 50% of your lungs are damaged, as seen on a chest CT scan, would one then be considered for admission to Delhi hospitals. Fortunately, this woman slowly recovered in spite of bad food (no surprise) and untrained "nurses" who reused needles. But what could a patient do in such a situation? She is now out of the hospital but still has low blood oxygen levels whenever she moves around.

Once people heard that I had been able to arrange for a patient to be transferred to Delhi, I got multiple calls from other patients. People that I know called me, gasping for air, asking how to get oxygen. I was sending prescriptions at midnight so they could get oxygen refilled at centers in Delhi. I couldn't help but feel a growing sense of desperation. Even our hospital was not being given the oxygen they needed — the suppliers said: "You do not have ICU capabilities, so you don't need oxygen." Our oxygen supplies were so limited that if 3 or 4 patients who needed oxygen were admitted, we likely could not have served them. We check our oxygen tanks daily to make sure we are ready.

As things worsened, we saw ambulances waiting outside hospitals with patients dying inside. People in rickshaws, propped against buildings, lying on the ground, all dying due to the lack of oxygen. Our local government stopped allowing private laboratories to do PCR (polymerase chain reaction) testing for COVID so that numbers would appear lower. Misinformation about fake treatments by fake doctors was flooding WhatsApp text messages, so too were claims about masks being infested by bugs. People were even shaving off their hair because they thought their hair was contaminated by the coronavirus. Friends of mine who were nurses were beaten up if they went out during the day, and police violence was not uncommon.

The fear lingers even now, as the second wave is decreasing. At any moment, we know it can get worse. Our vaccines are not close to 90% efficacious, so though I am vaccinated, I am afraid to visit my parents for fear of transmitting COVID to them. We know that our country is far away from everyone being vaccinated. We can only dream of removing our masks like the recent mandates in America. At any moment, any of us can get sick. They are predicting that a possible third wave may hit in October 2021. Who knows what will happen to me, my family, my country?

1 Making of a Pandemic

"The only thing the virus wants is targets."

Adam Elkus,
George Mason University

Contents

1. Introduction
2. Coronaviruses — Structure and Replication
3. Evolution of Human Coronaviruses
4. Differences Between Outbreaks, Epidemics and Pandemics
5. Factors Affecting the Severity of a Pandemic
6. Impact of Genetic Mutations on Viral Transmission and Mortality
7. Containment, Mitigation and Flattening the Curve
8. Pandemic Waves

1. Introduction

On November 17, 2019, a new coronavirus strain (SARS-CoV-2) caused a severe respiratory illness in a person living in Wuhan, China. Less than four months later, on March 11, 2020, the WHO upgraded the SARS-CoV-2 outbreak to a pandemic (designated COVID-19) because the virus had rapidly spread across the globe, with 55 countries across five continents reporting over 100,000 cases and 4,000 deaths.

Healthcare systems in some countries were overwhelmed with people needing care. Those infected with the virus were occupying many of the hospital beds, including those in intensive care units (ICUs). Hospitals were canceling elective admissions and surgeries and setting up temporary sites to care for patients. There was a severe shortage of personal protective equipment (PPE) for healthcare workers caring for patients. The WHO was overseeing a new collaborative global effort to increase the production of PPE, develop diagnostic tests in sufficient quantities to diagnose those who are infected, find drugs to treat patients, and develop vaccines to prevent the disease.

As countries tried to contain and mitigate the spread of the virus, the pandemic was having a major impact on the global economy. Unemployment rates were rising, and many people, especially those who are poor, were struggling. An intense debate continued on how to find the right balance between saving lives and helping the economy.

The WHO and many countries had been planning for the next pandemic for years. The planning focused mainly on influenza since based on previous history, it was a virtual certainty there would be future influenza pandemics. Why was the world not better prepared to deal with a pandemic? Why did this new strain of coronavirus cause a pandemic when two other new strains of coronavirus that first appeared in 2002 and 2012 caused serious respiratory disease outbreaks (Table 1.1), but not a pandemic? These are just two of the many key questions discussed in this book. A good place to begin is with a discussion on coronaviruses, including SARS-C0V-2, the cause of the current pandemic.

Table 1.1. Severe Acute Respiratory Disease (SARS) Outbreaks Due To Coronaviruses First Detected in Humans during the 21st Century

Disease Name	SARS	MERS	COVID-19
Coronavirus causing disease	SARS-CoV-2	MERS-CoV	SARS-CoV-2
Years of outbreak	2002–2004	2012, 2015, 2018	2019–Present
Location of initial case	Shunde, China	Jeddah, Saudi Arabia	Wuhan, China
Confirmed cases	~8,100	~2,500*	>80 million*
Confirmed deaths	774	858*	>1.8 million*
Case fatality rate	~9%	~35%	~2.3%

*Data as of December 30, 2020.

Key Point: Each pandemic teaches us new lessons. COVID-19 has proved to be a master teacher.

2. Coronaviruses — Structure and Replication

Coronaviruses are a large family of RNA viruses that have existed for thousands of years but were first discovered in the 1930s.[1,2] The structure of coronaviruses is spherical with a lipid envelope[2] (Figure 1.1). The nucleocapsid, contained within the envelope, is formed from multiple copies of the nucleocapsid (N) protein that binds to the positive-sense single-stranded RNA genome.[3] The lipid bilayer envelope (E), membrane (M) proteins, and N proteins provide protection for the virus when outside the host cell.[4] The E and M proteins are important in forming the viral envelope and maintaining its structural shape.[1] The coronavirus surface has club-shaped spikes that project from the membrane surface. Each spike contains three identical copies of the spike (S) protein, composed of S1 and S2 subunits. The S protein allows the virus to attach to and penetrate host cells.

The genome size of coronaviruses is large for an RNA virus and ranges from approximately 26 to 32 kilobases depending on the specific coronavirus strain.[5] The genome encodes the four major structural proteins: S, E, M and

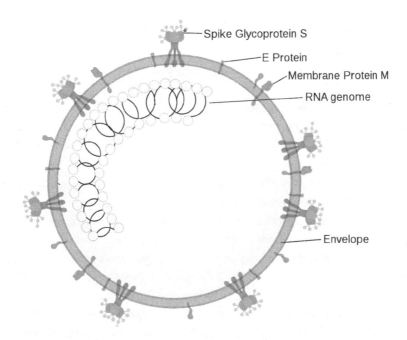

Figure 1.1. Structure of SARS-CoV-2.[2]

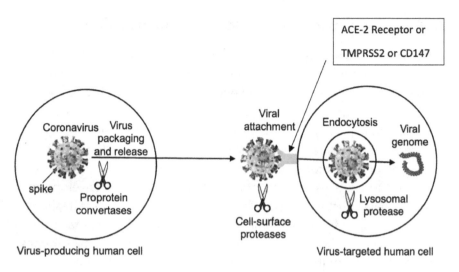

Figure 1.2. Replication cycle of SARS-COV-2.[1]

N.[6] It also encodes proteins necessary for virus replication and accessory proteins whose function can differ depending on the specific coronavirus.[1]

Infection begins when the viral spike protein attaches to its complementary host cell receptor[1] (Figure 1.2). Angiotensin-converting enzyme 2 (ACE2) receptors are the primary receptor for many coronaviruses, including SARS-CoV-2.[7,8] After attachment, a host cell protease such as transmembrane serine protease 2 (TMPRSS2) cleaves and activates the receptor-attached spike protein, allowing the virus to enter the host cell by endocytosis followed by a fusion of the viral envelope with the host endosome membrane.[9]

Once the virus is inside the cell, the RNA is replicated and becomes the genome of the newly created progeny virus synthesized in the cell. The genome also serves as messenger RNA (mRNA) for replicative and some of the accessory proteins, whereas other accessory proteins and viral structural proteins are translated from smaller mRNAs by the host's ribosomes associated with the endoplasmic reticulum.[1,9] The viral structural proteins S, E and M move along the secretory pathway into the Golgi compartment. There, the M proteins direct the protein interactions required for the assembly of viruses following its binding to the nucleocapsid. The release of progeny viruses from the host cell occurs via exocytosis through secretory vesicles. Once released, the viruses can infect other host cells.

3. Evolution of Human Coronaviruses

Coronaviruses are named for the crown-like spikes on their surface. There are four main subgroupings of coronaviruses, known as alpha, beta, gamma and delta. Coronavirus strains infect different species of animals, including swine, cattle, horses, camels, cats, dogs, rodents, spiny anteaters, birds and bats. In animals, these coronaviruses mainly cause intestinal disease. Infection is transmitted by the fecal-oral route.[10]

Each of the human coronaviruses shares a common ancestry with bat coronaviruses and emerges through bats that function as intermediary hosts. Prior to the 21st century, only four coronavirus strains caused disease in humans (i.e., NL63 alpha coronavirus, 229E alpha coronavirus, OC43 beta coronavirus and HKU1 beta coronavirus). These strains typically cause upper respiratory tract infections but are not associated with severe disease.

Three new strains of human coronaviruses have appeared since the turn of the 21st century and each can cause severe respiratory diseases,[2] including pandemics (Tables 1.1 and 1.2). In November 2002, a new strain of betacoronavirus (SARS-CoV-1) appeared in the Guangdong Province of China. Data suggest that SARS-related coronaviruses coevolved over a prolonged time. The ancestors of SARS-CoV-1 first infected leaf-nose bats and subsequently spread to horseshoe bats and then evolved through an intermediary host, Asian palm civets, before infecting humans.[11,12] The Asian palm civet lives throughout the jungles of Asia and some people consider them a food delicacy. Palm civets are sold in some wet markets where people also buy fruits, vegetables, seafood, meats, and other products (the role of wet markets in outbreaks is further discussed in Chapter 7). Epidemiologic data suggests that the initial outbreak may have started in a wet market in the Guangdong Province.[13]

Over the course of seven months, SARS-CoV-1 caused more than 8,000 people to develop severe acute respiratory syndrome (SARS) manifested by either pneumonia or respiratory distress syndrome.[13,14] Human-to-human transmission was the main mode of spread of the disease. Most of the cases occurred in southern China, Hong Kong, Singapore and Taiwan, but travel-related cases occurred in over 30 countries. Deaths occurred in 774 patients for a case fatality rate (CFR) of ~10%. Contact tracing and quarantine implemented by public health officials in affected countries were effective in eliminating the spread of the virus. By late July 2003, there were no new cases, and the WHO declared the global outbreak over. Since that time, there have been no new SARS-CoV-1 outbreaks.

In September 2012, a different betacoronavirus (MERS-CoV) appeared in Saudi Arabia and then spread to other countries in the Middle East and elsewhere.[15] MERS-CoV emerged in humans from bats through the intermediate host of camels.[16] MERS-CoV, although related to several bat coronavirus species, appears to have diverged from these other several centuries ago.[17]

Initially, human disease seemed to occur only in humans with contact with camels (as described in the next section). However, in May 2013, a case of human-to-human transmission occurred in France.[18] Despite documented cases of human-to-human spread of MERS, the virus has trouble spreading between humans. Nevertheless, there have been over 2,400 cases and 858 deaths for a case fatality rate of ~35%.[19] Indigenous MERS cases have occurred in various Middle East countries, including Bahrain, Iran, Jordan, Kuwait, Lebanon, Oman, Qatar, Saudi Arabia, United Arab Emirates (UAE), and Yemen. Additionally, travel-related cases have occurred in people from at least 17 countries. Outbreaks of this disease continue today in the Middle East. More information on MERS is contained in Chapter 8.

In December 2019, the most recent new betacoronavirus, SARS-CoV-2, was detected in Wuhan, China, where a large outbreak of pneumonia was occurring in the population.[20] This strain has approximately 70% genetic similarity to SARS-CoV-1 and appears to originate from bats.[21,22] Pangolins, a keratin-covered mammal wildlife sold in wet markets, have been proposed as the intermediate hosts of the virus, but further research is needed to determine if this is correct.[23]

Initially, SARS-CoV-2 seemed like it could be limited to an outbreak, but unfortunately, this turned out not to be the case. On March 11, 2020, SARS-CoV-2 had already caused over 118,000 confirmed cases and 4,300 deaths globally, and the WHO upgraded the status of the outbreak to a pandemic. The havoc that SARS-CoV-2 has triggered upon the world and why it was capable of doing this is the focus of this book.

> Key Point: Up until the turn of this century, there were only four human coronaviruses, and they caused mild respiratory tract infections. Since then, three new coronaviruses have emerged, and each has caused severe disease.

4. Differences Between Outbreaks, Epidemics and Pandemics

The term **Outbreak** refers to an increase, often sudden, in the number of cases of a disease above what normally occurs in a population within a limited geographic area. An **Epidemic** carries the same definition as an outbreak but in an expanded geographic area. A **Pandemic** refers to an epidemic that has spread over many countries or the entire globe and affects a very large number of people.[24] Thus, "outbreak", "epidemic", and "pandemic" are words describing the relative number of infections associated with a given organism. The former two terms are frequently used interchangeably, so there is no universally accepted definition for their relative size. (Chapters 7 and 8 contain a more detailed discussion of outbreaks, epidemics and pandemics and the microbes that cause them.)

Historically, influenza viruses are the most common cause of pandemics. The first clear description of an influenza pandemic dates back to 1580 when a virus spread from Asia to North Africa before moving to Europe and into North America, causing severe illness and death.[25,26] From this date, documentation of the history of pandemics is more reliable. The most lethal pandemic in recorded history occurred in 1918 due to a newly evolved influenza virus. Since that time, there have been three other pandemics in 1957, 1968 and 2009, each of them due to new strains of the influenza virus. Based on the certainty that influenza will continue to cause pandemics, the WHO published its first Global Influenza Plan in 1999, and subsequently, there have been multiple updates of this plan.[27] The influenza pandemic planning was occurring at the same time when the WHO was dealing with a four-fold increase in outbreaks due to various other microbes, many of which originated in animal species,including two new strains of coronavirus (i.e., SARS-CoV-1 and MERS).[28]

Key Point: "Outbreak", "epidemic" and "pandemic" are words that roughly describe the numbers of cases caused by an infectious agent. An approximation might be as follows: Outbreak (<1,000 people), epidemic (>1,000 to <1,000,000) and pandemic (>1,000,000) often involving many countries and continents.

---

5. Factors Affecting the Severity of a Pandemic

The two most important factors determining the severity of a pandemic are the transmission rate and fatality rate. If both the transmission rate and the mortality rate are high, then the pandemic is going to be severe. This was the case in 1918 when a new avian H1N1 virus killed between 50 and 100 million people.[27] In contrast, the 2009 influenza pandemic, caused by a new swine/avian H1N1, had a relatively low transmission and mortality rate.

Human coronaviruses mainly infect the epithelial cells of the respiratory tract, particularly the lungs, by binding to ACE2 receptors.[29] Those infected are able to shed the virus into the environment. Transmission between humans is mainly by aerosol or droplets, although infection via the fecal-oral route and contaminated objects or surfaces is possible.[30,31]

The likelihood of person-to-person transmission is expressed by R_0, spoken of as the R naught, previously called the basic reproduction number.[32] If R_0 is greater than one, the outbreak will continue. If it is less than one, it will end.

The estimated R_0 is based on laboratory and/or epidemiological data being gathered at the time of the outbreak or pandemic. For COVID-19, the estimated R_0 incorporated polymerase chain reaction (PCR) testing of people to confirm if they were infected and antibody

Table 1.2. Transmission and Mortality Rates of Previous Pandemics*

Transmission Route	Source	Infection Name	R_0**
Vectorborne	Mosquito	Yellow fever (1800s)	1.1–7.0
		Yellow fever (2000s)	
		Dengue	2.7–5.4
		Malaria (falciparum)	2.0–>1000
	Flea	Plague (14th century)	5–7
		Plague (2008–2016)	
Environment	Water	Cholera (1853)	1.9–551
		Cholera (2010)	
People	Body fluids	Syphilis (1500s)	N/A
		HIV	1.2–11.3
	Airborne or	COVID-19	1.2–6.5
	Droplet	Influenza (1918)	1.8
		Influenza (1957)	1.65
		Influenza (1968)	1.80
		Influenza (2009)	1.46
		TB (1900)	3.0
		Smallpox	3.5–6.0

*This table comes from Table 8.3 in Chapter 8, but is simplified to highlight the R_0 and mortality issues.

**R_0 = basic reproduction number, likelihood of person-to-person transmission.

testing to demonstrate a prior infection. Mathematical modeling using the laboratory data and epidemiologic data was also used to estimate the R_0.[32] The R_0 in the COVID-19 pandemic is estimated to be somewhere between 2 and 3, meaning that, on average, an infected person is likely to infect 2 to 3 additional susceptible people. The R_0, early on in the pandemic, when few public health interventions were ongoing, may have been closer to 4.[33]

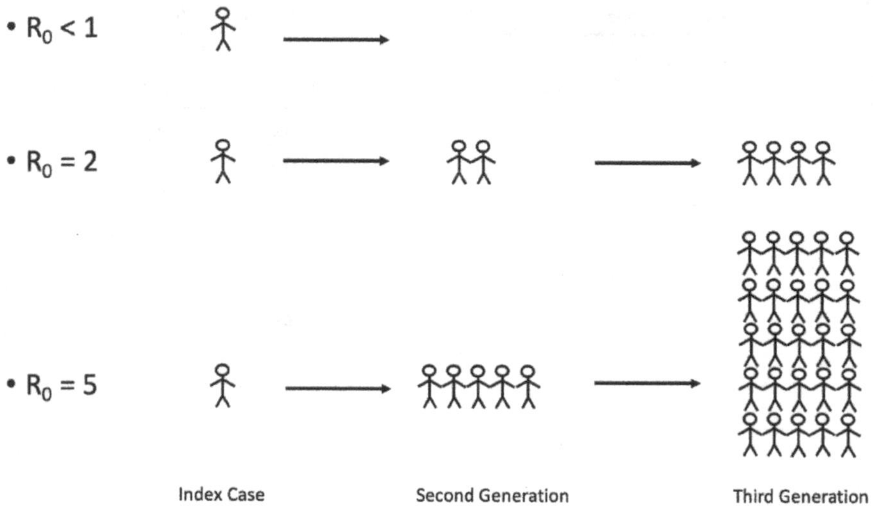

- $R_0 < 1$
- $R_0 = 2$
- $R_0 = 5$

Index Case · Second Generation · Third Generation

Figure 1.3. The effect of R_0 (basic reproduction number) on how many cases occur in the next generation of a propagated outbreak. If R_0 is less than one, the outbreak will end. If R_0 equals two, the number of cases can double each generation. If R_0 equals five, the number of cases can go up five times each generation. Source: R. Sherertz.

Figure 1.3 shows the importance of R_0 related to transmission; simply put, R_0 is the number of people that can be infected by one person but usually represents a population average. It can also be used to estimate what proportion of the population needs to have SARS-CoV-2 infection-induced immunity or be immunized to achieve adequate herd immunity (Figure 1.4). **Herd immunity** is the proportion of the population that needs to be immune to prevent a propagated outbreak. For example, the estimated R_0 of 2–3 for SARS-CoV-2 indicates that the proportion of the population needing to be immune to prevent propagation is >50%; whereas, if the R_0 is ~14, as is the case for the measles virus, then 95% of the population needs to be immune.[34,35]

The second major factor affecting the severity of a pandemic is the fatality rate. The estimated fatality rate uses one or more of the following calculations:

Population Fatality Rate (PFR) — To calculate the death rate, the number of deaths recorded is divided by the number of people in the population, and then multiplied by 100 to yield a percentage.[35]

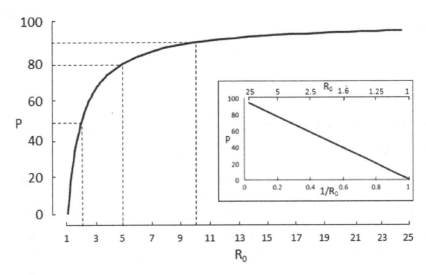

Figure 1.4. The relation between the basic reproduction number of a virus, R_0, and the proportion of the population that needs to be immunized to achieve herd immunity. For example, if R_0 equals 5, 80% of the population will need to be immunized to achieve herd immunity. With permission — jeffrey.aronson@phc.ox.ac.uk

Case Fatality Rate (CFR) — Calculated by dividing the number of deaths from a specified disease over a defined period of time by the number of individuals diagnosed with the disease during that time; the resulting **ratio** is then multiplied by 100 to yield a percentage.[35]

Infectivity fatality rate (IFR) — Calculated by dividing the number of deaths caused by the pathogen by the number of symptomatic or asymptomatic people infected by the pathogen.[36]

Fatality rates in pandemics occurring before the last century used PFR and/or CFR because the laboratory capability to detect infected patients who were not ill was unavailable. However, the IFR is a particularly important measure of fatality for the COVID-19 pandemic because a large percentage of those infected never develop symptoms.[37,38] The actual rate of asymptomatic infection appears to be between 20 and 40% (Chapter 4). The result is that the COVID-19's global CFR (~2.3%), is substantially higher than the global IFR (~0.6%).[39]

Key Point: The major determinants of the severity of a pandemic are the transmission rate and mortality rate. The higher the transmission and mortality rate the worse the pandemic.

6. Impact of Genetic Mutations on Viral Transmission and Mortality

The role of genetic mutations in causing a virus to become more transmissible or lethal remains an issue studied by researchers across the globe. RNA viruses are more prone to a high rate of mutations than DNA viruses.[40] Mutations often have no effect or are deleterious to the virus; the later may negatively influence viral adaptation to the host. Furthermore, interactions between different mutations can negate some adaptations. However, viruses with mutations that enhance the ability of the virus to replicate or be transmitted become the prevalent strains in circulation. Particularly troubling in the case of influenza viruses and coronaviruses are those mutations that expand the host range from animals to humans. Despite intense investigation, the genetic mutations that can change an avian or other animal virus into a human pathogen capable of causing a pandemic remain unclear.[40]

Influenza viruses mutate at a particularly high rate. Most studies examining which genetic mutations might affect transmissibility and lethality have focused on influenza viruses[40] due in large part to the multiple pandemics occurring every century due to this virus. Influenza viruses infect a large number of animals as well as humans, have high mutation rates, and frequently undergo reassortment.[41] Reassortment is a process of genetic recombination in which co-infection of a host cell with multiple viruses may result in the shuffling of gene segments to generate progeny viruses with novel genome combinations. Indeed, the ability of influenza viruses to adapt and jump from animals to humans caused the 2009 pandemic, where a unique blend of influenza viruses underwent reassortment. This created a virus similar to an H1N1 strain found in European and Asian birds and a North American H1N1 virus that has genes from avian, human, and swine influenza viruses to form the HIN1 pandemic influenza strain.[42] Additionally, H5N1 and H7N9 avian influenza viruses have caused limited human disease outbreaks in Asia with high mortality.[43] However, these latter two viruses have not mutated in a way that has allowed them to transmit easily between humans and therefore have not resulted in pandemics.

Coronaviruses, including the initial SARS-CoV-2 strain causing the current pandemic, mutate at a marginally slower rate than influenza viruses.[44] Since SARS-CoV-2 started causing disease in humans, virologists have followed the rate of appearance of virus mutations across the globe. In the first six months since its emergence, the circulating virus has averaged about two genomic mutations per month.[45] The estimated evolution rates for these two RNA viruses are 0.7×10^{-3} base pair substitutions/site/year for the coronavirus and 1.8×10^{-3} for influenza A viruses, which is close enough to raise the concern that the SARS-Cov-2 virus may evolve fast enough that annual vaccination may be needed similar to influenza viruses. (See Chapter 5 for a discussion of the impact of SARS-CoV-2 variants on vaccines.)

At the whole-genome level, SARS-CoV-2 shares an 88% sequence identity with the bat-SL-CoVZC45 and 87% sequence identity with the bat-SL-CoVZXC2. SARS-CoV-2 is somewhat less genetically similar to the SARS-CoV (~79%) and MERS-CoV (~50%).[46,47] The mutations that allowed SARS-CoV-1 to jump from bats to humans involved an intermediary host, most likely palm civets, and likely occurred over many years. The origin of SARS-CoV-2 is further discussed in Chapter 7.

On December 14, 2020, the United Kingdom reported a SARS-CoV-2 variant of concern (VoC) — lineage B.1.1.7[48] (the methodology the WHO uses to name SARS-CoV-2 variants and decide which ones are considered VoC is noted towards the end of this section). This B.1.1.7 variant appears to have emerged in September 2020 and subsequently became the dominant circulating SARS-CoV-2 variant in England. By the end of 2020, this variant had been detected in over 30 countries on multiple continents, including Asia, Africa, the Americas, and Europe. The evidence to date suggests that this variant is more transmissible between people, and it therefore could increase the percentage of population immunity required for pandemic control.[49] Similar concerns have been raised about some other variants, including the B.1.351 variant first reported in South Africa and the P.1 variant initially reported from Brazil.

One problem with naming variants is the nomenclature since three different systems are used — Gisaid, Pango and Nextstrain.[50] Each of these makes sense to those who use a particular nomenclature method but are hard for other people to understand. The WHO appointed a group to come up with a system that non-biologists could understand and that did not stigmatize groups (e.g., "Chinese virus" or "UK variant"). A modification to the nomenclature for variants was announced by the WHO in May 2021. The new nomenclature system uses the Greek alphabet to make it easier for the public to follow the evolution of VoC.

These three viruses were labeled VoC by the WHO, and it is very likely that as the pandemic continues, other variants will be given this label because they cause increased transmissibility and/or severity of disease. A fourth VoC, Delta (B.1.617.2) that emerged in India posed an increased risk to global public health and was categorized as a VoC in 2021. This Delta virus was determined to have a markedly increased transmission rate (estimated to be 40–60% higher than the other three VoCs.[51,52] The question of whether this variant also causes more severe disease is actively being studied. The WHO, US CDC and other health organizations have also classified some of the other evolving SARS-CoV-2 viruses as variants of interest, which are viruses where the genetic changes suggest they may be associated with increased transmission and/or disease severity.[53] The SARS-CoV-2 strains given the VoC classification are the ones spreading across the globe, and therefore the most impactful. As of mid-2021, the delta (B.1.617.2) SARS-CoV-2 strain was the predominant SARS-Cov-2 virus causing disease in most countries. The clinical and public health implications of SARS-CoV-2 variants are further discussed in Chapters 4 and 5. Towards the end of 2021 a new variant, omicron, emerged that appears to be more transmissible than any of the previous VoC (see Chapter 5 for further discussions on the impact of VoC).

Key Point: It is likely that genetic mutations occurring in viruses can decrease or increase the transmissibility and lethality of the disease, but the ability to forecast what mutations will lead to remains elusive. While tracking variants by continuing sequencing of SARS-CoV-2 on a large scale across the globe, it is critical that we develop a more complete understanding of which mutations are critical to affecting transmission and lethality. Until this occurs, we will continue to rely on epidemiologic studies to retrospectively look at which variants are important.

7. Containment, Mitigation and Flattening the Curve

Containment and mitigation policies are used to stop or slow down the spread of a pandemic, and both can be instituted at the same time.[54] Containment includes a number of steps used to stop the spread of the virus within and outside of the outbreak area. One of the strongest containment steps utilizes a lockdown of affected areas, which includes everyone staying in their homes and only going outside for essential activities (e.g., grocery shopping) or if they provide essential services (e.g., healthcare workers).

If containment has not worked, mitigation policies can still be effective at slowing the spread of the virus. Two of the most effective mitigation steps are the use of masks and social distancing (people separate by at least 3–6 feet).[54] One of the main purposes of mitigation is to stop the healthcare systems in countries from being overwhelmed with patients. Public health officials use the term "flattening the curve"[55] (Figure 1.5) to help explain why they are recommending mitigation steps. By flattening the curve, hospitals can avoid being overwhelmed by patients and can provide better care to those who are sick. An extensive discussion of the impact that containment and mitigation had on the COVID-19 pandemic in various countries is contained in Chapters 2 and 3.

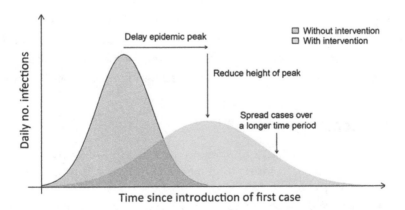

Figure 1.5. Flattening the curve.[55]

8. Pandemic Waves

Some pandemics associated with respiratory diseases, especially influenza, have episodic waves of disease. Each wave is associated with an increased incidence of disease followed by decreasing incidence.[56] The lull between waves is likely not devoid of disease, but the incidence is low enough that it gives the appearance that the disease is going away. In the 1918 and 2009 influenza pandemic, the first wave occurred in the spring in the northern hemisphere, and then the incidence of disease substantially decreased in the summer only to come back in the fall. In the 1918 pandemic, the fatality rate was high (~2.5%), and the second wave was more intense than the first wave.[56] In the 2009 pandemic, the mortality rate was lower (~0.4%), and both waves were less intense than in 1918.[57]

Influenza virus waves tend to be worse in the colder months. Various mechanisms could explain the low incidence of disease in the summer. One is that influenza viruses like cold and dry weather and do not thrive as well in hot, humid weather.[58] Additionally, children are the main transmitters of influenza viruses, and when schools are closed for the summer, there is less transmission of the virus to family members and others.[59]

Initially, it was hoped that SARS-CoV-2 might behave similarly to influenza, resulting in a lull in disease activity in the summer.[60] While the endemic coronaviruses cause seasonal upper respiratory tract infections mainly in the winter, the SARS-CoV-1 and MERS viruses have not spread widely enough to determine if they were also seasonal viruses. However, the large wave of COVID-19 disease occurring during the summer of 2020 throughout the southern US, Mexico, and other locales indicates that hot, humid weather is not enough to slow down the pandemic. Chapter 2 discusses how the SARS-CoV-2 virus spread the disease across the globe.

References

1. Shang J, Wan Y, Luo C. (2020) Cell entry mechanisms of SARS-CoV-2. *Proceedings of the National Academy of Sciences* **117**:11727–11734. DOI:10.1073/pnas.2003138117
2. Wikipedia. (nd) Coronavirus. https://en.wikipedia.org/wiki/Coronavirus Accessed: April 19, 2021.

3. Chang CK, Hou MH, Chang CF, *et al.* (2014) The SARS coronavirus nucleocapsid protein — forms and functions. *Antiviral Research* **103**:39–50. DOI:10.1016/j.antiviral.2013.12.009

4. Neuman BW, Kiss G, Kunding AH, *et al.* (2011) A structural analysis of M protein in coronavirus assembly and morphology. *Journal of Structural Biology* **174**:11–22. DOI:10.1016/j.jsb.2010.11.021

5. Woo PC, Huang Y, Lau SK, Yuen KY. (2010) Coronavirus genomics and bioinformatics analysis. *Viruses* **2**:1804–1820. DOI:10.3390/v2081803.

6. Snijder EJ, Bredenbeek PJ, Dobbe JC, *et al.* (2003) Unique and conserved features of genome and proteome of SARS-coronavirus, an early split-off from the coronavirus group 2 lineage. *Journal of Molecular Biology* **331**:991–1004. DOI:10.1016/S0022-2836(03)00865-9

7. Zhang B, Yixin Li, Zhang AZ, *et al.* (2020) Identifying airborne transmission as the dominant route for the spread of COVID-19. *Proceedings of the National Academy of Sciences* **117**(26):14857–14863. DOI:10.1073/pnas.2009637117

8. Shin JY. (2020) Overlooked receptors in Covid-19: What ACE2 alone cannot explain. *Microbial Instincts.* https://medium.com/microbial-instincts/overlooked-receptors-could-explain-quirks-of-covid-19-that-ace2-alone-cannot-9470817f59d0

9. Simmons G, Zmora P, Gierer S, *et al.* (2013) Proteolytic activation of the SARS-coronavirus spike protein: Cutting enzymes at the cutting edge of antiviral research. *Antiviral Research* **100**:605–614. DOI:10.1016/j.antiviral.2013.09.028

10. Murphy FA, Gibbs EP, Horzinek MC, Studdart MJ. (1999) *Veterinary Virology. Academic Press, Boston,* pp. 495–508.

11. Gouilh MA, Puechmaille SJ, Gonzalez JP, *et al.* (2011) SARS-Coronavirus ancestor's foot-prints in South-East Asian bat colonies and the refuge theory. *Infection, Genetics and Evolution* **11**:1690–1702. DOI:10.1016/j.meegid.2011.06.021

12. Cui J, Han N, Streicker D, *et al.* (2007) Evolutionary relationships between bat coronaviruses and their hosts. *Emerging Infectious Diseases* **13**:1526–1532. DOI:10.3201/eid1310.070448

13. CDC. (nd) Severe Acute Respiratory Disease (SARS). Centers for Disease Control and Prevention. https://www.cdc.gov/sars/index.html. Accessed: April 19, 2022.

14. WHO. (2004) Guidelines for the global surveillance of severe acute respiratory syndrome (SARS). Updated recommendations, October 2004. World

Health Organization. https://www.who.int/csr/resources/publications/WHO_
CDS_CSR_ARO_2004_1/en/

15. Azhar EI, El-Kafrawy SA, Farraj SA, *et al.* (2014) Evidence for camel-to-hu-
man transmission of MERS Coronavirus. *New England Journal of Medicine*
370:2499–2505. DOI:10.1056/NEJMoa1401505

16. Forni D, Cagliani R, Clerici M, Sironi M. (2017) Molecular evolution of human
coronavirus genomes. *Trends in Microbiology* **25**:35–48. DOI:10.1016/j.
tim.2016.09.001

17. Lau SK, Li KS, Tsang AK, *et al.* (2013) Genetic characterization of Betacoronavirus lineage C viruses in bats reveals marked sequence divergence in the
spike protein of pipistrellus bat coronavirus HKU5 in Japanese pipistrelle:
Implications for the origin of the novel Middle East respiratory syndrome
coronavirus. *Journal of Virology* **87**:8638–8650. DOI:10.1128/JVI.01055-13

18. Ministry of Solidarites and Health. (2013) Nouveau coronavirus — Point de
situation: Un nouveau cas d'infection confirmé (Novel coronavirus — Status
report: A new case of confirmed infection), May 12. www.social-sante.gouv.fr

19. WHO. (2018) Middle East respiratory syndrome coronavirus (MERS-CoV) WHO
MERS global summary and assessment of risk. World Health Organization.
https://www.who.int/csr/disease/coronavirus_infections/risk-assessment-
august-2018.pdf

20. WHO. (nd) Timeline of WHO's response to COVID-19. World Health Organization. https://www.who.int/news-room/detail/29-06-2020-covidtimeline. Updated:
June 30, 2020.

21. Cohen J. (2020) Wuhan seafood market may not be source of novel virus
spreading globally. *ScienceMag*. Retrieved: January 29.

22. Eschner K. (2020) We're still not sure where the COVID-19 really came from.
Popular Science. Retrieved: January 30.

23. Liu P, Jiang JZ, Wan XF, *et al.* (2020) Are pangolins the intermediate host of
the 2019 novel coronavirus (SARS-CoV-2)? *PLOS Pathogens* **16**:e1008421.
https://doi.org/10.1371/journal.ppat.1008421

24. CDC. (nd) Lesson 1: Introduction to epidemiology, Section 11: Epidemic disease occurrence. Level of disease. Centers for Disease Control and Prevention. https://www.cdc.gov/csels/dsepd/ss1978/lesson1/section11.html

25. Saunders-Hastings PR, Daniel Krewski D. (2016) Reviewing the history of pandemic influenza: Understanding patterns of emergence and transmission.
Pathogens **5**:66. DOI:10.3390/pathogens5040066

26. Jordan D, Tumpey T, Jester B. (nd) The deadliest flu: The complete story
of the discovery and reconstruction of the 1918 Pandemic Virus. Centers

for Disease Control and Prevention. https://www.cdc.gov/flu/pandemic-resources/reconstruction-1918-virus.html

27. WHO. (nd) Pandemic plan: Influenza. World Health Organization. https://www.who.int/influenza/preparedness/pandemic/en/. Last update: 2018.

28. The Lancet. (2020) Zoonosis: Beyond the human–animal–environment interface. *Lancet* **396**:1. DOI:10.1016/S0140-6736(20)31486-0

29. Li F, Li W, Farzan M, Harrison SC. (2015) Structure of SARS coronavirus spike receptor-binding domain complexed with receptor. *Science* **309**:1864–1868. DOI:10.1126/science.1116480

30. Decaro N. (2011) *Alphacoronavirus. The Springer Index of Viruses*, eds. Tidona C, Darai G. Springer, pp. 371–383. DOI:10.1007/978-0-387-95919-1_56

31. Decaro N. (2011) *Betacoronavirus. The Springer Index of Viruses*, eds. Tidona C, Darai G. Springer, pp. 385–401. DOI:10.1007/978-0-387-95919-1_57

32. Delamater PL, Street EJ, Leslie TF, *et al.* (2019) Complexity of the basic reproduction number (R_0). *Emerging Infectious Diseases* **25**:1–4.

33. Katul GG, Mrad A, Bonetti S, *et al.* (2020) Global convergence of COVID19 basic reproduction number and estimation from early-time SIR dynamics. *PLOS One* **15**:e0239800. https://doi.org/10.1371/journal.pone.0239800

34. Gani R, Leach S. (2001) Transmission potential of smallpox in contemporary populations. *Nature* **414**:748–751.

35. CDC. (2012) *Principles of Epidemiology in Public Health Practice: An Introduction to Applied Epidemiology and Biostatistics*, 3rd edition, Center for Disease Control and Prevention. https://www.cdc.gov/csels/dsepd/ss1978/lesson3/section3.html

36. Condit R. (2020) Infection fatality rate — A critical missing piece for managing Covid-19. https://www.virology.ws/2020/04/05/infection-fatality-rate-a-critical-missing-piece-for-managing-covid-19/

37. CDC. (nd) Unexplained respiratory disease outbreaks: Defining an outbreak of unexplained respiratory illness. Centers for Disease Control and Prevention. https://www.cdc.gov/urdo/outbreak.html. Accessed: July 28, 2020.

38. CDC. (nd) Coronavirus disease 2019 (COVID-19). Centers for Disease Control and Prevention. Accessed: July 28, 2020. https://www.cdc.gov/coronavirus/2019-ncov/cases-updates/about-epidemiology/studying-the-diesease.html

39. WHO. (2020) Transmission of SARS-CoV-2: Implications for infection prevention precautions. Scientific Brief, World Health Organization, July 9. https://www.who.int/news-room/commentaries/detail/transmission-of-sars-cov-2-implications-for-infection-prevention-precautions

40. Lyons DM, Lauring AS. (2018) Mutation and epistasis in influenza virus evolution. *Viruses* **10**:407. DOI:10.3390/v10080407

41. Shao W, Li X, Goraya MU, *et al*. (2017) Evolution of influenza A virus by mutation and re-assortment. *International Journal of Molecular Sciences* **18**:1650. DOI:10.3390/ijms18081650

42. CDC. (2009) Origin of 2009 H1N1 flu (Swine flu): Questions and answers. Centers for Disease Control and Prevention. https://www.cdc.gov/h1n1flu/information_h1n1_virus_qa.htm

43. Chatziprodromidou IP, Malamatenia A, Guitian J, *et al*. (2018) Global avian influenza outbreaks 2010–2016: A systematic review of their distribution, avian species and virus subtype *Systematic Reviews* **7**:17. DOI:10.1186/s13643-018-0691-z

44. John Hopkins Center for Health Security. (2020) SARS-CoV-2 genetics. Updated: April 16. https://www.centerforhealthsecurity.org/resources/COVID-19/COVID-19-fact-sheets/200128-nCoV-whitepaper.pdf

45. Kupferschmidt K. (2020) The pandemic virus is slowly mutating. But is it getting more dangerous? *Science*, July 14.

46. Wang H, Li X, Li T, *et al*. (2020) The genetic sequence, origin, and diagnosis of SARS-CoV-2. *European Journal of Clinical Microbiology & Infectious Diseases* **39**:1–7. DOI:10.1007/s10096-020-03899

47. Lu R, Zhao X, Li J, *et al*. (2020) Genomic characterization and epidemiology of 2019 novel coronavirus: Implications for virus origins and receptor binding. *Lancet* **395**:565–574. DOI:10.1016/S0140-6736(20)30251-8

48. Public Health England. (2020) PHE investigating a novel variant of COVID-19., December 14. https://www.gov.uk/government/news/phe-investigating-a-novel-variant-of-covid-19

49. CDC. (2021) Emergence of SARS-CoV-2 B.1.1.7 lineage — United States, December 29, 2020 — January 12, 2021. *MMWR* **70**:95–99. https://www.cdc.gov/mmwr/volumes/70/wr/mm7003e2.htm?s_cid=mm7003e2_e

50. Lisa Winter. (2021) WHO updates the nomenclature of SARS-CoV-2 variants. *Science*, June 1. https://www.the-scientist.com/news-opinion/who-updates-the-nomenclature-of-sars-cov-2-variants-68837

51. WHO. (2021) Tracking SARS-CoV-2 variants, May 31. World Health Organization. https://www.who.int/en/activities/tracking-SARS-CoV-2-variants/

52. Public Health England. (2021) Vaccines highly effective against hospitalization from Delta variant, June 14. https://www.gov.uk/government/news/vaccines-highly-effective-against-hospitalisation-from-delta-variant

53. CDC. (2020) SARS-CoV-2 variant classifications and definitions. Centers for Disease Control and Prevention, June 15. https://www.cdc.gov/coronavirus/2019-ncov/science/about-epidemiology/index.html

54. Walensky RP, del Rio C. (2020) From mitigation to containment of the COVID-19 pandemic: Putting the SARS-CoV-2 genie back in the bottle. *JAMA* **323**:1889–1890. DOI:10.1001/jama.2020.6572

55. CDC. (nd) Nonpharmaceutical measures for pandemic influenza in nonhealth-care settings — Social distancing measure. Centers for Disease Control and Prevention. https://wwwnc.cdc.gov/eid/article/26/5/19-0995-f1. Accessed: April 12, 2021.

56. Jeffery K, Taubenberger JK, Morens DM. (2006) 1918 Influenza: The mother of all pandemics. *Emerging Infections* **12**:15–22. https://wwwnc.cdc.gov/eid/article/12/1/05-0979_article

57. Kamigaki T, Oshitani H. (2009) Epidemiological characteristics and low case fatality rate of pandemic (H1N1). *PLOS Currents*. https://www.ncbi.nlm.nih.gov/pmc/articles/PMC2797432/

58. Foster H. (2014) The Reason for the season: Why flu strikes in winter. *SITN Blog*. http://sitn.hms.harvard.edu/flash/2014/the-reason-for-the-season-why-flu-strikes-in-winter/

59. Lee BY, Shah M. (2012) Prevention of influenza in healthy children. *Expert Review of Anti-Infective Therapy* **10**:1139–1152. DOI:10.1586/eri.12.106. https://earthobservatory.nasa.gov/features/covid-seasonality

60. Voiland A. (2020) Could COVID-19 have seasons? Searching for signals in earth data earth observatory. July 14. https://earthobservatory.nasa.gov/features/covid-seasonality

2 Path of Destruction

"If the basics aren't followed, there is only one way this pandemic is going to go. It is going to get worse and worse and worse."

Tedros Adhansom Ghebreyesus,
WHO Director-General,
July 13, 2020

Contents

1. The SARS-CoV-2 Outbreak Begins and Spreads Across the Globe (December 2019–March 11, 2020)
   a. Spread through all regions
   b. Initial attempts to contain and mitigate the spread of SARS-Cov-2 vary across regions and countries
   c. WHO Director General declares the COVID-19 pandemic
2. The COVID-19 Pandemic Intensifies (March 12, 2020–December 31, 2020)
   a. WHO develops the Solidarity Call to Action and the Access to COVID-19 Tools Accelerator programs to help create equity in supplies, drugs and vaccine availability
   b. Formation of the WHO Task Force to investigate the origins of SARS-CoV-2
3. Success of Containment and Mitigation Policies Vary Across Regions and Countries
   a. Asian region with spotlight comparing China and India
   b. European region with spotlight comparing Sweden and Norway
   c. Americas regions with spotlight comparing the United States and Canada
   d. African region with spotlight comparing South Africa and the rest of the region
   e. Eastern Mediterranean region with spotlight comparing Iran and Jordan
   f. Antarctica

1. The SARS-CoV-2 Outbreak Begins and Spreads Across the Globe (December 2019–March 11, 2020)

The outbreak caused by a new coronavirus, SARS-CoV-2, is first detected in China towards the end of 2019 and spread across the globe over the next few months, leading the WHO to declare a pandemic on March 11, 2020. The timeline of many of the events that led to the declaration of the pandemic is well documented.[1,2]

The spread of the SARS-CoV-2 virus into each WHO region is noted in Figure 2.6. The WHO has 194 member countries divided into the following six regions: (1) African (47 countries), (2) Americas (includes all 35 countries in North America, South America, Latin America, and the Caribbean), (3) European (53 countries), (4) Eastern Mediterranean (21 countries), and (5) Southeast Asia and (6) Western Asia (27 countries). The number of countries reporting SARS-CoV-2 cases at the time the pandemic was declared are noted in Figure 2.7.

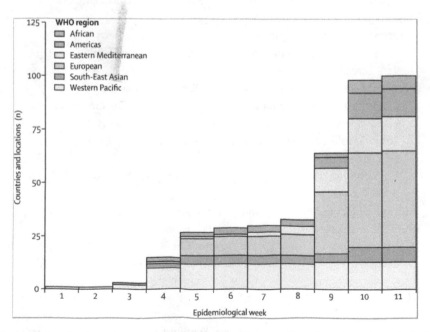

Figure 2.6. Confirmed cases of COVID-19, by WHO region and epidemiological week, from Dec 31, 2019 to March 10, 2020.[1]

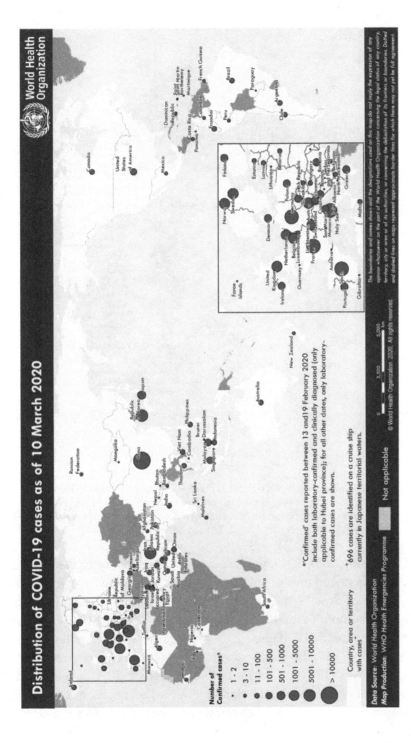

Figure 2.7. Countries, territories or areas with reported confirmed cases of COVID-19, as of March 10, 2020.[1]

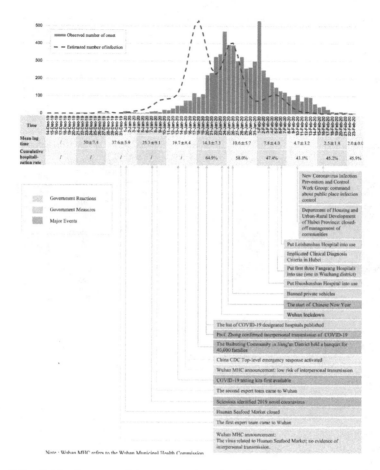

Figure 2.8.   Epidemic curves of the estimated number of infections and observed number of new cases, along with the weekly mean lag time between the date of diagnosis, cumulative hospitalization rate and government reactions, measures, and major events in Wuhan from December 14, 2019 to February 23, 2020.[3] With permission.

On December 31, 2019, the Chinese government informs the WHO of an outbreak of pneumonia of unknown cause in 44 people living in Hunan, China, a city of over 11 million people. Retrospective investigations by the Chinese authorities identify human cases with the onset of symptoms in early December 2019[3] (Figure 2.8). Among the first 425 patients with confirmed COVID-19, the median age is 59 years, and 56% are males. The majority of cases (55%) with onset before January 1, 2020, are linked to the Huanan Seafood Wholesale Market. Officials suspect that the source of this new disease is the market since many of the patients presenting with this illness worked there. Whether or not the market was the original site for the first cases of COVID-19 remains unclear.[4]

A week after reporting the outbreak to the WHO, Chinese investigators working in a Shanghai Laboratory identify the cause of the disease to be a new coronavirus that is eventually given the name SARS-CoV-2. On January 10, 2020, the gene sequencing data is posted on Virological.org, a hub for the pre-publication of data designed to assist with public health activities and research.[5]

The outbreak spreads further in Wuhan and the surrounding province of Hubei and it is established that transmission of the disease is occurring between humans by mid-January. There are now over 200 cases, including infections among healthcare workers. Chinese authorities also report four deaths. Detection of cases in Chinese travelers occurs in Japan, Thailand and South Korea.

By the end of the third week of January, there are more than 580 cases of COVID-19 and 17 deaths in China, all in the Hubei province. The Chinese government shuts down public transportation, including the airport and railway stations in Wuhan and soon thereafter in Ezhou and Huanggang, two smaller cities in the Hubei Province. The government cancels plans for Chinese New Year festivities. All these steps are done in the hope of containing the spread of the virus.

The WHO Director-General, Tedros Adhanom Ghebreyesus, convenes a meeting of the International Health Regulation (IHR) committee on January 22 to decide whether this outbreak constitutes a Public Health Emergency of International Concern (PHEIC). A PHEIC is an extraordinary event that is determined to constitute a public health risk to other countries through the international spread of disease that will potentially require a coordinated international response. A PHEIC implies a situation that is serious, sudden, unusual or unexpected, carries implications for public health beyond the affected countries' national border, and may require immediate international action.[6]

The declaration of a PHEIC will help empower the Director-General to utilize the International Health Regulation (IHR). The IHR, created in 2005, represents a binding international legal agreement involving 196 countries across the globe, including all the WHO member states. The aim of the IHR is to help the international community prevent and respond to acute public health risks that have the potential to cross borders and threaten people worldwide. The IHR is meant to prevent, protect against, control, and provide a public health response to the international spread of disease in ways that are commensurate with and restricted to public health risks, and avoid unnecessary interference with international traffic and trade.[6] Based on the information they have at that time, the Emergency Committee defers a decision.

By the last week in January, the number of cases in China increases to over 7,700, with more than 170 deaths. Additionally, the disease spreads to at least 10 other countries, most of them in Asia, but cases also occur in travelers from Europe, Scandinavia, the Middle East, and the Americas (Figure 2.6).

The IHR Emergency Committee is reconvened on January 29 and based on its recommendation the Director-General declares the COVID-19 outbreak a PHEIC the next day. This is the sixth time the WHO has declared a PHEIC since the concept originated in 2005. Prior PHEICs were declared to help deal with the 2009 influenza pandemic, complete the goal of eradicating wild type polio from the world (2014), the Ebola virus outbreak in Western Africa (2014), the Zika virus outbreak in the Americas (2016), and the Ebola virus outbreak in the eastern region of the Democratic Republic of the Congo (2018).[6]

By the beginning of February, China has over 20,000 COVID-19 cases and 400 deaths. The healthcare system in Wuhan is overwhelmed with patients requiring hospitalization and care in intensive care units (ICUs). Temporary hospitals are rapidly constructed, often within ten days. China initiates the first therapeutic trial using the antiviral drug, remdesivir, an investigational nucleotide analog drug with a broad-spectrum antiviral activity that had not been approved for use by any regulatory agency. The decision to try remdesivir is based on its *in vitro* and *in vivo* activity in animal models against the viral pathogens SARS-CoV-1 and MERS. The limited preclinical data on remdesivir in MERS and SARS-CoV-1 suggests that the drug may have potential activity against SARS-CoV-2.[7]

Increasing numbers of countries are dealing with COVID-19 cases, and some implement travel bans for travelers from China and/or quarantining their own citizens upon their return from China. Japan reports 10 cases of COVID-19 on a cruise ship and has the second highest number of cases in the world.[8] The spread of SARS-CoV-2 on cruise ships will soon become a recurrent problem.

By the second week of February, there are over 40,000 confirmed cases of COVID-19, with approximately 6,500 considered severe. The death toll of victims from SARS-COV-2 is now over 1,000, surpassing the death toll of the SARS outbreak in 2002–2003 that killed 773 people and the MERS outbreak that has claimed the lives of over 850 people to date. The WHO Director-General notes the increasing incidence of transmission between people with no travel history to China is very concerning and calls the outbreak a very grave threat for the world.

On February 13, China reports a huge overnight spike of 14,840 cases in Hubei province. However, this really represented a change in how its government reported cases, switching from reporting only confirmed cases to including both laboratory-confirmed cases and clinically diagnosed cases. These additional cases include medical professionals classifying a confirmed case based on chest imaging. The WHO and most other countries are still only reporting laboratory-confirmed cases. Later in the month, the WHO switches methods for reporting confirmed COVID-19 cases, now aligning with how the Chinese government had reported cases since February 13. Later in the month, China goes back to reporting only laboratory-confirmed cases. The changing case definitions make it even more difficult to track the global impact of the pandemic.

The Chinese CDC publishes a paper with detailed information on 72,414 COVID-19 patients, of which more than 44,672 are confirmed.[9] The data appears to show that the case fatality rate (CFR) for COVID-19 is less than SARS and MERS. Approximately 85% of COVID-19 patients had mild to moderate disease, 15% developed more severe diseases, including pneumonia, and 5% were critically ill with respiratory failure, septic shock, and/or multi-organ failure, with 2% of all reported cases dying. Mortality rates were higher in older patients, with few deaths among children.

By the middle of February, there is a lull in the outbreak within China. The number of new COVID-19 cases in the Hubei province is declining, and over 36,000 patients have recovered. How was China able to contain the outbreak when many other countries were not? The short answer is that the Chinese government imposed a very strict lockdown on January 23.[10] The lockdown included stopping movement in and out of Wuhan, the center of the epidemic, and 15 other cities in the Hubei province that is home to more than 60 million people. Travel by plane or train was suspended, and roads were blocked. People were told to stay at home and venture out only to get food or medical help. Expansion of the initial lockdown in Hubei was rapidly extended to other parts of China and eventually included ~760 million people (~50% of China's population). The lockdown lasted over two months, with some easing along the way. The number of new cases went down to about 20 per day compared to thousands per day at the peak. Unlike in some other countries, there were very few violations of the lockdown by Chinese citizens (Chapter 3 further discusses how different countries tried to contain or mitigate the spread of SARS-CoV-2).

By the fourth week of February, there are over 3,000 confirmed COVID-19 cases in 44 countries, with at least 50 deaths, including the first case in the African continent reported from Ethiopia (Figure 2.6). The WHO's concern is increasing over the number of cases with no clear epidemiological links, such as travel history to China or contact with a confirmed case. In a press conference on February 24, the Director-General notes that the window of opportunity to contain the outbreak is getting shorter. His message to each country is clear: now is the time to aggressively act to contain the COVID-19 outbreak, otherwise many more people will develop the disease.[11]

The WHO raises the global risk of the spread of COVID-19 from high to very high, but still does not declare COVID-19 a pandemic.[12] When asked why at a press conference at the end of February, Dr. Michael Ryan, Executive Director of the WHO Health Emergencies Program stated: "To declare a pandemic — it is unhelpful to do that when you are still trying to contain a disease... China has clearly shown that this is not necessarily the natural outcome of this event if we take action, if we move quickly, if we do the things we need to do." He also noted that of the 46 countries reporting cases, eight had not reported new cases over the past two weeks and 23 reported fewer than 10 cases.

a. Spread through all regions

However, Europe is experiencing a marked increase in COVID-19 cases at this point.[13,14] Italy has over 1,000 COVID-19 cases, the third most of any country, behind only China and South Korea. Furthermore, new cases originating from Italy have spread to 14 other countries. The SARS-CoV-2 virus was thought to have entered Italy in January, but a report published in late 2020 notes that the virus was isolated from a child in November 2019.[15] The European Commission requests member states to review pandemic preparedness plans and inform the commission of how they plan to implement them.[14] The commission also announces an initiative to launch a joint procurement procedure to support its member states in obtaining personal protective equipment (PPE) as COVID-19 cases rise in the region.

Towards the end of February, a report from the US CDC notes that 14 COVID-19 cases have occurred within the US, in addition to 39 cases in repatriated persons from high-risk settings outside the US. Dr. Nancy Messonnier, Director of the National Center for Immunization and Respiratory Diseases holds a press briefing[16] where she indicates: "It's not so much of a question of if this will happen anymore, but rather more of a question of exactly when this will happen." She further warns: "Prepare for the expectation that this might be bad." President Trump makes clear his unhappiness about what she said and reportedly tries to have her fired,[17] but she proves to be right (see Chapter 3 for further discussion of the impact that politics has on the COVID-19 pandemic). Some of the other countries in the Americas are now dealing with travel-related cases.

At this point, Africa is the least affected of all the WHO regions (Figure 2.6), and the virus has spread at different rates within various parts of Africa (Figure 2.9). Between February and mid-March, efforts focus on ways to both

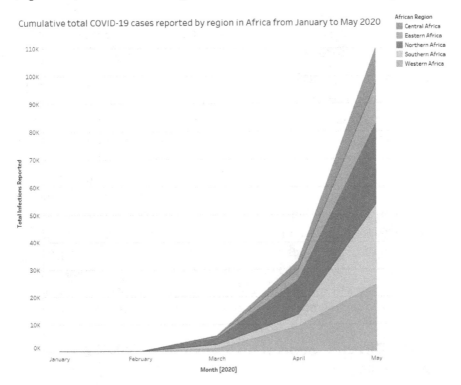

Figure 2.9. Cumulative total COVID-19 cases reported by region in Africa from February 16 to May 22, 2020. Modified from reference 18.

contain and mitigate the impact of COVID-19, especially by increasing the capacity of African Union member states to detect cases.[18] A collaboration between the African CDC, the WHO, and the West African Health Organization, with support from outside funding organizations, help provide the expertise and funding to create an African Task Force for Coronavirus to leverage existing continental expertise through technical working groups aligned to priority areas. The technical working groups review the latest evidence and best practices, adapting them into policies and technical recommendations to help inform public-health action against COVID-19 and to foster coordinated preparedness and responses across the continent. These groups focus on ways to increase testing capacity across each of the African countries and to strengthen emergency operations centers, effective surveillance, and contact tracing and isolation on the continent.[19] Additional efforts involve increasing the capacity to manufacture PPE and other medical equipment in Africa.

b. Initial attempts to contain and mitigate the spread of SARS-Cov-2 vary across regions and countries

By the first week in March, 38 countries have instituted various travel restrictions, including travel bans of visitors from China and other countries reporting transmission of COVID-19, visa restrictions, quarantine of foreigners, and self-isolation of returning citizens. Trade restrictions between countries have not occurred at this point, and the WHO's PHEIC guidance usually advises against travel or trade restrictions.[20] The guidance notes that travel and trade bans to affected areas or denial of entry to passengers coming from affected areas are usually not effective in preventing the importation of cases and may have a significant economic and social impact. The WHO guidance does indicate that countries can temporarily justify significant travel restrictions at the beginning of an outbreak to give the country time to implement outbreak preparedness measures or in settings with few international connections and limited response capacity.

c. WHO Director General declares the COVID-19 pandemic

On March 11, 2020, the WHO changes its course. At a press conference, the Director-General notes that the worsening conditions caused by

SARS-CoV-2 could now be characterized as a pandemic.[21] In his opening statement to the press, he states:

> "In the past two weeks, the number of cases of COVID-19 out-side China has increased 13-fold, and the number of affected countries has tripled. There are now more than 118,000 cases in 114 countries, and 4,291 people have lost their lives. Thousands more are fighting for their lives in hospitals. In the days and weeks ahead, we expect to see the number of cases, the number of deaths, and the number of affected countries climb even higher.
>
> WHO has been assessing this outbreak around the clock, and we are deeply concerned both by the alarming levels of spread and severity and by the alarming levels of inaction.
>
> We have therefore made the assessment that COVID-19 can be characterized as a pandemic. Pandemic is not a word to use lightly or carelessly. It is a word that, if misused, can cause unreasonable fear or unjustified acceptance that the fight is over, leading to unnecessary suffering and death. Describing the situation as a pandemic does not change the WHO's assessment of the threat posed by this virus. It does not change what the WHO is doing, and it does not change what countries should do.
>
> We have never before seen a pandemic sparked by a corona-virus. This is the first pandemic caused by a coronavirus. And we have never before seen a pandemic that can be controlled at the same time. The WHO has been in full response mode since we were notified of the first case. And we have called every day for countries to take urgent and aggressive action. We have rung the alarm bell loud and clear.
>
> As I said on Monday, just looking at the number of cases and the number of countries affected does not tell the full story. Of the 118,000 cases reported globally in 114 countries, more than 90% of the cases are in just four countries and two of those — China and the Republic of Korea — have significantly declining epidemics. Eighty-one countries have not reported any cases, and 57 countries have reported 10 cases or less.
>
> We cannot say this loudly enough, or clearly enough, or often enough: all countries can still change the course of this pandemic. If countries detect, test, treat, isolate, trace, and mobilize

their people in the response, those with a handful of cases can prevent those cases from becoming clusters, and those clusters becoming community transmission. Even those countries with community transmission or large clusters can turn the tide on this virus. Several countries have demonstrated that this virus can be suppressed and controlled.

The challenge for many countries who are now dealing with large clusters or community transmission is not whether they **can** *do the same — it is whether they* **will**. *Some countries are struggling with a lack of capacity. Some countries are struggling with a lack of resources. Some countries are struggling with a lack of resolve.*

We are grateful for the measures being taken in Iran, Italy and the Republic of Korea to slow the virus and control their epidemics. We know that these measures are taking a heavy toll on societies and economies, just as they did in China.

All countries must strike a fine balance between protecting health, minimizing economic and social disruption, and respecting human rights. The WHO's mandate is public health. But we are working with many partners across all sectors to mitigate the social and economic consequences of this pandemic. This is not just a public health crisis, it is a crisis that will touch every sector — so every sector and every individual must be involved in the fight. I have said from the beginning that countries must take a whole-of-government, whole-of-society approach, built around a comprehensive strategy to prevent infections, save lives and minimize impact.

Let me summarize it in four key areas.

First, prepare and be ready.

Second, detect, protect and treat.

Third, reduce transmission.

Fourth, innovate and learn.

I remind all countries that we are calling on you to activate and scale up your emergency response mechanisms.

Communicate with your people about the risks and how they can protect themselves — this is everybody's business.

Find, isolate, test and treat every case and trace every contact.

Ready your hospitals.

Protect and train your health workers.

And let us all look out for each other, because we need each other.

There has been so much attention on one word.

Let me give you some other words that matter much more, and that are much more actionable.

Prevention.

Preparedness.

Public health.

Political leadership.

And most of all, people.

We are in this together, to do the right things with calm and protect the citizens of the world. It is doable."

It is clear for several weeks that many high, middle and low-income countries are either unable or unwilling to take the steps, including locking down parts of (or all) of their population to contain the spread of SARS-CoV-2. It is thus uncertain whether it would have made a substantial difference in the impact of the pandemic had the WHO declared COVID-19 a pandemic on March 11 versus weeks earlier. Further discussion on why countries were unable to contain the COVID-19 outbreak can be found in Chapter 3.

> Key Point: Infection of people with SARS-CoV-2 occurred 17 years after the outbreak of SARS-CoV-1. Unfortunately, the outbreak due to SARS-CoV-2 proved much more difficult to contain. While both viruses arose in Asia, SARS-CoV-1 was contained, and a pandemic did not ensue. SARS-CoV-2 containment was not successful and resulted in the current pandemic. Some experts believe the pandemic should have been declared prior to March 11, 2020.

2. The COVID-19 Pandemic Intensifies (March 12, 2020–December 31, 2020)

<u>Global view</u>

Following the WHO declaring COVID-19 a pandemic, the number of confirmed cases and deaths increases rapidly over the following months[22,23] (Figure 2.10).

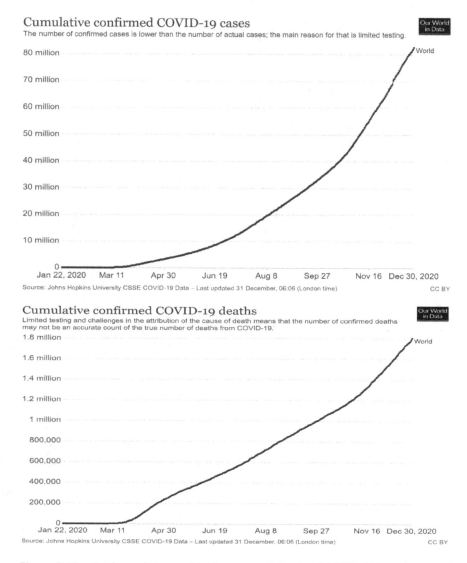

Figure 2.10. Total cumulative worldwide cases and deaths of COVID-19 from January 22 to December 30, 2020.[22,23]

a. WHO develops the Solidarity Call to Action and the Access to COVID-19 Tools Accelerator programs to help create equity in supplies, drugs and vaccine availability

The WHO collaborates with various outside organizations to develop plans and funding to create a unified global effort to increase the global capacity to produce sufficient quantities of PPE and other types of needed medical equipment, provide access to SARS-CoV-2 antigen and antibody testing, and to develop drugs to treat COVID-19 patients and vaccines to prevent COVID-19 disease. To achieve this, the WHO develops two new interconnected programs to help respond to the pandemic — The Solidarity Call to Action and the Access to COVID-19 Tools (ACT)-Accelerator.

The Solidarity Call to Action initiative is created to decrease the impact of the COVID-19 pandemic across the globe by creating mechanisms for equitable global access to COVID-19 health technologies through the pooling of knowledge, intellectual property, and data.[24] Previous pandemics and the initial first few months of the COVID-19 pandemic demonstrated the fallibility of traditional ways of working when it comes to equitable access to essential health technologies. The initiative calls on governments, research organizations, and development funders to commit to urgently undertaking the following:[25-29]

- Take action to promote innovation, remove barriers, and facilitate open sharing of knowledge, intellectual property, and data necessary for COVID-19 detection, prevention, treatment and responses, including through national legal and policy measures, and international collaboration on regulatory practices, to ensure availability, affordability and quality of these products.
- Promote that all COVID-19 publicly funded and donor-funded research outcomes are affordable, available and accessible to all on a global scale through appropriate provisions in funding agreements, and include specific provisions regarding access to and affordability of resulting COVID-19-related health products through global non-exclusive voluntary licensing and other mechanisms as needed.

- Encourage all research outcomes to be published under open licenses that would allow access free of charge, use, adaptation, and redistribution by others with no or limited restrictions.
- Encourage open and collaborative approaches in pre-competitive drug discovery and working together with international organizations towards equitable distribution and access to products needed for COVID-19.
- Ensure that research results are registered and published in line with the WHO's joint statement on public disclosure of results from clinical trials.
- The UN creates a Supply Chain Task Force to coordinate procurement and distribution of medical supplies. The supply chain will need to cover more than 30% of the world's needs in the acute phase of the pandemic and would need to ship at least 100 million medical masks and gloves, up to 25 million N95 masks, gowns, and face shields, up to 2.5 million diagnostic tests, and other equipment every month. Hubs will be located in one or more countries in each region. The estimated cost for storing and moving supplies is US$280 million.

The Solidarity concept is needed due to the lack of global sharing of needed tests, drugs and vaccines during the 2009 influenza pandemic. The WHO Director-General warns against a repeat of "nationalism" for vaccines and other products needed to combat this pandemic and requests that countries sign the Solidarity Call to Action by the end of May 2020. However, by July 2020, only 39 countries have signed on.[24] These countries are a mix of low, middle and high-income countries and this lack of widespread endorsement needs further resolution.

The most urgent immediate problem is a shortage of PPE and SARS-CoV-2 tests. While some countries are participating in the Solidarity Call to Action, many other countries are experiencing shortages of PPE and are attempting to work out individual deals with companies across the globe to meet their needs. This individual country approach causes the European Commission to implement restrictions on selling PPE supplies, such as masks, face shields, and protective garments, outside the European Union. Any exports of this equipment require authorization by EU member states.[30] Similarly, the US government places a moratorium on the USAID's (United States Agency for International Development) global shipments of PPE.[31]

The problems with inadequate supplies extend well beyond PPE and include equipment such as ventilators and oxygen concentrators, which many countries are having trouble getting from the small number of companies that produce them. The WHO is able to buy 14,000 oxygen concentrators to be sent to 120 countries and identify 170,000 additional concentrators that could be available over the next six months.[32]

The funding for the Solidarity effort is inadequate, and the WHO, in conjunction with the UN, launches an independent grant-making foundation to broaden its contributor base for the COVID-19 Solidarity Response Fund.[33] The Director-General notes that the idea for the foundation started more than two years ago as a way to help the WHO deal with a constrained budget where the majority of its funding is designated for specific programs, making it difficult to respond to new problems. The foundation aims to increase flexible global health funding for the WHO through nontraditional sources, such as the general public, individual major donors, and corporate partners. The foundation is a legally separate entity that collaborates with the WHO global health program.

The WHO, in collaboration with other Global Alliance Partners (i.e., Bill and Melinda Gates Foundations [BMGF], Coalition for Epidemic Preparedness Innovation [CEPI], Gavi, The Global Fund, Unitaid, Wellcome Trust, World Bank, Global Financing Facility, and others), launches the ACT-Accelerator at the end of April 2020.[34] This global initiative focuses on speeding up the development and production of diagnostic tests, therapeutics and vaccines to respond to the COVID-19 pandemic. The purpose of the ACT-Accelerator is to bring together governments, scientists, businesses, civil society, philanthropists, and global health organizations to speed up the development of tools needed to end the pandemic. The ACT-Accelerator supports the development and equitable distribution of the tests, treatments and vaccines. This effort focuses on reducing mortality and severe disease, restoring full societal and economic activity globally in the near term, and facilitating high-level control of COVID-19 disease in the medium term.

Towards the end of June, the WHO publishes an investment case for the four pillars of the ACT-Accelerator initiative.[35] The WHO notes that the international community needs to raise US$27.9 billion of the US$31.3 billion needed over the next 12–18 months to ensure the development and delivery of critical tools in the fight against COVID-19. The amount will cover investment needs for COVID-19 diagnostics, vaccines and therapeutics.

It does not yet include the estimates for the health systems connection component of the initiative that will help ensure the efficient use of these tools in all participating countries.

Prior to the pledging summit to support this initiative, Dr. Ngozi Okonjo-Iweala, the Chair of the Gavi Board and special envoy for the initiative, notes in a press briefing that the amounts needed are huge, but "they are not when we think of the alternative. If we spend billions now, we'll be able to avoid spending trillions later."[36] The following day, the summit, hosted by the European Commission and Global Citizen, raises nearly US$7 billion for the development of COVID-19 vaccines, tests and treatments, as well as to help ensure their equitable access.[37] The summit participants include the European Investment Bank, the European Commission, and 40 governments.

b. Formation of the WHO Task Force to investigate the origins of SARS-CoV-2

The World Health Assembly (WHA) has an annual meeting at the WHO, where all 194-member countries provide guidance and feedback to the WHO Director-General on global health topics of concern. The agenda for the 73rd annual WHA meeting includes topics related to the pandemic and a variety of other issues. The meeting occurs virtually on May 18–19, but on the first day, the issue of the origins of the SARS-CoV-2 virus and China's initial response to the outbreak dominates the meeting. The WHA members request that the WHO send a group of experts to investigate this matter.[38]

In response to this request, the WHO Director-General announces in July 2020 the formation of the Independent Panel for Pandemic Preparedness and Response that will go to China to investigate the origin of the COVID-19 pandemic.[39] The co-chairs of the Panel are former New Zealand Prime Minister Helen Clark and former Liberian President Ellen Johnson Sirleaf. The panel is asked to present an interim report by November 2020 and a full report at the WHA in May 2021. Subsequently, at the 75th session of the UN General Assembly in September 2020, the Lancet COVID-19 Commission issues a statement noting that the evidence to date supports that the SARS-CoV-2 is a naturally occurring virus rather than the result of a laboratory creation and release.[40] However, China has still not allowed the

Independent Panel to enter their country, and during the rest of 2020 this issue keeps coming up. During the first week of 2021, the Director-General takes the unusual step of publicly criticizing China for hindering access of the Independent Panel into the country.[41] The Independent Panel is finally allowed to travel to China in March 2021 and reports that the possibility that SARS-CoV-2 escaped from a laboratory is unlikely. The Panel also tells the Director-General that their access to data was limited. The Director-General once again criticizes China by saying: "I expect future collaborative studies to include more timely and comprehensive data sharing."

Key Point: China's government was not forthcoming about the severity of disease caused by SARS-CoV-2 during the initial outbreak of disease. Their opaqueness and strict lockdown and other containment and mitigation policies implemented in their population led the WHO to believe that the disease might be controlled, as well as the WHO delay in declaring the COVID-19 outbreak a pandemic. The WHO issued a substantial number of technical reports on how SARS-CoV-2 outbreak could be stopped. Some countries proved up to the task, but most were not.

---

3. Success of Containment and Mitigation Policies Vary Across Regions and Countries

<u>Regional view</u>

This section looks at how SARS-CoV-2 spread across the WHO regions through the end of 2020. Figures 2.11 and 2.12 show this number of cases and deaths in 2020 by region.[42,43] The Americas region is inclusive of the North and South America areas, and the WHO Southeast Asian and Western regions are inclusive of the Oceania and Asia regions.

In each WHO region, we give an overview of how the region has done during the first year of the pandemic, along with an example of a country that was relatively successful in containing/mitigating the spread of SARS-CoV-2 and one that was less successful. Potential reasons for the disparity in the impact of the containment and mitigation steps on the spread of the pandemic in the two comparison countries in each region are briefly noted

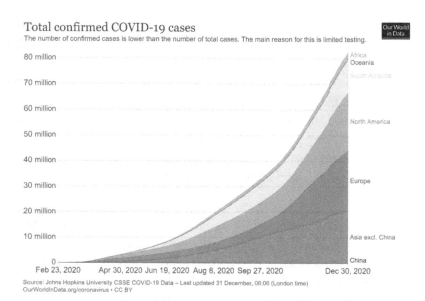

Figure 2.11. Total confirmed COVID-19 cases from February 23, 2020 to December 30. 2020.[42] The WHO Americas region is inclusive of the North and South America areas noted on the figure, and the WHO Southeast Asian and Western regions are inclusive of the Oceania and Asia/China areas noted in this figure.

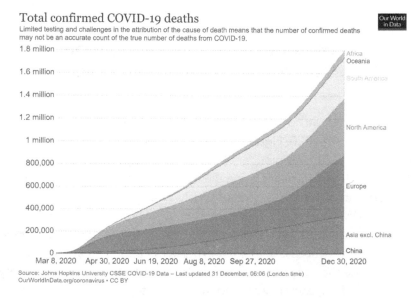

Figure 2.12. Total cumulative deaths from COVID-19 by WHO region from March 8, 2020 to December 30, 2020.[43] The WHO Americas region is inclusive of the North and South America areas noted on the figure, and the WHO Southeast Asian and Western regions are inclusive of the Oceania and Asia/China areas noted in this figure.

in this section. A more in-depth discussion on issues affecting containment and mitigation attempts and the impact this has had on people's lives are discussed in Chapter 3. Most of the figures in this chapter are from the *Our World in Data Statistics and Research COVID-19 Pandemic* website, where a wide array of data is available on how various countries responded to the pandemic and how successful they were in containing or mitigating the impact of COVID-19.

a. Asian region with spotlight comparing China and India

Despite the rapid global rise in cases, some Asian countries have been able to contain, or effectively mitigate, the spread of the virus during 2020. The control measures used by these countries include SARS-CoV-2 testing, contact tracing, quarantine, and lockdown, with each country using these techniques to varying degrees. Asian countries that were reasonably successful in containing or mitigating the spread of the virus during 2020 include China, Singapore, Taiwan, South Korea, Hong Kong, Vietnam, New Zealand, and Australia. Other Asian countries, including India, were less successful in slowing the spread of the virus. Figures 2.13 and 2.14

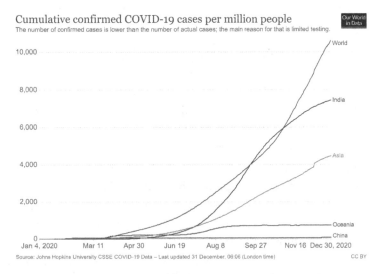

Figure 2.13. Cumulative confirmed COVID-19 cases per million population. Comparison of China, India, Asia, and the World from January 2020 to December 30, 2020.[44] The WHO Southeast Asian and Western regions are inclusive of the Oceania and Asia/China areas noted in this figure.

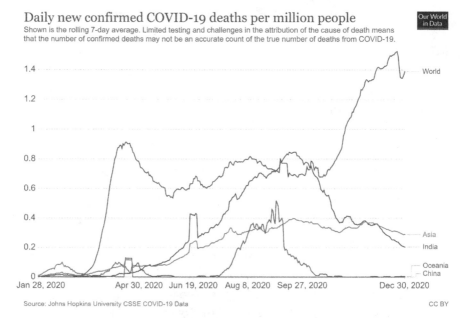

Figure 2.14.   Daily new confirmed COVID-19 deaths per million population. Comparison of China, India, Asia, and the World from January 2020 to December 30, 2020.[45] The WHO Southeast Asian and Western regions are inclusive of the Oceania and Asia/China areas noted in this figure.

compare the total number of daily confirmed cases[44] and deaths[45] per million population in the world, the continent of Asia, China and India.

By the time the COVID-19 pandemic is affirmed in March, China is starting to ease its lockdown while India begins to see a marked increase in COVID-19 cases and deaths. The Indian government responds on March 24 by initiating a 3-week countrywide lockdown. The lockdown initially slows the increase in COVID-19 cases but soon new cases and deaths surge in various parts of the country. India extends its lockdown several times, but becomes geographically more specific based on the number of cases occurring in a given area. By mid-May, the number of confirmed COVID-19 cases in India has surpassed China. By the end of August, India has the third most number of cases and deaths in the world, behind only the US and Brazil, and by the end of 2020, India is second only to the US in the total number of confirmed cases and deaths.[46]

Local outbreaks are still occurring almost every month in China during this period, but the number of COVID-19 cases in China markedly decreases, and there are weeks when there are no new reports of cases. However, on May 17, the Chinese government quarantines over 8,000 people in the northeastern part of the country due to the detection of a cluster of seven cases.[47] Other relatively small outbreaks continue throughout the year despite the intense public health responses.[48] Although both China and India introduced lockdowns, the ability of the Chinese government to effectively enforce this was greater than in India (see Chapter 3 for a more in-depth discussion of the differing responses and outcomes in China versus India).

b. European region with spotlight comparing Sweden and Norway

By March 2020, Europe has become the epicenter of the COVID-19 pandemic, with more reported cases and deaths than the rest of the world combined, apart from China. The CFR approaches 9% during this time, with Italy and Spain recording the highest CFRs. Europe continues to have the highest rate of cases and deaths through mid-May (Figures 2.11 and 2.12).

To counter this increase in COVID-19 cases, different European countries introduce various policies to try to contain or mitigate the spread of the virus. Figures 2.15 and 2.16 compare the number of confirmed cases and deaths per capita in the world, the continent of Europe, Sweden and Norway throughout 2020. The number of COVID-19 cases per million population is substantially higher in Sweden compared to Norway. The major difference between these two countries is their different approaches to mitigating the spread of the virus. While Sweden educated the public about the use of masks, social distancing, and other mitigation measures, it did not enforce them, while Norway did.[49] The differences between Sweden and Norway are further discussed in Chapter 3.

c. Americas regions with spotlight comparing the United States and Canada

The global epicenter of the COVID-19 pandemic switches to North America in the spring of 2020 (Figures 2.11 and 2.12). Figures 2.17 and 2.18 compare

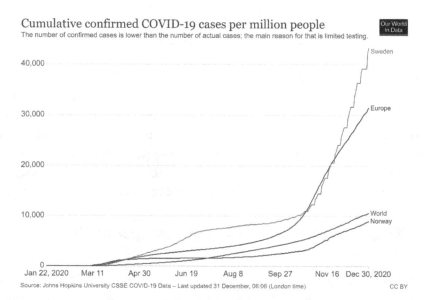

Figure 2.15. Cumulative confirmed COVID-19 cases per million population. Comparison of Norway, Sweden, Europe, and the World from January 22, 2020 to December 30, 2020.[44]

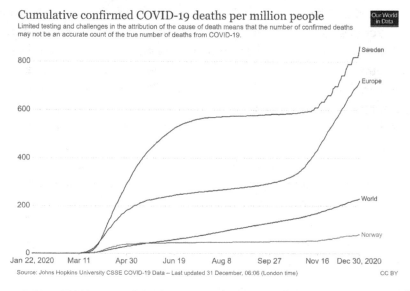

Figure 2.16. Cumulative confirmed COVID-19 deaths per million population. Comparison of Norway, Sweden, Europe, and the World from January 22, 2020 to December 30, 2020.[45]

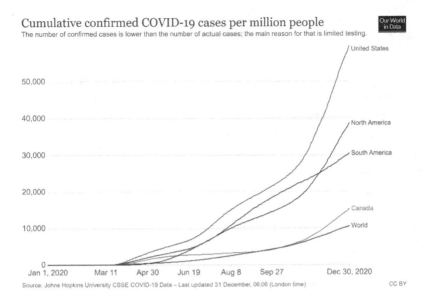

Figure 2.17. Cumulative confirmed COVID-19 cases per million population in the US, Canada, and the World from January 1, 2020 to December 30, 2020.[44] The WHO Americas region is inclusive of the North and South America areas noted in the figure.

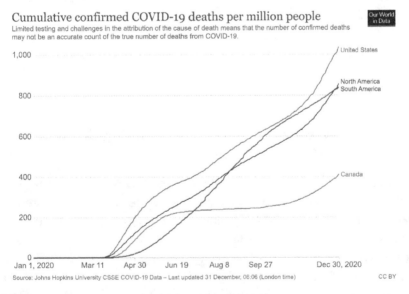

Figure 2.18. Cumulative confirmed COVID-19 deaths per million population in the US, Canada, and the World from January 1, 2020 to December 30, 2020.[45] The WHO Americas region is inclusive of the North and South America areas noted in the figure.

the total number of confirmed cases and deaths per capita in the world, North America, the US and Canada, with the US by far having the most number of cases.

The majority of cases that occur in the US through June are in the northeast and west coasts, with New York City particularly hard hit with emergency rooms, hospital ICUs, and morgues becoming overwhelmed. Similar to the US, Canada has an initial surge in disease through May but is able to flatten the curve after that.[50] Both countries initially employ lockdown procedures to mitigate the pandemic, but Canada's cabinet members and public health officials, along with provincial and indigenous population leaders, do a much better job of devising public policy measures to slow the infection rate to prevent the outbreak from overwhelming the healthcare systems.[51]

From June through August, the highest incidence of disease within the US is in its southern states. The disease is also spreading rapidly within Mexico, but the Presidents of both countries repeatedly downplay the seriousness of the pandemic.[51] The impact of downplaying the seriousness of the pandemic is further discussed in Chapter 3.

The third wave of the COVID-19 pandemic in the US is underway by the fall of 2020, and by end of 2020, the US has greater than 24% of the global COVID-19 cases and 19% of the deaths, despite having only 4% of the world's population.[46] The average number of new cases during the last week of December is 183,287, and at least 1 in 17 of those living in the US have been infected, and 1 in 969 die.[52]

d. African region with spotlight comparing South Africa and the rest of the region

The last region to feel the impact of the pandemic is Africa. Only a relatively small number of cases and deaths per capita are detected before April 2020 (Figures 2.11 and 2.12),[42,43] and Africa appears to have the fewest cases even as 2020 ended.[53] However, pandemic data from Africa is the least reliable because of the low level of testing for SARS-CoV-2 in many of these countries. As noted in Figure 2.19, only South Africa is doing a substantial amount of testing in Africa.[54] Those countries noted in Figure 2.19 as having "no data" are usually the ones doing very low levels of

Total COVID-19 tests per 1,000 people, Dec 28, 2020
The figures shown relate to the closest date for which we have data, with a maximum of 10 days' difference.

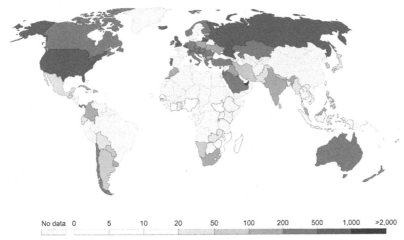

No data 0   5   10   20   50   100   200   500   1,000 >2,000

Source: Official sources collated by Our World in Data   OurWorldInData.org/coronavirus • CC BY
Note: Comparisons of testing data across countries are affected by differences in the way the data are reported. Details can be found at our
Testing Dataset page.

Figure 2.19. Total COVID-19 tests done per 1,000 population from January 1, 2020 to December 28, 2020.[54]

testing (in China and a few other countries where the map indicates there is no data, testing is being done but not reported outside the country).

Due to the lack of reliable data in most other countries in Africa, the total number of confirmed cases and deaths in South Africa is compared to the African region as a whole rather than another individual country (Figures 2.20 and 2.21). The incidence of disease in Africa starts to increase in April, and by July, the rate of disease and deaths in South Africa approaches the rate seen in the US. However, while the number of cases in the rest of Africa is increasing, the death rate appears to be lower than expected, even when factoring in the lower testing rate (Figure 2.21). In addition to the low amount of testing per capita in the rest of Africa, another reason for the apparent lower death rate is likely related to the much lower median age of the population on the African continent[55] and the increasing risk of death with increasing age caused by SARS-CoV-2.[56] This and other potential reasons are discussed further in Chapter 3.

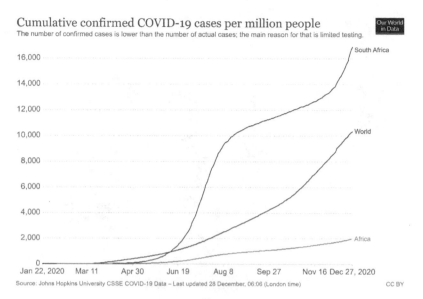

Figure 2.20. Cumulative confirmed COVID-19 cases per million population. Comparison of South Africa, all other African countries, and the World from January 22, 2020 to December 27, 2020.[44]

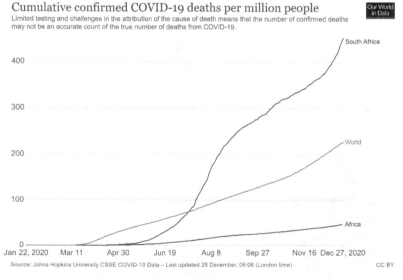

Figure 2.21. Cumulative confirmed COVID-19 deaths per million population. Comparison of South Africa, all other African countries and the World from January 22 2020 to December 27, 2020.[45]

e. Eastern Mediterranean region with spotlight comparing Iran and Jordan

The data from all Middle Eastern countries do not appear in *Our World in Data* as a region, but it is important to examine the impact of the pandemic on countries in this region. There are 21 countries in the WHO Eastern Mediterranean region. There is substantial concern about the accuracy of the data reported in some of these countries. During the early part of the pandemic, there were reports of some governments suppressing or falsifying COVID-19 data due to concerns that the actual data would cause public fear and unrest.[57,58] The number of reported cases and deaths are shown in Figures 2.22 and 2.23. Actual numbers are likely to be substantially higher than those reported for not only those countries that are suppressing data but also in Yemen and Syria, where the longstanding armed conflicts have a very large impact on their capacity to respond to the medical and other needs of their citizens.

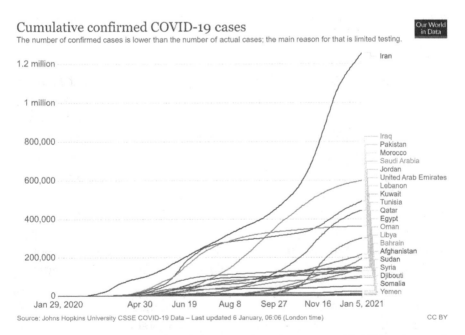

Cumulative confirmed COVID-19 cases

The number of confirmed cases is lower than the number of actual cases; the main reason for that is limited testing.

Source: Johns Hopkins University CSSE COVID-19 Data – Last updated 6 January, 06:06 (London time) CC BY

Figure 2.22. Cumulative confirmed COVID-19 cases from January 29, 2020 to January 5, 2021.[44] The cumulative data for the Middle East region is not available in Our World in Data.

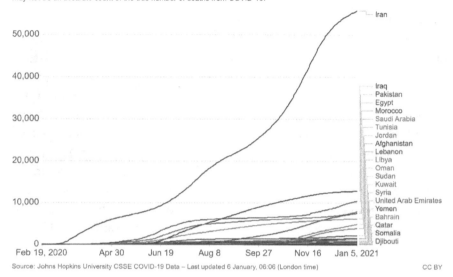

Figure 2.23. Cumulative confirmed COVID-19 deaths from January 29, 2020 to January 5. 2021.[45] The cumulative data for the Middle East region is not available in Our World in Data.

This section looks specifically at Iran and Jordan since the WHO provided help to Iran, and the World Bank did the same for Jordan. Iran does considerably worse than Jordan and many of the other Middle East countries in controlling the number of cases and deaths per capita during the first half of 2020 (Figures 2.24 and 2.25), despite the fact that there is no ongoing armed conflict within the country.[59-61] Iran requires substantial assistance from the WHO even during the early months of the pandemic.[61] The negative impact of the US sanctions on Iran's economy that have been in place since 2017 is a major reason why Iran did worse than Jordan during the first pandemic wave.[61] In contrast, Jordan was able to get international funding to help deal with the first wave of the pandemic.[60] During the second half of 2020, the pandemic causes substantial disruption in many countries in the region. Jordan's case rate exceeds that of Iran, but its fatality rate remains per capita lower than in Iran. Chapter 3 contains a further discussion of how Iran and Jordan did during the first year of the pandemic.

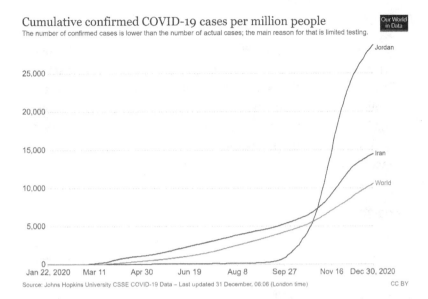

Figure 2.24. Cumulative confirmed COVID-19 cases per million population. Comparison of Jordan and Iran from January 22, 2020 to December 30, 2020.[44]

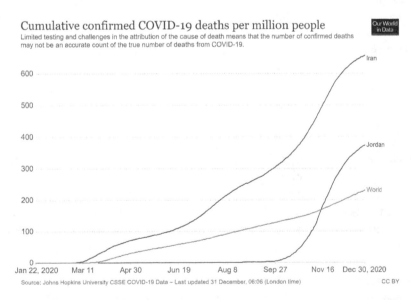

Figure 2.25. Cumulative confirmed COVID-19 deaths per million population. Comparison of Jordan and Iran from January 22, 2020 to December 30, 2020.[45] Cumulative data for the entire Middle East region is not available.

f. Antarctica

Although Antarctica is not a region of the WHO, it is worth noting that even this sparsely populated continent was not able to remain free of SARS-Cov-2. Towards the end of December 2020, 26 members of the Chilean military and ten maintenance personnel at the General Bernardo O'Higgins Riquelme Antarctica base were the first to be infected with the virus with some developing disease.[62] A total of 60 personnel at the base were evacuated back to Chile for care and isolation.

References

1. WHO. (nd) Timeline of WHO's response to COVID-19. World Health Organization. https://www.who.int/news-room/detail/29-06-2020-covidtimeline. Accessed: April 19, 2020.

2. Ravelo JL, Jerving S. (nd) COVID-19 — A timeline of the coronavirus outbreak. Devex. https://www.devex.com/news/covid-19-a-timeline-of-the-coronavirus-outbreak-96396

3. Li W-Y, Yong D, Chau P-H, Yip PSF. (2021) Wuhan's experience in curbing the spread of coronavirus disease (COVID-19), *International Health*, **13**(4):350–357. https://urldefense.com/v3/__https://doi.org/10.1093/inthealth/ihaa079__; !!GA8Xfdg!3oSpNQ974QkJvP97b-FZ-5WwSGbxbnk15gNWrq9ZziCLzfc3l 1PHXSonA-ENq_TyN8mgEjltGUlSi1rgVYxr$"

4. Cohen J. (2020) Wuhan seafood market may not be source of novel virus spreading globally. *Science Magazine*, January 26. https://www.sciencemag.org/news/2020/01/wuhan-seafood-market-may-not-be-source-novel-virus-spreading-globally

5. Holmes E. (2020) Novel 2019 coronavirus genome. https://virological.org/t/novel-2019-coronavirus-genome/319

6. WHO. (nd) What are the International Health Regulations and Emergency Committees? World Health Organization. https://www.who.int/news-room/q-a-detail/what-are-the-international-health-regulations-and-emergency-committees

7. Gilead. (2020) Description of remdesivir. https://www.gilead.com/purpose/advancing-global-health/covid-19/about-remdesivir

8. Nakazawa E, Ino H, Akabayashi A. (2020) Chronology of COVID-19 cases on the Diamond Princess cruise ship and ethical considerations: A report

from Japan. *Disaster Medicine and Public Health Preparedness*, pp. 1–8. DOI:10.1017/dmp.2020.50

9. Wu Z, McGoogan JM. (2020) Characteristics of and important lessons from the coronavirus disease 2019 (COVID-19) outbreak in China: Summary of a report of 72 314 cases from the Chinese Centers for Disease Control and Prevention. *JAMA* **323**(13):1239–1242. DOI:10.1001/jama.2020.2648

10. Pan A, Liu L, Wang C, *et al.* (2020) Association of public health interventions with the epidemiology of the COVID-19 outbreak in Wuhan, China. *JAMA* **323**(19):1915–1923. DOI:10.1001/JAMA.2020.6130

11. WHO. (2020) WHO Director-General's opening remarks at the media briefing on COVID-19 — 24 February 2020. World Health Organization. https://www.who.int/dg/speeches/detail/who-director-general-s-opening-remarks-at-the-media-briefing-on-covid-19---24-february-2020

12. WHO. (2020) Coronavirus disease (COVID-19) Press Conference, 28 February 2020. World Health Organization. https://www.who.int/docs/default-source/coronaviruse/transcripts/who-audio-emergencies-coronavirus-press-conference-full-28feb2020.pdf?sfvrsn=13eeb6a4_2

13. Spiteri G, Fielding J, Diercke M, *et al.* (2020) First cases of coronavirus disease 2019 (COVID-19) in the WHO European Region, 24 January to 21 February 2020. *Eurosurveillance* **25**(9):2000178. DOI:10.2807/1560-7917.ES.2020.25.9.2000178

14. Cheng SO, Khan S. (2020) Europe's response to COVID-19 in March and April 2020 — A letter to the editor on "World Health Organization declares global emergency: A review of the 2019 novel coronavirus (COVID-19)". *International Journal of Surgery* **78**:3–4. DOI:10.1016/j.ijsu.2020.04.011

15. Wilson R. (2020) Coronavirus identified in Italy months before first confirmed case. *The Hill*, December 10. https://thehill.com/policy/healthcare/529627-coronavirus-identified-in-italy-months-before-first-confirmed-case

16. Thielking M, Braswell H. (2020). CDC expects "community spread" of coronavirus, as top official warns disruptions could be 'severe'. *STAT*, February 25. https://www.statnews.com/2020/02/25/cdc-expects-community-spread-of-coronavirus-as-top-official-warns-disruptions-could-be-severe/

17. Panetta G. (2020) Trump reportedly threatened to fire a top doctor at the CDC for sounding the alarm about the coronavirus in February. *Business Insider*, April 22. https://www.businessinsider.com/trump-wanted-to-fire-cdc-doctor-for-raising-alarm-on-coronavirus-wsj-2020-4

18. Loembé MM, Tshangela A, Salyer SJ, *et al.* (2020) COVID-19 in Africa: The spread and response. *Nature Medicine* **26**(7):999–1003. doi:10.1038/s41591-020-0961-x

19. Nkengasong J. (2020) Let Africa into the market for COVID-19 diagnostics. *Nature*, April 28. https://doi.org/10.1038/d41586-020-01265-0

20. WHO. (2020) WHO advice for international travel and trade in relation to the outbreak of pneumonia caused by a new coronavirus in China. World Health Organization, January 10. https://www.who.int/news-room/articles-detail/who-advice-for-international-travel-and-trade-in-relation-to-the-outbreak-of-pneumonia-caused-by-a-new-coronavirus-in-china

21. WHO. (2020) WHO Director-General's opening remarks at the media briefing on COVID-19 — 11 March 2020. World Health Organization. https://www.who.int/dg/speeches/detail/who-director-general-s-opening-remarks-at-the-media-briefing-on-covid-19---11-march-2020

22. Richie H, Ortiz-Opsina E, Bellekian, *et al.* (nd) What is the total number of confirmed cases? https://ourworldindata.org/covid-cases

23. Richie H, Ortiz-Opsina E, Bellekian, *et al.* (nd) What is the total number of confirmed deaths? https://ourworldindata.org/covid-deaths

24. WHO. (2020) Endorsements of the Solidarity Call to Action. World Health Organization, July 31. https://www.who.int/emergencies/diseases/novel-coronavirus-2019/global-research-on-novel-coronavirus-2019-ncov/covid-19-technology-access-pool/endorsements-of-the-solidarity-call-to-action

25. WHO. (nd) Making the response to COVID-19 a public common good: Solidarity Call to action. World Health Organization. https://www.who.int/emergencies/diseases/novel-coronavirus-2019/global-research-on-novel-coro-navirus-2019-ncov/covid-19-technology-access-pool/solidarity-call-to-action

26. WHO. (2017) International Clinical Trials Registry Platform (ICTRP) Joint statement on public disclosure of results from clinical trials. World Health Organization. https://www.who.int/ictrp/results/jointstatement/en/

27. WHO. (nd) Global Observatory on Health R&D. World Health Organization. https://www.who.int/research-observatory/why_what_how/en/

28. WHO. (nd) COVID-19 technology access pool. Commitments to share knowledge, intellectual property and data. World Health Organization. https://www.who.int/emergencies/diseases/novel-coronavirus-2019/global-research-on-novel-coronavirus-2019-ncov/covid-19-technology-access-pool

29. United Nations Department of Global Communications. (2020) Supply chain and COVID-19: UN rushes to move vital equipment to frontlines. May 15. https://www.un.org/en/coronavirus/supply-chain-and-covid-19-un-rushes-move-vital-equipment-frontlines

30. WHO. (nd) Commission Implementing Regulation (EU) 2020/402 of 14 March 2020, making the exportation of certain products subject to the production of

an export authorization. World Health Organization. https://www.legislation.
gov.uk/eur/2020/402/contents

31. Bertrand N, Orr G, Lippman D, Toosih N. (2020) Pence task force freezes
    coronavirus aid amid backlash. *Politico*, March 31. https://www.politico.com/
    news/2020/03/31/pence-task-force-coronavirus-aid-157806

32. WHO. (2020) WHO Director-General's opening remarks at the media brief-
    ing on COVID-19 — 24 June 2020. World Health Organization. https://www.
    who.int/dg/speeches/detail/who-director-general-s-opening-remarks-at-the-
    media-briefing-on-covid-19---24-june-2020

33. WHO. (2020) WHO launches an independent grant-making foundation. World
    Health Organization, May 27. https://www.who.int/news-room/detail/27-05-
    2020-who-foundation-established-to-support-critical-global-health-needs

34. WHO. (2020) The Access to COVID-19 Tools (ACT)-Accelerator. World Health
    Organization, April. https://www.who.int/initiatives/act-accelerator

35. WHO. (2020) ACT-Accelerator update. Publication of investment cases.
    World Health Organization, June 25. https://www.who.int/publications/m/
    item/act-a-investment-case

36. UN. (2020) Global partners require $31 billion to speed up COVID-19 medicines
    for all. *UN News*, June 26. https://news.un.org/en/story/2020/06/1067282

37. Global Citizen. (2020) Global goal: Unite for our future', Global Citizen and
    the European Commission mobilize $1.5 billion in cash grants, and $5.4
    billion in loans and guarantees — For a total of $6.9 billion pledged — To
    combat the disproportionate impact of COVID-19 on vulnerable and dis-
    advantaged communities. *CISION PR Newswire*, June 27. https://www.
    prnewswire.com/news-releases/global-goal-unite-for-our-future-global-
    citizen-and-the-european-commission-mobilize-1-5-billion-in-cash-grants-
    and-5-4-billion-in-loans-and-guarantees--for-a-total-of-6-9-billion-pledged--
    to-combat-the-disproportionate-im-301084708.html

38. Schnirring L. (2020) World Health Assembly opens amid pandemic tensions,
    calls for probe. Center for Infectious Disease Research and Policy, May 18.
    https://www.cidrap.umn.edu/news-perspective/2020/05/world-health-
    assembly-opens-amid-pandemic-tensions-calls-probe

39. WHO. (2020) Independent evaluation of global COVID-19 response
    announced. World Health Organization, July 9. https://www.who.int/
    news-room/detail/09-07-2020-independent-evaluation-of-global-covid-19-
    response-announced

40. The Lancet. (2020) Lancet COVID-19 Commission statement of the occasion
    of the 75th session of the UN General Assembly. *Lancet* **396**:1102–1124.

41. The New York Times. (2021) The WHO criticizes China for not letting its experts into the country. NY Times Coronavirus Briefing, January 5. https://www.nytimes.com/2021/01/05/us/coronavirus-today.html

42. Richie H, Ortiz-Opsina E, Bellekian, *et al.* (nd) What is the total number of confirmed cases? https://ourworldindata.org/grapher/total-covid-cases-region

43. Richie H, Ortiz-Opsina E, Bellekian, *et al.* (nd) What is the total number of confirmed deaths? https://ourworldindata.org/grapher/total-covid-deaths-region

44. Richie H, Ortiz-Opsina E, Bellekian, *et al.* (nd) What is the total number of confirmed cases per million population? https://ourworldindata.org/coronavirus-data-explorer?

45. Richie H, Ortiz-Opsina E, Bellekian, *et al.* (nd) What is the total number of confirmed deaths per million population? https://ourworldindata.org/coronavirus-data-explorer?

46. JHU. (nd) COVID-19 dashboard, Center for Systems Science and Engineering, Johns Hopkins University. https://www.arcgis.com/apps/opsdashboard/index.html#/bda7594740fd40299423467b48e9ecf6

47. Reuters. (2020) China reports seven new coronavirus infections. *Reuters*, May 17. https://www.reuters.com/article/us-health-coronavirus-china-cases/china-reports-seven-new-coronavirus-infections-idUSKBN22U01R

48. Bloomberg. (2020) Beijing locks down part of city after virus outbreak at market. *Bloomberg News*, June 13. https://www.bloomberg.com/news/articles/2020-06-13/beijing-shuts-biggest-vegetable-market-after-45-covid-19-cases?srnd=prognosis

49. Holroyd M. (2020) Coronavirus: Sweden stands firm over its controversial COVID-19 approach. *Euro News*, August 4. https://www.euronews.com/2020/04/06/coronavirus-sweden-stands-firm-over-its-controversial-covid-19-approach

50. Ramírez MS. (2020) Canada's response to coronavirus. Wilson Center. https://www.wilsoncenter.org/article/canadas-response-coronavirus

51. Rivers M, Gallon N. (2020) Why are these three presidents downplaying coronavirus warnings? CNN, March 25. https://www.cnn.com/2020/03/24/americas/coronavirus-latin-america-presidents-intl/index.html

52. The New York Times (2020) Coronavirus tracker NY Times December 31, 2020. https://www.nytimes.com/interactive/2020/us/coronavirus-us-cases.html

53. Nordlin L. (2020) The pandemic appears to have spared Africa so far. Scientists are struggling to explain why. *Science*. https://www.sciencemag.org/

news/2020/08/pandemic-appears-have-spared-africa-so-far-scientists-are-struggling-explain-why?

54. Richie H, Ortiz-Opsina E, Bellekian, *et al.* (nd) What is the total number of COVID tests done per 1,000 population?

55. Desjerdine J. (2019) Mapped: The median age of the population on every continent. World Economic Forum in coolaboration with Visual Capitalist. February 15, 2019. https://www.weforum.org/agenda/2019/02/mapped-the-median-age-of-the-population-on-every-continent/

56. Richie H, Ortiz-Opsina E, Bellekian, *et al.* (2020) Coronavirus (COVID-19) deaths August 18, 2020. OurWorldinData.org. https://ourworldindata.org/covid-deaths

57. BBC News. (2020) Coronavirus: Iran cover-up of deaths revealed by data leak. *BBC News*, August 3. https://www.bbc.com/news/world-middle-east-53598965

58. Grace R. (2020) COVID-19 prompts the spread of disinformation across MENA. Middle East Institute, March 20. https://www.mei.edu/publications/covid-19-prompts-spread-disinformation-across-mena

59. Alterman JB. (2020) Covid hasn't crushed the Middle East yet. Centers for Strategic and International Studies, November 18. https://www.csis.org/analysis/covid-hasnt-crushed-middle-east-yet

60. Relief Web. (2020) The impact of Covid-19 on the Middle East and North Africa. April 12. https://reliefweb.int/report/world/impact-covid-19-middle-east-and-North-africa.

61. WHO. (2020) In Middle East COVID-19 hotspot Iran, WHO walks the talk. World Health Organization, December 23. https://www.who.int/news-room/feature-stories/detail/in-middle-east-covid-19-hotspot-iran-who-walks-the-talk

62. With first positive tests in Antarctic, no continent is untouched by the virus. December 23, 2020. The Indian Express from the NY Times. https://indianexpress.com/article/world/with-first-positive-tests-in-antarctica-no-continent-is-untouched-by-coronavirus-7115835/

3 Disorganized Global Response

"It is discomfiting but true that most people still underestimate the true impact of the COVID-19 pandemic. Its immediate effects are so shocking that we are all caught up in them. But the longer-term implications may be more profound still. If we are not careful, they will shake the world order to its foundations."

Jeremy Farrar, Director of the Wellcome Trust,
Financial Times interview,
June 20, 2020
https://www.ft.com/video/24bb768e-5292-4703-baed-275ce1a578e4

Contents

1. Overview
   a. WHO issues technical reports on how countries can contain and mitigate the spread of SARS-CoV-2
   b. Effectiveness of various containment and mitigating steps
      i. Government policies
2. Lessons Learned from How Various Regions/Countries Responded to the Pandemic
   a. Asia
      i. China vs. India
   b. Europe
      i. Sweden vs. Norway
   c. Americas
      i. US vs. Canada

d. Africa
    i. South Africa vs. the African Region
e. Eastern Mediterranean Region
    i. Iran vs. Jordan
3. Conclusions

1. Overview

a. WHO issues technical reports on how countries can contain and mitigate the spread of SARS-CoV-2

The WHO issued various technical reports providing advice on steps countries could take to contain and mitigate the spread of SARS-CoV-2.[1,2] The guidance was developed in conjunction with many experts in various fields and covered multiple topics including:

1) Critical preparedness, readiness and response actions for COVID-19.
2) Country-level coordination, planning and monitoring.
3) Serology and early investigation protocols.
4) Risk communication and community engagement.
5) Naming the coronavirus disease (COVID-19).
6) Surveillance, rapid response teams, and case investigation.
7) Clinical care.
8) Essential resource planning.
9) Virus origin and reducing animal-to-human transmission.
10) Humanitarian operations, camps, refugees/migrants in non-camps and other fragile settings.

During a press conference on April 13, 2020, the WHO Director-General notes six steps countries should take as they go into lockdown mode[3]:

1) Expand, train, and deploy a health care workforce to deal with COVID-19.
2) Create systems to find all suspected case at community levels.
3) Increase production and availability of testing.
4) Identify and equip facilities needed to treat and isolate patients.

5) Develop plans on how to quarantine contacts.

6) Focus the whole government on the suppression and control of the pandemic.

He urges countries to only ease control efforts, such as stay-at-home orders, if the right public health measures are in place, including "significant capacity" for contact tracing. Furthermore, if countries are going to make this move, they must do it slowly.

The WHO guidance is designed to help countries develop their own COVID-19 response policies that take into account logistical, financial and other issues specific to their country. Early in the pandemic, many countries implemented a range of stringent policies, including lockdowns with stay-at-home orders, work and school closures, cancellation of public gatherings (e.g., sporting events, political rallies, etc.), and restrictions on public transportation (e.g., decreasing availability of buses and subways). These measures were implemented to slow the spread of the virus by decreasing the number of interactions between people and urging physical distance between people. Various interventions that can help to contain and mitigate the impact of COVID-19 are noted in Table 3.3.[1,2,4]

Table 3.3. Interventions that can help enable effective containment and mitigation of COVID-19.*

Activity Restriction	Public Health interventions	Governments and Political
Stay at home	SARS-CoV-2 virus and antibody testing	Political leadership support for science-based interventions
Business and school closures	Contact tracing	Balance between saving lives and impact on economy
Limiting public gatherings	Isolation and quarantine of those exposed or infected	National cohesive programs for providing needed supplies
Limiting public transport	Wearing masks and social distancing	Income support and debt protection for individuals and businesses
Limiting national and International travel	Clear communications	Clear and truthful communications
Public's response to restrictive policies	Public's willingness to accept interventions	Don't politicize the pandemic

*Table derived from several references.[1,2,4]

The rest of this chapter examines the varying ability of countries to contain and mitigate the pandemic based on how they implemented their policies and the response of their population to those policies.

b. Effectiveness of various containment and mitigating steps

i. *Government policies*

Each government must consider how strictly to enforce the various components of the containment and mitigation policy components noted in Table 3.3. These policies can have a marked effect on the health and economic well-being of their citizens and vary substantially between countries. In part, this is because the policies need to be compliant with the laws of the specific country and attempt to consider the likelihood that most of the population will be compliant with the specific recommended components. Therefore, the policies need to include input from a wide array of people, including those involved not only in public health and healthcare sectors but also other sectors such as business, education and religion. The degree to which each country implemented and enforced its own policies varied substantially. Furthermore, how well these policies impact the severity of the pandemic requires additional validation. These considerations will be highlighted in this chapter by continuing to focus on the nine countries that were highlighted in Chapter 2.

To help understand which policies were most effective in controlling the pandemic, we use the policy datasets available in *Our World in Data*[4] in conjunction with other published information. *Our World in Data's* Policy Section is from the Oxford Coronavirus Government Response Tracker (OxCGRT) and is maintained by researchers from the Blavatnik School of Government, University of Oxford.[5] The OxCGRT presents data collected from public sources by a team of over 100 Oxford University students and staff from around the world and is updated as needed.

The OxCGRT collects publicly available information on 17 indicators of government responses that span containment and closure policies (e.g., school closures and restrictions in movement), economic policies, and health system policies (e.g., testing regimes). The OxCGRT project calculates a Government Stringency Index, a composite measure of nine of the response metrics. The nine metrics used to calculate a Government's

Stringency Index are: school closures, workplace closures, cancellation of public events, restrictions on public gatherings, closures of public transport, stay-at-home requirements, public information campaigns, restrictions on internal movements, and international travel controls.

The index is calculated as the mean score of the above nine metrics and is scored on a scale of 0 to 100. Countries with higher scores suggest they have implemented stricter control overall. A higher score also suggests a stricter government response (i.e., 100 is the strictest response). If policies vary at the subnational level, the index score notes the response level of the strictest sub-region. The score does not indicate how effective the government was in instituting their policies. Therefore, conclusions about the impact of these policies are based on our review of additional data, and not just from the OxCGRT group.

Figure 3.26 notes the overall Stringency Index of Government Polices for COVID-19 as of December 29, 2020.[4] Scoring of some of the individual metrics within the overall score are noted in Figures 3.27 to 3.34.[4] The metrics

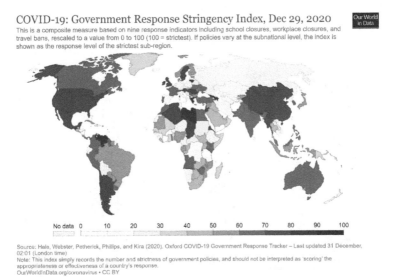

COVID-19: Government Response Stringency Index, Dec 29, 2020

This is a composite measure based on nine response indicators including school closures, workplace closures, and travel bans, rescaled to a value from 0 to 100 (100 = strictest). If policies vary at the subnational level, the index is shown as the response level of the strictest sub-region.

No data 0   10   20   30   40   50   60   70   80   90   100

Source: Hale, Webster, Petherick, Phillips, and Kira (2020). Oxford COVID-19 Government Response Tracker – Last updated 31 December, 02:01 (London time)
Note: This index simply records the number and strictness of government policies, and should not be interpreted as 'scoring' the appropriateness or effectiveness of a country's response.
OurWorldInData.org/coronavirus • CC BY

Figure 3.26. The overall Stringency Index of Government Polices for COVID-19, as of December 29, 2020.[4] The Index is based on nine metrics that include school closures, workplace closures, cancellations of public events, restrictions of public gatherings, closure of public transport, stay at home requirements, public information campaigns, restrictions on internal movements, and international travel controls. The index is scored from 0 to 100 and countries with higher scores suggest that they implemented stricter control overall. Scoring of some of the individual metrics within the overall score is noted in Figures 3.27 to 3.34.

Stay-at-home requirements during the COVID-19 pandemic, Dec 31, 2020

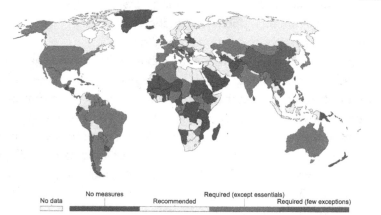

Source: Hale, Webster, Petherick, Phillips, and Kira (2020). Oxford COVID-19 Government Response Tracker – Last updated 31 December, 02:01 (London time)
Note: There may be sub-national or regional differences in restrictions. The policy categories shown may not apply at all sub-national levels. A country is coded as having these restrictions if at least some sub-national regions have implemented them.
OurWorldInData.org/coronavirus • CC BY

Figure 3.27. Stay at home component metric of the Stringency Index for COVID-19 from January 21, 2019 to December 31, 2020. This metric is broken into four levels: no measures, recommended, required except for essential activities, and required with a few exceptions.[4]

Workplace closures during the COVID-19 pandemic, Dec 31, 2020

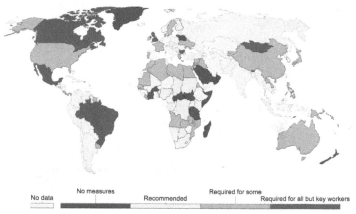

Source: Hale, Webster, Petherick, Phillips, and Kira (2020). Oxford COVID-19 Government Response Tracker – Last updated 31 December, 02:01 (London time)
Note: There may be sub-national or regional differences in policies on workplace closures. The policy categories shown may not apply at all sub-national levels. A country is coded as 'required closures' if at least some sub-national regions have required closures.
OurWorldInData.org/coronavirus • CC BY

Figure 3.28. Stringency of workplace closure policy metric of the Stringency Index from January 21, 2019 to December 31, 2020. This metric is broken into four levels: no measures, recommended, required except for essential activities, and required with a few exceptions.[4]

Public transport closures during the COVID-19 pandemic, Sep 30, 2020

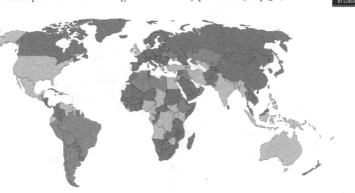

Source: Hale, Webster, Petherick, Phillips, and Kira (2020). Oxford COVID-19 Government Response Tracker – Last updated 30 September, 15:30 (London time)
Note: The policies shown may not apply at all sub-national levels. A country is coded as having these restrictions if at least some sub-national regions have implemented them.
OurWorldInData.org/coronavirus • CC BY

Figure 3.29. Stringency of public transport closure policy metric of the Stringency Index from January 21, 2019 to December 31, 2020. This metric is broken into four levels: no measures, recommended, required except for essential activities, and required closing for most people.[4]

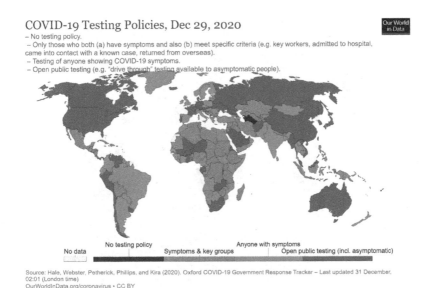

Source: Hale, Webster, Petherick, Phillips, and Kira (2020). Oxford COVID-19 Government Response Tracker – Last updated 31 December, 02:01 (London time)
OurWorldInData.org/coronavirus • CC BY

Figure 3.30. Stringency of testing people for evidence of COVID-19 infection metric of the Stringency Index from COVID-19 from January 21, 2019 to December 29, 2020. This metric is broken into four levels: no testing, symptoms and key groups, anyone with symptoms, and open public testing, including asymptomatic cases.[4]

Which countries do COVID-19 contact tracing?, Dec 29, 2020

'Limited' contact tracing means some, but not all, cases are traced. 'Comprehensive' tracing means all cases are traced.

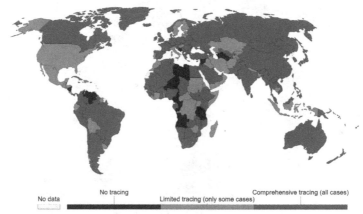

| No data | No tracing | Limited tracing (only some cases) | Comprehensive tracing (all cases) |

Source: Hale, Webster, Petherick, Phillips, and Kira (2020). Oxford COVID-19 Government Response Tracker – Last updated 31 December, 02:01 (London time)
OurWorldInData.org/coronavirus • CC BY

Figure 3.31. Stringency of contact tracing policy metric for the Stringency Index from January 21, 2019 to December 29, 2020. This metric notes those who had contact with a person who tested positive for COVID-19 and how likely they were to have been traced. This metric is broken into three categories: no tracing, tracing of only some people, and comprehensive tracing.[4]

Face covering policies during the COVID-19 pandemic, Dec 29, 2020

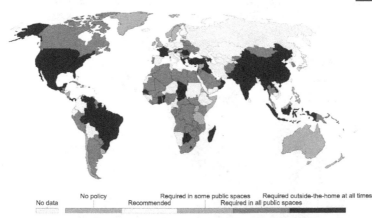

| No data | No policy | Recommended | Required in some public spaces | Required in all public spaces | Required outside-the-home at all times |

Source: Hale, Webster, Petherick, Phillips, and Kira (2020). Oxford COVID-19 Government Response Tracker – Last updated 31 December, 02:01 (London time)
Note: There may be sub-national or regional differences in restrictions. The policy categories shown may not apply at all sub-national levels. A country is coded as having these restrictions if at least some sub-national regions have implemented them.
OurWorldInData.org/coronavirus • CC BY

Figure 3.32. Stringency of face covering policy metric of the Stringency Index from January 21, 2019 to December 29, 2020. This metric is broken into five categories: no policy, recommended, required in some specified instances, required in all shared/public outside the home with other people present, or all situations when social distancing is not possible.[4]

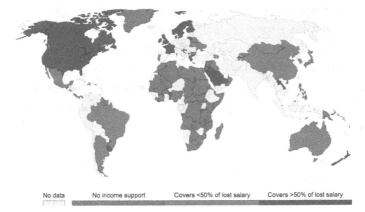

Figure 3.33. Government support of an individual's income metric of the Stringency Index from January 21, 2019 to December 31, 2020. This metric is broken into three categories: no relief, covers <50% of salary, and covers >50% of salary.[4]

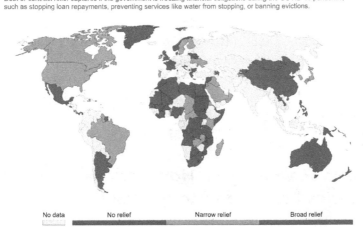

Figure 3.34. Government support of debt or contract relief for citizens Stringency Index from January 21, 2019 to December 31, 2020. This metric is broken into three categories: no relief, narrow relief, and broad relief.[4]

that are included in these figures help provide insight into the differences between various highlighted countries and offer potential reasons why some of the counties were better at flattening the curve of the COVID-19 pandemic so that their medical facilities did not become overwhelmed. A few of the metrics were not shown in the accompanying figures because they did not appear to differentiate countries (e.g., one of the OxCGRT stringency criteria was the Google mobility trends that examined how the pandemic changed the movement of people around the world; however, it did not appear to differentiate mitigation policies between countries in a way that correlated with how well the countries handled the pandemic).

Globally, the different approaches of countries to implementing containment and mitigation policies can be thought of in three overlapping different categories — the hard approach (e.g., the shutdown of non-essential business, restricting the movement of citizens outside their homes, etc.), quick approach (e.g., rapidly shutting down borders, extensive contact testing, etc.), and soft approach (e.g., relying on recommendations rather than a requirement for mitigation steps such as masks, social distancing, etc.). Each approach has its potential pros and cons.[7]

The rest of Chapter 3 uses the countries highlighted in Chapter 2 to examine why these three approaches did better in some countries than others.

Key Point: The containment and mitigation practices that countries used had variable impacts in different countries. In the rest of this chapter, we examine these practices, but an accurate assessment that can be used for future pandemics will take years to really understand what practices worked and why.

---

2. Lessons Learned from How Various Regions/Countries Responded to the Pandemic

a. Asia

1) What determines how effective lockdown is in decreasing deaths due to the pandemic?

2) Can SARS-CoV-2 testing and contact tracing contain the spread of the pandemic?
3) Why are some countries better able to contain a pandemic?

Asia, as a region, has been the most successful in containing and mitigating COVID-19 to date (Chapter 2, Figures 2.13 and 2.14). Many of the Asian countries implemented restrictions on population movement to slow the spread of COVID-19 and prevent health systems from becoming overwhelmed; some have even been able to eliminate COVID-19 from their country for substantial periods of time using the hard approach of a strict lockdown and/or the quick approach by rapidly implementing testing of all contacts in conjunction with intense contact tracing and quarantine. China, Hong Kong, Japan, New Zealand, Singapore, and South Korea had early success in limiting the impact of the pandemic using one or both of these approaches. For example, early during the pandemic, China relied on the hard approach, including a lockdown of large geographical areas, in conjunction with testing, while Korea used the quick approach that included high levels of testing and contact tracing.[8]

i. *China vs. India*

Some Asian countries attempted to use the hard or quick approach, but were less successful. The marked variation in the effectiveness of lockdown policies on containment of the pandemic is illustrated by comparing China and India.

China has an authoritarian government with the ability to institute and strictly enforce a lockdown. In the city of Wuhan where the SARS-CoV-2 virus was first detected in January 2020, the R_0 was initially estimated to be in the 3–4 range,[9] people were only allowed to leave their homes for essential activities (e.g., grocery shopping) or if they were considered essential workers (e.g., food market employees). The government prohibited travel into or out of the city and surrounding province. Within weeks the number of new cases started to decrease, and by the second week of March 2020, new COVID-19 cases were very infrequent.[10]

Since that time through most of 2021, there have been a relatively small number of new outbreaks for which the government rapidly instituted

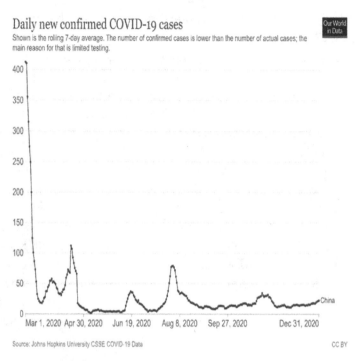

Figure 3.35. Reported outbreaks of COVID-19 in China in 2020.

similar measures in areas that were affected (Figure 3.35). In June 2020, a COVID-19 outbreak started in the Beijing China Xinfadi Agricultural Market, after almost two months of no reported cases since the outbreak ended in Wuhan.[11] This time, the city was not locked down, but all market workers, visitors and close contacts were sought and tested for COVID-19. During this outbreak, there were 335 confirmed cases, along with a substantial number of asymptomatic cases. All were isolated, and those needing care were sent to one specific hospital designated for the care of COVID patients. By July 5, no further cases were detected. In October 2020, locally transmitted symptomatic COVID-19 disease occurred in 12 people in the city of Qingdao.[12] The government responded by putting the hospital in lockdown and running a 5-day campaign to test all 9.5 million people living in Qingdao.

The government's extremely tight control over the information that is made public and the inability of its citizens to communicate freely makes it hard to gauge the response of the public to the lockdown. The central government suppressed information early on in the pandemic and punished those who warned about the severity of the outbreak. Two doctors in Wuhan, Li Wenliang and Xie Linka, messaged colleagues and friends via WeChat, a Chinese social media platform with over a billion users, warning of possible "SARS" cases and urging people to stay away from the Huanan Seafood Wholesale Market, where the patients said they had gone. China's state censors rapidly clamped down on various reports related to the outbreak of a new coronavirus, removing local news reports that exposed the dire circumstances in the city of Wuhan.[13] Those restrictions were put to the test after the death of Dr. Li Wenliang, who contracted SARS-CoV-2 and died on February 7, 2020. Less than 90 minutes after his death, the hashtag "I want freedom of speech" went viral on Weibo, a popular Chinese blogging site, with nearly 2 million posts. The posts were gone by sunrise. The government used various techniques to control the public opinion on their handling of the pandemic, including ordering the news media to downplay the crisis along with informants and trolls to monitor the internet.[14]

India's ability to contain the pandemic stands in stark contrast to what China was able to do. The first COVID-19 case was reported on January 30, 2020, but India waited until March 25 to initiate a 2-month lockdown. At that point, India initiated policies to help contain the pandemic, but compared to China, the lockdown was delayed. Furthermore, the policies were not as stringent (Figure 3.26) and were less successful (see Chapter 2, Figures 2.13 and 2.14).

There are multiple reasons why India was much less successful in controlling the spread of the pandemic. Individual Indian states have substantial decision-making authority compared to provincial governments in China. Another major factor is that over 85% of India's workforce is part of an informal economy.[15] These workers do not get government benefits and need to work on a daily basis to provide food for themselves and their families. Additionally, since the government often does not know where these people are living, it makes it very difficult to do contact tracing. While the number of daily new cases and deaths slowed down during the initial 2-month lockdown, the number of daily new cases and deaths went up dramatically soon thereafter (Figures 2.13 and 2.14).

Further efforts by the Indian government to contain the virus caused a public backlash against the government. By October 2020, India had the second-highest number of reported infections in the world (7.1 million cases, compared with 7.6 million in the United States [US]) and was adding about 30,000 more cases a day than the US.[16] The surge stems at least in part from India's strict lockdown in the spring, which prompted millions of migrant laborers to leave urban areas that they could no longer afford to live in. Their exodus back to India's rural communities where they came from helped the virus spread across the country. Many hospitals, especially those in rural areas, were overwhelmed with patients and struggled to provide adequate care for them.[17,18] Furthermore, while the Chinese government tested a high percentage of its population wherever COVID-19 cases were detected in an area,[9] the extent of testing in India varied widely between individual states.[18]

The economic impact in 2020 of COVID-19 on China[19] (Figure 3.36) and India[20] (Figure 3.37) was substantial for both countries. However, China provided partial income support and debt relief for its population while India

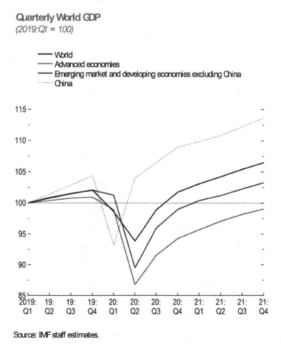

Quarterly World GDP
(2019:Q1 = 100)

— World
— Advanced economies
— Emerging market and developing economies excluding China
···· China

Source: IMF staff estimates.

Figure 3.36. Impact of the COVID-19 pandemic on China's economy when comparing the pre-pandemic period in 2019 and during the pandemic in 2020.[19]

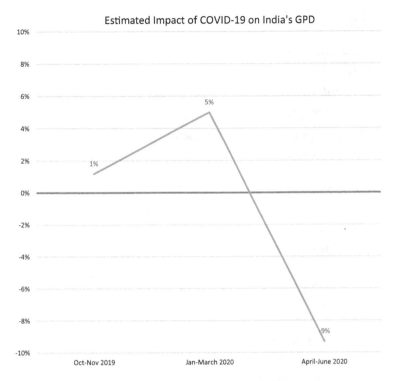

Figure 3.37. Impact of the COVID-19 pandemic on India's GDP from October 2019 to June 2020. Figure modified from reference 20.

did not (Figures 3.33 and 3.34). China's economy is already recovering, but this has not been true for India, which during the first half of 2021 had seen the greatest number of COVID-19 cases and deaths of any country in the world.

Key Point: China and India are the two most populated countries in the world but have very different forms of government. China has a central-ized autocratic government that was able to rapidly enforce very stringent containment policies throughout the country. After the initial outbreak in Wuhan, the government has been able to limit the number of cases and thereby decrease the severity of the COVID-19 pandemic within its borders. In contrast, India's democratic government is less centralized, with individual states having greater authority on how to deal with the pandemic. Thus, India's attempt to mitigate the impact of the pandemic was slower, and its policies were more difficult to enforce due to less central government control and a very large underground workforce/economy.

b. Europe

1) Can herd immunity to SARS-CoV-2 be achieved rapidly enough to decrease the overall number of deaths?

2) Do more stringent mitigation policies save lives at the cost of public physical and mental health?

3) Do more stringent mitigation policies negatively impact the economy during and after the pandemic?

In Europe, the first wave of COVID-19 peaked in April 2020, and by June, the incidence of disease had substantially decreased. However, in September, a second wave occurred, and the incidence of COVID-19 rapidly increased (Chapter 2, Figures 2.15 and 2.16). Many European countries reinstated restrictions, including the closure of bars and sports centers.[21] Italy, the European country that had been most impacted during the first wave, made masks mandatory, and those who did not wear a mask faced a €1,000 fine. By the fall of 2020, the per capita number of new cases in Europe exceeded the number in the US for the first time since March 2020.

Multiple factors influenced the severity of the second wave. Countries across Europe were desperately trying to hold at bay the rapidly growing number of COVID-19 cases, employing targeted closures and travel restrictions to avoid the large-scale lockdowns that damaged their economies in the spring. However, the movement of people indoors due to cooler weather, the negative impact these restrictions had on the economy, and increasing anger from some citizens about these restrictions contributed to governments lifting restrictions between the first and second waves.[22-24]

The European Union adopted new guidelines in October 2020 aimed at coordinating the varying travel policies of member countries.[25] It used a single map with a color-coded system to denote the scale of outbreaks from "low end" to "high". Other measures included unifying how quarantines and testing were done to smooth travel between European Union countries and ensuring ample warning when national travel advisories are about to change to help ensure that travelers are not left stranded. However, the measures were not mandatory, and individual countries were able to take unilateral actions, including stepping up restrictions or changing the risk category for regions based on their own assessments.

The public response to the tightening of restrictions during this second wave was less accepting than during the first wave. In part, this was due to the substantial economic and emotional distress some families experienced during the first wave. Furthermore, some business leaders were issuing dire warnings that whole industries could collapse if restrictions go too far. This public pushback was not only true for Europe during the second wave, as many governments throughout the globe received greater pushback from their citizens.[26]

The WHO was concerned with the increasing pushback and issued guidance on dealing with "pandemic fatigue", which makes interventions more difficult to enforce.[26] As exhaustion and frustration with pandemic restrictions set in, many governments tried to tread a middle-of-the-road course between keeping the virus in check and determining what the public could tolerate.

This is especially difficult in democracies, where governments are ultimately answerable to voters. Public attention often focuses on those who shout the loudest. There were a number of widely covered protests in countries that called for an end to the restrictions, including outside the Reichstag in Berlin and in London's Trafalgar Square. Some protestors called the pandemic a hoax and a government-driven plot. Court challenges to these restrictions were also increasing. In perhaps the most telling indication that people are either confused or no longer listening to guidance, COVID-19 cases continued to explode through Europe, including in places where new measures had already been promulgated. In some countries, particularly England, new rules were often changed, causing confusion and interfering with efforts to slow the transmission of the virus.[24,27]

Slowing the spread of the virus, which thrives on human contact, still depends on individuals changing their behavior. Surveys in countries across Europe showed that a majority of people were willing to comply with regulations if they are well-explained and easy to follow.[22,23] While issues around wearing masks and other individual behaviors remain less politicized in Europe, especially when compared to the US, the prospect of a winter under tight restrictions stirred new frustration and divided political parties. About 20% of people were against regulations, presumably for personal, emotional and financial reasons, but the WHO's European research group also found that roughly half the population is ambivalent about the regulations.[26] They appear to be open to regulations but their concerns need to be heard, and they need to be educated on why the interventions are important. Unclear communication by public health officials and politicians adds to the problem.

i. *Sweden vs. Norway*

Some of the major issues concerning how different governments responded to the pandemic are highlighted by the different approaches Sweden and Norway took to helping the public through the COVID-19 pandemic.

As the pandemic spread across Europe in the spring of 2020, Sweden took a very different approach to the pandemic than most other European countries. The Swedish government followed the advice of their public health advisors, led by Anders Tegnell, and rejected the concept of lockdowns, even those specifically aimed at hot spots.[28] Schools were closed to children over 16, and gatherings of more than 50 people were discouraged, but bars, restaurants, and other public spaces remained open, and citizens were trusted to distance appropriately. Furthermore, public health officials discouraged the use of masks based on what was felt to be inadequate evidence that they helped protect people from infection.[29]

Sweden believed their approach would rapidly cause a large proportion of its population being infected (>50%), and this would result in herd immunity for the rest of the population. They recognized that this approach might cause more deaths among vulnerable people but believed they could minimize the number of deaths while decreasing the pandemic's impact on their economy. They felt that this approach would be more sustainable over time than the tougher measures used by other countries.[30]

Initially, this approach appeared to be working. In late April, Anders Tegnell announced that the rise in infections was beginning to flatten and had reached a plateau in Stockholm, where most of the cases were occurring, as well as in other parts of the country.[30] He indicated that approximately 20% of Sweden's population had already been infected, and in a few weeks, they would achieve herd immunity.

Cumulative confirmed COVID-19 deaths per million people

Limited testing and challenges in the attribution of the cause of death means that the number of confirmed deaths may not be an accurate count of the true number of deaths from COVID-19.

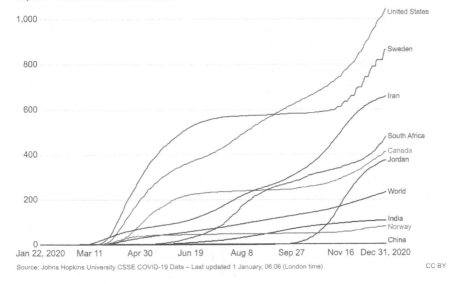

Figure 3.38. Cumulative confirmed COVID-19 deaths per million population from January 22, 2020 to December 31, 2020 in the World and the nine countries highlighted in Chapter 3.[31]

However, the following months would tell a very different story. The number of deaths per capita far exceeded what happened in Norway and in most of other countries, including those highlighted in this chapter, except for the US (Figure 3.38).[31] Sweden recorded the most coronavirus deaths per capita in Europe. The peak number of daily deaths per capita occurred in mid-April and was >4-fold higher in Sweden compared to Norway. Furthermore, the plateauing of deaths from the first wave of the pandemic occurred over a month later in Sweden compared to Norway. More than half the deaths in Sweden occurred in care homes for older people, something that Tegnell admitted was a "failure", especially since a cornerstone of Sweden's strategy was protecting those over 70 years of age.[32] He went on to argue that only time would tell if the overall strategy was the right one for Sweden.

A nationwide study conducted by the Public Health Agency of Sweden found that just 7.3% of Stockholm residents had developed COVID-19 antibodies by late April and that was the largest number of positive results found anywhere in the country.[33] Thus, Sweden, like the other countries, had not come close to achieving herd immunity. In May, the WHO reported that global studies had found antibodies in only 1–10% of the global population, with similar findings seen in studies from Spain and France. The WHO warned against any country waiting on the disease-induced herd immunity as a strategy for controlling the pandemic.[34]

There was also substantial pushback against other aspects of the Swedish strategy. The Public Health Agency of Sweden's website stated, "as long as siblings or other members of the family do not show symptoms of the disease, they can go to school, preschool, or their workplace". Anders Vahlne, a professor of virology at Karolinska, along with various other experts, argued that this advice misled the public by implying that those who do not have symptoms are not contagious, and this resulted in further spread of the virus to those at high risk.[35] The Health and Social Care Inspectorate reported that 75% of the complaints received from the public and healthcare workers were about the lack of protective equipment such as face masks in homes or institutions that provided care to people. Furthermore, the guidelines kept changing, adding to the confusion of not only the public but also healthcare workers.[28]

Testing and contact tracing were other areas where Sweden fell behind. Until April, only high priority groups — patients in hospitals, high-risk groups such as people over 70 or with underlying health problems, healthcare staff, and key workers were being tested, and even then, only for those with severe symptoms. Sweden had carried out 23.6 tests per 1,000 people as of May 24, 2020, as compared to 44.8 in Norway.[36] Meanwhile, contact tracing had largely been abandoned since the beginning of March. Anders Tegnell said in a June 3 press conference that there had initially been problems with laboratory capacity, but also healthcare capacity, because testing is a very complicated chain of events because you need to have staff and resources in each part of the chain. He noted that while the laboratory issue has now been fixed, the resources and training are still lacking.

In an interview by Sverige Radio, Tegnell admitted there was "quite obviously a potential for improvement in what we have done… If we were to encounter the same disease again, knowing exactly what we know about it today, I think we would settle on doing something in between what Sweden did and what the rest of the world has done".[32]

By mid-November, Sweden was in the midst of its second wave, and the number of cases and deaths were substantially higher than in Norway (Figures 2.15 and 16). In December, Sweden's Prime Minister announced that the government was limiting public gatherings (e.g., theaters, religious services, etc.) to no more than eight people, but there would be no limit on private gatherings.[37] The government also drafted legislation that would close shops, gyms and public transport, but if passed, it would not take effect until March 2021. Masks were still not required because of the continuing belief by Tegnell and others that there was not enough evidence to recommend them. Despite the fact that Figure 3.26 gives Sweden a higher score for stringency policies than Norway, Sweden had no mask policy (Figure 3.32), and enforcement of some of the other mitigation activities was lax (Figure 3.31).

The government-appointed commission to assess Sweden's pandemic strategy issued its first report in mid-December 2020, and noted that the government was responsible for the weakness in its eldercare program, and this contributed to the high number of deaths in this population.[38] The King of Sweden strongly criticized the overall response to the pandemic, noting that too many lives have been lost.[39] Towards the end of December, Sweden abandoned this approach and employed a modified lockdown.

Some experts from other countries have a view similar to that expressed by Tegnell. Dr. Kulldorff (a Harvard University biostatistician and epidemiologist with expertise in infectious disease outbreaks), Dr. Sunetra Gupta (an Oxford University epidemiologist with expertise in immunology, vaccine development and mathematical modeling in infectious disease), and Dr. Jay Bhattacharya (a Stanford University physician and epidemiologist with expertise in economics and public health that focuses on infectious diseases and vulnerable populations) wrote the declaration they named the **Great Barrington Declaration** on October 4, 2020. In this declaration, they state their "grave concerns about the damaging physical and mental health impacts of the prevailing COVID-19 policies, and recommended an approach they call 'focused protection'".[40] The idea behind this declaration was that containment and mitigation policies are detrimental, and a better approach would be to let the virus spread and produce herd immunity as quickly as possible. The focused protection would be aimed at the old and infirm who are the most vulnerable population. They put the Great Barrington Declaration on the Internet with a request for other healthcare professionals to sign it if they agreed with what was written. The full declaration is 514 words, and by the end of 2020, more than 10,000 people have signed onto the Declaration that can be found at https://gbdeclaration.org/.

In contrast to Sweden, Norway went into a fairly restrictive lockdown on March 10, 2020, closing schools, restaurants, cultural events, gyms, and tourist attractions. It also banned outside travelers. By mid-April, Norway started easing restrictions and relied mainly on testing, contact tracing, and home isolation. Norway had significantly fewer COVID-19 cases (Figure 2.15) and deaths (Figure 2.16) per capita than Sweden.

Whether those countries with more restrictive containment policies will have a larger negative impact on their economies is an important one. Comparing the economic impact of the Swedish and Norwegian pandemic policies provides some interesting insights into this question. An expert committee was charged by Norway's government to do a cost-benefit analysis of the lockdown measures they used during the first wave. The report indicated that their policy substantially decreased the number of COVID-19 cases and deaths and the cost to Norway was approximately US$3 billion per month.[41] The committee recommended

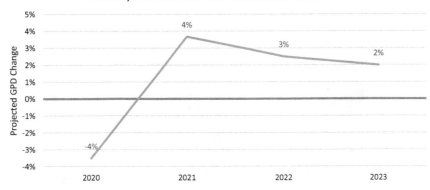

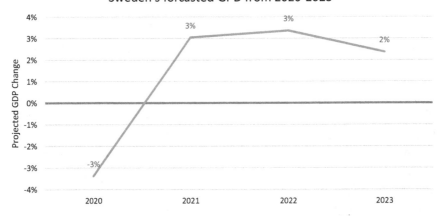

Figure 3.39. Norway's and Sweden's predicted GDP growth in 2020–2023. Figure modified from reference 42.

avoiding a total lockdown at a national level if a second wave occurred and instead employing mitigation at an individual level in infected areas. However, if this did not prevent a surge, then a "brake strategy" should be used to suppress the rate of transmission but should not try to bring the R_0 below 1. Modeling the impact of Norway's more stringent policy did not appear to have a greater negative impact on its economy compared to Sweden[42] (Figure 3.39). The International Money Fund also predicted

IMF DataMapper   Real GDP growth (Annual percent change, 2021)

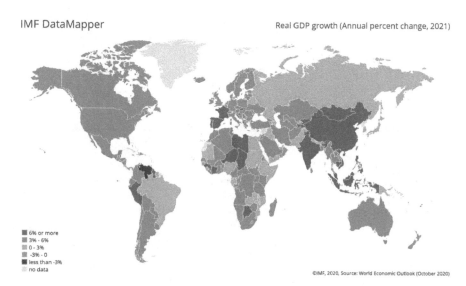

Figure 3.40.   International Money Fund (IMF)-predicted GDP growth in 2021 for each country.[43]

that the economies of these two countries would compare favorably to other countries across the globe[43] (Figure 3.40).

A final note is that after the US CDC examined the relationship of mortality to the OxCGRT containment and mitigation stringency index for each of the European countries during the first wave,[44] it found that those countries that implemented more stringent policies (Figure 3.41) had the fewest COVID-19 deaths per capita (Figure 3.40). The CDC data helps validate the usefulness of the stringency index as a way to predict the mortality in a country caused by the pandemic. Additionally, early implementation of these policies also appeared to decrease deaths.

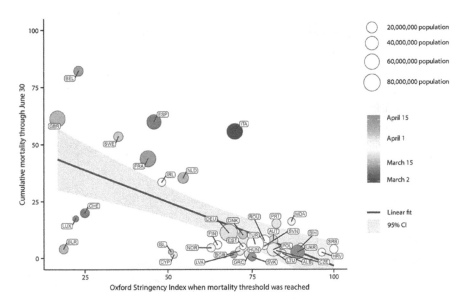

Figure 3.41. Early policy stringency* and cumulative mortality† from COVID-19 — 37 European countries, January 23 to June 30, 2020.[44]

Abbreviations: ALB = Albania; AUT = Austria; BEL = Belgium; BGR = Bulgaria; BIH = Bosnia and Herzegovina; BLR = Belarus; CHE = Switzerland; CI = confidence interval; COVID-19 = coronavirus disease 2019; CYP = Cyprus; CZE = Czechia; DEU = Germany; DNK = Denmark; ESP = Spain; EST = Estonia; FIN = Finland; FRA = France; GBR = United Kingdom; GRC = Greece; HRV = Croatia; HUN = Hungary; IRL = Ireland; ISL = Iceland; ITA = Italy; LTU = Lithuania; LUX = Luxembourg; LVA = Latvia; MDA = Moldova; NLD = Netherlands; NOR = Norway; POL = Poland; PRT = Portugal; ROU = Romania; SRB = Serbia; SVK = Slovakia; SVN = Slovenia; SWE = Sweden; TUR = Turkey; UKR = Ukraine.

*Based on the Oxford Stringency Index (OSI) on the date the country reached the mortality threshold. The OSI is a composite index ranging from 0 to 100 based on the following nine mitigation policies: (1) cancellation of public events, (2) school closures, (3) gathering restrictions, (4) workplace closures, (5) border closures, (6) internal movement restrictions, (7) public transport closure, (8) stay-at-home recommendations, and (9) stay-at-home orders. The mortality threshold is the first date that each country reached a daily rate of 0.02 new COVID-19 deaths per 100,000 population based on a 7-day moving average of the daily death rate. The color gradient represents the calendar date that each country reached the mortality threshold.

†Deaths per 100,000 population.

Key Point: Sweden and Norway took different approaches to mitigate the impact of the pandemic. Sweden's *laissez-faire* policy resulted in a high rate of deaths, while Norway's firmer enforcement of its containment policy resulted in a substantially lower disease incidence and mortality. Future studies will examine the balance between lives saved and the physical and mental toll of strict containment measures, but a definitive answer is unlikely. This more stringent approach did not appear to cause a greater negative impact on Norway's economy.

c. Americas

1) What is the impact on public health and the economy when national leadership ignores science-based recommendations?
2) Are mitigation policies more effective if implemented at the national level vs. state/local level?
3) Are there effective ways to deal with citizens who refuse to follow mitigation policies?

The Americas region had the highest deaths per capita of any region in 2020[45,46] (Figure 3.42). The US was the country with the highest number of total and per capita cases and deaths, and this would remain true throughout the rest of 2020. However, the US was not the only country in the Americas having very high numbers of cases and deaths. Several other countries also had high case and deaths rates (Figure 3.42). Furthermore, in the first four months of 2021, Brazil was particularly hard hit, in part due to the increased rate of transmission of the γ (P.1) variant and also due to President Bolsonaro's downplaying the severity of the pandemic (see Chapter 3 Conclusion section for further discussion regarding President Bolsonaro's impact on COVID-19 in Brazil).

i. *US vs. Canada*

In this section, the US is compared to Canada because the political leadership of these two governments dealt with the pandemic in very different ways, and this helps us understand the impact of their differing approaches on the impact of the pandemic on the health of their citizens (see Chapter 2,

Cumulative confirmed COVID-19 deaths per million people, Dec 31, 2020
Limited testing and challenges in the attribution of the cause of death means that the number of confirmed deaths
may not be an accurate count of the true number of deaths from COVID-19.

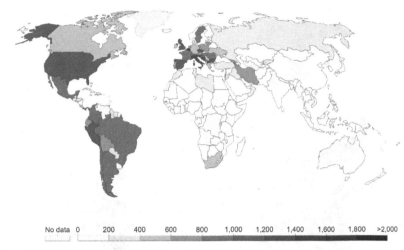

No data 0   200   400   600   800   1,000 1,200 1,400 1,600 1,800 >2,000

Source: Johns Hopkins University CSSE COVID-19 Data – Last updated 4 February, 15:00 (London time)   CC BY

Figure 3.42. Cumulative confirmed map of COVID-19 deaths per million population, as of December 31, 2020.[45]

Figures 2.17 and 2.18). By mid-December, nearly 900 of 938 US cities and more than 2,000 of 3,270 US counties were considered COVID-19 hotspots, and almost 50 counties had a greater than 500% increase in deaths compared to the previous weeks[47] (Figure 3.43).

The first pandemic wave in the US occurred during the first three months of 2020 and resulted in high numbers of cases and deaths in the northeast. The intensity of the pandemic was decreasing by April, but by the end of May, a second wave was impacting the US. It soon became clear that the earlier predictions that a second wave would not occur until the winter were wrong. The second wave peaked towards the end of July, but by early October, a third wave was spreading across the US, and unlike the previous two waves, rural areas were being hit as hard, if not harder, than urban settings. From late November through December, the third wave caused the highest numbers of cases and deaths seen in any nation, and the healthcare capacity in many places throughout the country was insufficient to care for all these patients.[47-49] The description by several

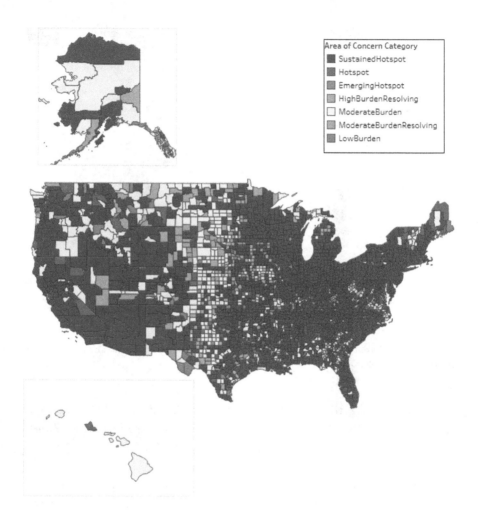

Figure 3.43.   This map shows areas of concern around the US on December 16, 2020. Red counties are "sustained hotspots" with high sustained caseloads and a higher risk of health care capacity issues. Figure is modified from reference 47.

physicians in the Prologue section of this book poignantly details what happens when a medical center is overwhelmed provides a disturbing description of what happens in locations when mitigation steps are inadequate to flatten the curve.

The WHO's Global Preparedness Monitoring Board 2019 Annual Report on Global Preparedness for Health Emergencies listed the US as the number one most prepared country amongst the 194 countries.[50] The obvious question is why did the US end up with the highest number of COVID-19 cases and deaths per million population in 2020? The answer to this has very little to do with US healthcare capabilities. Rather, it relates to the political situation in the US where the Trump administration believed that stringent mitigation steps would damage the economy to the point that it would affect the November 2020 presidential elections. The Trump administration, therefore, decided to downplay the consequences on public health and rejected much of the science-based approach recommended by experts.

A number of reviews of the federal government's response to the pandemic highlight many of the major problems that occurred.[48-51] During the initial weeks of the first pandemic wave, the Trump administration treated the SARS-CoV-2 outbreak as a minor problem that would soon go away. However, it soon became clear that the virus was continuing to spread in the US. Towards the end of January 2020, the White House announced the creation of the President's Coronavirus Task Force and named Health and Human Services Secretary Alex Azar as the Chair. The stated mission of the Coronavirus Task Force was to monitor, contain and mitigate the spread of SARS-CoV-2. The initial people appointed to the Task Force included subject matter experts from various US government agencies, including Dr. Robert Redfield, Director of the US CDC, and Dr. Anthony Fauci, Director of the National Institute of Allergy and Infectious Diseases at the National Institutes of Health (NIH).

Crucial to the response to limit the spread of the virus was the development of SARS-CoV-2 testing. Various countries had developed SARS-CoV-2 tests by early February. However, the US CDC encountered problems with developing the SARS-CoV-2 tests for the US, and through most of February, little testing was done, which artificially lowered the number of cases and hindered contact tracing (see Chapter 4 for more about SARS-CoV-2 tests). During this time, the Trump administration continued to claim that adequate testing was available.

A great deal of criticism was directed at the federal government's response to the pandemic, particularly around the shortage of protective equipment, SARS-CoV-2 tests, and other supplies. At the end of February 2020, President Donald Trump replaced Alex Azar with Vice-President Mike Pence and added Dr. Deborah Brix to the Task Force to be the response coordinator.

During March, the federal government appeared to have a new sense of urgency regarding the seriousness of the pandemic. Much of the country was essentially in lockdown and the governors of the states most affected by the virus finally convinced the administration that the federal government should be coordinating the efforts to fix problems with insufficient numbers of tests, protective equipment, ventilators, and other supplies. Congress passed a US$8.6 billion supplemental appropriation bill to provide money for various aspects of the pandemic response. This improved the availability of medical supplies and helped fix the problem caused by individual states bidding against each other for these types of items and thereby driving up their purchase costs.

The number of daily cases and deaths from the first wave of COVID-19 started to decrease by mid-April. By then, the Trump administration had decided that opening the economy was to be its top priority and the federal government could now let the individual states handle the pandemic. They referred to this as "state authority handoff", and this policy was likely a major contributor to the increase in cases and deaths per capita compared to most countries.

Mark Meadows, the newly appointed White House Chief of Staff, created his own small group of aides to shift the responsibility to the states, and they were, for the most part, ignoring the advice of the Coronavirus Task Force.[48,49,52] This group was focused on improving the economy and minimizing the impact of the pandemic on Trump's chance for re-election in November 2020. They chose to ignore the advice of most of those serving on the Coronavirus Task Force, including Dr. Fauci, who emphasized that the number of cases would go back up quickly if social distancing, wearing masks, and other mitigation steps were not kept in place. Instead, they pointed to Dr. Deborah Birx, the only member of the Coronavirus Task Force who was asked to be part of the Meadows group. Dr. Brix reportedly held the minority view that the pandemic would not worsen until the winter. Her conclusion was based on a model from the University of Washington that was on the low end for predicting the number of cases and deaths, but these numbers were based on the assumption that the general population would continue to comply with the recommended mitigation techniques.[53] However, other models from Harvard[54] and other academic centers predicted substantially higher numbers of cases and deaths. Dr. Redfield would later note in a press conference that they had greatly underestimated the number of people who had been infected during the first wave and this mistake was contributing to the unanticipated second wave.[55] Dr. Brix would later say that some of the data that Trump showed at press conferences that was attributed to her was not data she had previously seen.[56] Furthermore, Dr. Brix stated that the restrained response by the Trump administration may have cost hundreds of thousands of lives.[56a]

Trump kept pushing for reopening the economy at press conferences, and at other public venues he would say that the virus would soon fade away. For those who disagreed with him, he would often use public humiliation and/or fabrication to argue why he was correct. The US CDC had been preparing detailed guidelines for when states should open their economies. However, the Trump administration would not allow these guidelines to be published, and instead, a document containing much less stringent guidelines was made available.[57] Some of the governors who continued to follow the previous CDC guidelines about when to curtail lockdowns were publicly disparaged by Trump.

The disagreements went way beyond the question of whether to open the economy. Trump would frequently make misleading statements about public health and medical issues. In press conferences, he would recommend treatments for COVID-19 that were not based on scientific data, or even worse, went against what the data showed. Dr. Fauci would sometimes publicly disagree with Trump during or after press conferences or when asked by the press at other times about what he thought. This resulted in Trump rebuking him on various occasions, including at his election campaign rallies. This public disagreement resulted in Dr. Fauci and his family being the recipients of many death threats from Trump supporters and requiring around the clock protection by the Secret Service.[58]

Trump tried to bolster his argument that enforcing mitigation was not the correct approach to dealing with the pandemic by appointing Dr. Scott Atlas, a neuroradiologist from Stanford Medical Center with no experience in epidemiology or infectious disease, to the Coronavirus Task Force in August 2020.[59] Dr. Atlas, a proponent of the Great Barrington Declaration,[40] believed it was better to let the virus spread as rapidly as possible in the hopes it would quickly result in herd immunity. Therefore, he believed that people should not adhere to mitigation steps such as wearing masks or undergoing SARS-CoV-2 testing unless they were at high risk for severe disease, as these mitigation actions would worsen the pandemic by delaying the development of herd immunity (see the above Europe region section for more details on the Great Barrington Declaration).

Throughout the first year of the pandemic, Trump repeatedly told the public the pandemic was not serious, the virus would go away within a few months, and there was no need to wear masks or practice social distancing. Indeed, his own actions, including not wearing masks and discouraging the public and people around him from wearing masks, resulted in super-spreader events involving those attending White House ceremonies and large indoor 2020 reelection campaign events.[60] Studies have shown that the risk of SARS-CoV-2 transmission between people is much higher during events that occur indoors, but the transmission of the virus can also happen outdoors if recommendations on social distancing and wearing masks are not followed.[61] Chapter 8 has a more detailed discussion of the risk of virus transmission indoors versus outdoors.

The Trump administration's interference with US CDC recommendations eventually resulted in more than 1,000 current and former CDC employees signing a public letter in October 2020, objecting to the politicization of their agency.[62] The US Food and Drug Administration (FDA) regulatory authority was also politicized with pressure to issue Emergency Use Authorization (EUA) for tests, drugs and vaccines that had not been adequately studied at the time Trump wanted them approved.[63] Some of his recommended treatments proved to be detrimental and two of them, disinfectants that some people mistakenly injected and bleach that was swallowed, resulted in deaths.[64–66]

An editorial written by the editors of the *New England Journal of Medicine* (NEJM) on October 8, 2020, a month before the Presidential election, laid out the case for why Trump and his administration failed the most important obligation of any US president, i.e., to protect American citizens.[67] The editors highlighted the following points:

- The US per capita mortality rate due to COVID-19 is higher than almost all other countries, including those that have a democratic system of government.

- Successful countries used early intensive testing, contact tracing, and isolation as needed. Despite the early warning, the US had an inadequate capacity to do this, and even later in the pandemic, the number of tests done per infected person was much lower than in many countries, and the test results were delayed. This made contact tracing essentially useless for disease control.
- Initially the US was unable to provide personal protective equipment (PPE) for healthcare workers and the public.
- Trump discouraged two of the most effective mitigation steps, social distancing and wearing masks, and this resulted in increased numbers of COVID-19 cases and deaths.
- The federal government had mostly abandoned disease control to the states despite the fact that the necessary expertise and tools to control the pandemic are within the federal government.
- The Trump administration chose to ignore and even denigrate healthcare experts and undermined public trust in science.
- While the federal government invested heavily in vaccine development, their rhetoric politicized vaccine development and increased public distrust.

The NEJM editors concluded by noting that many thousands of additional lives had been lost because of the weak, inappropriate and incompetent federal leadership and policies, and they should not be allowed to continue to hold their positions after the November 2020 election.[67]

A significant proportion of the US public refused to comply with recommendations to wear masks and socially distance. The actual numbers fluctuated over time[68] (Figures 3.44 and 3.45).

Not everyone who refused to wear masks and socially distance did this because of Trump's statements. Another major factor is described by the term "pandemic fatigue", which occurred to some extent in all countries and has been well described in previous pandemics. The WHO defines pandemic fatigue as demotivation to follow recommended protective behaviors that emerges over time and elicits a number of different emotions.[69] In some countries, pandemic fatigue manifests as angry public demonstrations. After months of dealing with COVID-19,

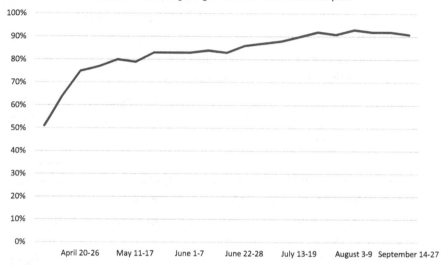

% Americans wearing masks

Figure 3.44. The percentages of Americans who have worn masks from April to September 2020. Currently, 91% of Americans say they have used a mask from September 14 to 27, 2020 — Americans' mask use has been at 90% or higher since mid-July 2020. Figure modified from reference 68.

the increasing incidence of pandemic fatigue is not unexpected. Finding ways to keep those with pandemic fatigue committed to wearing masks, social distancing, and other mitigation steps is difficult. The WHO guidance suggests that clear risk communication in combination with community engagement is key to keeping the public engaged.[69] However, even when risks are well communicated, some people still feel that the risk of being infected by the virus is outweighed by personal, social and economic consequences and so they forsake the restrictions.

Whether pandemic fatigue is worse in the US than elsewhere is difficult to determine, but some of the most public demonstrations of anger against government restrictions and individuals who request compliance with the restrictions have occurred in the US. Two of the most flagrant examples are

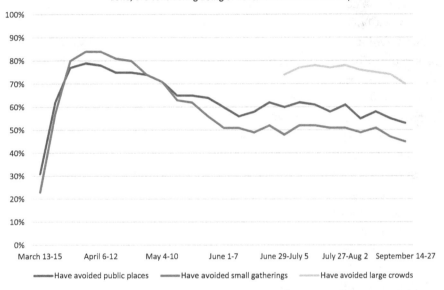

America's Social Distancing Habits

Prompt: "There are some things people may do because of their concern about the coronavirus. For each of the following, please indicate if this is something you have done, are considering doing or have not considered in the past

Figure 3.45. Americans' social distancing habits from March to September 2020. From September 14 to 27, 2020, 70% of Americans have avoided large crowds. 53% have avoided public places, and 45% have avoided small gatherings. Figure modified from reference 68.

the planned kidnapping of Michigan Governor Gretchen Whitmer[70] and armed protestors forcing their way into the Oregon Statehouse building.[71]

The anger is not only within those who feel that the restrictions infringe upon their freedom. Many people are also angry at those who are not complying with the restrictions, such as the wearing of masks in public, thereby putting them and others at risk.[72] At times, this results in attempts to confront and shame those who are not complying with public health recommendations. However, trying to make someone feel guilty is often counterproductive, whether it is done in person or on the Internet. While research is ongoing to find better ways to increase the number of people who are compliant with mitigation recommendations, it often comes down to how individuals and families judge risk versus benefit as it applies to their own situation. This point is highlighted by the following: the US CDC recommended avoiding travel and family gatherings during the 2020 Thanksgiving and Christmas holidays. The recommendation was based on the concern that if this was not done, many more people would develop COVID-19, and the health systems would become overwhelmed. While travel (plane, car and bus) was down during the weeks of Thanksgiving and Christmas holidays compared to the same period in 2019, it increased compared to other weeks since the start of the pandemic.[73,74] Subsequent to these two holidays, the number of COVID-19 cases and deaths increased dramatically.

The number of COVID-19 cases and deaths per capita in Canada was much lower than in the US (Chapter 2, Figures 2.17 and 2.18). One of the major reasons for this was that Canada implemented more stringent travel restrictions than the US. Early during the pandemic, Canada's travel restrictions included all people coming in and out of the country, while US travel restrictions did not apply to US citizens and their immediate families.[75,76]

Another factor that helped Canada was that the country had substantially improved its infectious disease tracking procedures after the SARS-CoV-1 outbreak in 2003–2004 that caused over 400 cases and 44 deaths in their country.[76] The outbreak resulted in Canada developing a centralized public health testing and tracking system along with protocols for responding to future outbreaks. Canada's testing and tracking response was better prepared than the US, where the initial response fell heavily on individual states. This public health response allowed the Canadian healthcare system to avoid being overwhelmed during the first year of the pandemic, unlike the US. Other factors that helped the Canadian government included their universal healthcare system, little political discord over the mitigation restrictions, and acceptance by most of its citizens of the restrictions that had been imposed.[76,77] The economic impact of the COVID-19 pandemic on both countries was similar. Based on the first half of 2020, the IMF estimated that the 2020 GDP would decrease by 5.3% and 5.7% for the US and Canada, respectively.[78] However, during the last half of 2020, the GDP estimates improved for the US and Canada, and both countries are expected to have a substantial rebound (>6%) in their gross domestic product (GDP) in 2021[43] (Figure 3.40). Thus, when compared to the US, the more stringent mitigation policy in Canada saved more lives while not resulting in a more pronounced negative impact on their economy.

Key Point: The US provides a case study on the negative impact of poor national leadership. The Trump administration was concerned that implementing stringent mitigation policies would further damage the economy and affect his reelection chances. President Trump's rejection of scientific advice, suppression of the truth, the purposeful fracturing of public opinion, and lack of concern for lives lost are the major reasons why the US had very high numbers of COVID-19 cases and deaths per capita as compared to Canada and most other countries. The mitigation policies of the US were left to individual states, and this led to further confusion and more fracturing of public opinion. In contrast, Canada's more stringent policies were supported by all the provinces and a larger majority of the public. The impact of the pandemic on their economy was similar to the US. Dealing with pandemic fatigue requires consistent national leadership, clear and transparent communication along with engagement of communities. The failure of the US leadership during the first year of the pandemic to protect its citizens and help the world respond to the pandemic is impossible to justify.

d. Africa

1) How important is data quality for determining the impact of COVID-19 on African countries?

2) Why did Africa do better than other regions during the first wave of the pandemic?

3) What are the major concerns for Africa during the second and potential future pandemic waves?

Africa was the last region to have confirmed COVID-19 cases and deaths, with the first wave starting in April 2020 and then slowing down in the summer. A noticeable increase in cases occurred towards the end of September, and by December, most African countries were experiencing a second wave. (Chapter 2, Figures 2.11, 2.12, 2.20, 2.21).

The data for the number of COVID-19 cases and deaths in Africa is the least reliable of all regions. This should not be a surprise since Africa has a long history of trouble with collecting accurate and timely data, including substantial problems with undocumented births and deaths.[79] By the end of December 2020, the WHO central office reported 1,919,903 COVID-19 cases and 42,697 deaths.[80] In contrast, the African CDC reported 2,759,313 cases and 65,160 deaths in the African region.[81]

This variance in data makes it difficult to determine the intensity of COVID-19 in the African region. One major reason for this is that early on in the pandemic, there was little availability of SARS-CoV-2 testing except in South Africa (Figure 2.19) and, therefore, the number of reported cases and deaths in most African countries likely substantially underestimated the actual numbers. Therefore, in this section, we decided to highlight South Africa and compare it to the African region as a whole.

i. *South Africa vs. the African Region*

Starting in March 2020, South Africa was the first country in the African region to experience sustained increases in cases and deaths and this continued throughout the rest of the year (Chapter 2, Figure 2.9). By November, the number of COVID-19 cases considerably increased in other African countries, with substantial variation across the region. The biggest rates of increase were mainly in the North African region where Nigeria, DR Congo and Uganda had sustained increases in cases. During the first few months in 2021, most other countries in Africa experienced a second wave.[81,82]

Based on data available at the end of 2020, South Africa accounted for more than a third of the confirmed cases detected in the African region and almost half of the confirmed deaths (Chapter 2, Figures 2.20 and 2.21). This high proportion of deaths in South Africa compared to the rest of the region is likely an overestimate given the higher levels of testing and greater availability of intensive care capabilities in South Africa compared to other countries in the region. Another potential explanation for the disproportionately high number of cases in South Africa is the emergence of a new SARS-CoV-2 variant, B.1.351, which appears to be approximately 50% more transmissible. This variant was first reported on December 18, 2020, from South Africa.[83,84] While the variant does not appear to be more lethal, as the number of cases increases, so will the deaths.

The total number of reported deaths in the African region (Chapter 2, Figure 2.12) and the deaths per capita were substantially lower than the rest of the world (Figure 3.42). In addition to the low amount of testing per capita in the African region, another important reason for the apparent lower death rate relates to the much lower median age of the population on the African continent and the increasing risk of death with increasing age caused by SARS-CoV-2. The median age in this region is 18 years compared to other continents, where the median age ranges from 31 to 42 years.[85] The risk of death due to SARS-CoV-2 is approximately 90 times higher in those >65 years of age as compared to those between the ages of 18 and 29 years,[86] and this lower median age helps explain the lower per capita death rate in Africa. Other factors such as lower rates of international travel and a greater proportion of time outdoors may also contribute to the lower number of deaths per capita in the African region.

The risk of a severe second pandemic wave in Africa is very high despite the seemingly favorable outcome during the first wave. Most of the first wave was in urban areas, but the second wave is spreading into rural areas where medical care is harder to access.[87] Furthermore, if the number of cases increases at a rate similar to South Africa, most of the other African countries will not have the healthcare capacity to deal with it. Only a few drug treatments have been found to help people with SARS-CoV-2 (steroids, remdesivir and mono/polyclonal antibodies), and these drugs are likely to be unavailable or in short supply in Africa (see the treatment section in Chapter 4 for a detailed discussion of COVID-19 drugs).

The best hope for Africa is COVID-19 vaccines, several of which have been shown to be highly effective in preventing severe disease. The WHO, working with various Global Alliance partners, had developed the ACT-Accelerator plan to provide vaccines to all countries (see Chapter 2 for details on this plan). However, by the end of 2020, only a few COVID-19 vaccines had received the emergency use authorization (EUA) from one or more regulatory agencies, and these vaccines were unavailable in most African countries. The WHO issued its first-ever vaccine EUA for the Pfizer COVID-19 RNA vaccine on December 31, 2020,[88] and it was not until late February 2021 that any African country had access to these vaccines. The WHO hopes that by the end of 2021, there would be sufficient quantities of COVID-19 vaccines to vaccinate at least 30% of the African population[89] (see Chapter 5 for a detailed discussion of COVID-19 vaccines, including the Global Alliance plans for purchase and distribution to all participating countries).

To a large extent, the ability of the African region to mitigate the subsequent pandemic wave will depend on the availability of COVID-19 vaccines and the acceptance of these vaccines by the various populations to be vaccinated. On this latter point, the recent experiences of some African countries with yellow fever and Ebola have afforded various governments the ability to learn how to better communicate and interact with different communities, which hopefully will help them develop an effective implementation program for the COVID-19 vaccines.[87]

Key Point: The African region appears to have done relatively well during the first wave of the COVID-19 pandemic, but it is difficult to be certain, given the low levels of SARS-CoV-2 testing and other problems with data acquisition. The reported low number of deaths per capita compared to other regions is plausible, given that the median age of the African population is much lower than any other region and the mortality due to COVID-19 is increased in older populations. The ability of the African region to mitigate the impact of the second pandemic wave will be heavily dependent on the ability of the Global Alliance to provide COVID-19 vaccines to a large percentage of the population so that the healthcare capacity of countries is not overwhelmed.

e. Eastern Mediterranean Region

1) Why was the impact of the COVID-19 pandemic harder on Iran compared to Jordan and many other countries in the Middle East region?
2) Why was Iran unable to contain the COVID-19 first wave?
3) How much did US economic sanctions impact the ability of Iran to respond to the pandemic?

When SARS-CoV-2 started spreading in the Middle East in February 2020, most countries instituted fairly stringent containment policies that were reasonably effective in controlling the spread of the disease.[90] However, Iran was unable to contain the initial outbreak, and the numbers of cases and deaths continued to increase throughout 2020 (Chapter 2,

Figures 2.23 and 2.24). The failure of Iran to mitigate the pandemic would seem surprising given that Iran has a strong authoritarian national government and in 2018 had the third-largest GDP of all the Middle Eastern countries (the GDP data is from the World Bank and for most countries is from 2019, but Iran's data was for 2018). In this section, Iran is compared to Jordan, a country with one of the lowest GDPs in this region,[91] to examine why Iran did worse than other Middle Eastern countries.

i. *Iran vs. Jordan*

Jordan, unlike Iran, was able to contain the spread of the virus during the first half of 2020 (Figures 2.23 and 2.24). The real numbers of cases and deaths in Iran were grossly underreported, especially early on when the Iranian government appeared to be in denial about the disease.[90,92] In February, the Deputy Minister of Health was diagnosed with COVID-19, and the next month, a vice president and two ministers were infected. With the situation rapidly worsening in Iran, the WHO country office had to devise its own standard operating procedures, often weeks ahead of the WHO Geneva headquarters. The national government lacked an overall plan for dealing with the pandemic countrywide despite its longstanding control over the population. Furthermore, the economy, already severely hurt by US-imposed economic sanctions, was rapidly worsening.

In March, WHO public health experts went to Iran and met with various people, including government and health officials, to help develop plans to scale up the response to the escalating epidemic. The experts prioritized areas for implementing control measures and pinpointed measures to strengthen the response in areas that had not yet been affected.[92] The WHO team observed that misinformation about COVID-19 was spreading quickly throughout the country and causing harm. For example, hundreds of people in Iran died from drinking methanol alcohol after reading false information on social media that it was a coronavirus cure. They developed a plan to help ensure that factual information was used when available and how to identify and counter false information. Before the pandemic, the WHO Iran country office did not have a communications officer, so a number of people with these skills were hired to work with the Iran Ministry of Health to develop locally relevant risk communication strategies to promote social distancing and other public health activities, and to counter false rumors. The WHO helped the government implement effective SARS-CoV-2 testing, contact tracing, and isolation policies. The WHO was able to help acquire PPE and other supplies despite worldwide shortages.

Previously, Iran's economy had been much stronger than Jordan's since it is an oil-producing country, and this commodity had generated many billions of dollars for the government. However, the decreased demand for oil caused by the COVID-19 pandemic in conjunction with US sanctions on Iran had a large impact on the country. In November 2018, the Trump administration re-imposed sanctions on Iran, which limited the country's ability to do business with other countries.[93] Previously, in 2015, these sanctions had been lifted by the Obama administration when an agreement had been reached with Iran to stop its efforts in producing nuclear weapons. Since the re-implementation of the sanctions, most European and other international banks had left the country because the US had threatened to sanction them. The net effect of these sanctions was to greatly limit the ability of Iran to import and export products, most importantly, their sale of oil, from which Iran's government generated much of its budget.

During the first two months of the pandemic, the Iranian government had imposed a lockdown, but this was lifted in April 2020. Thereafter, the number of cases and deaths continued to increase. The economic effect of the pandemic was substantial, and Iran applied to the IMF for a US$5-billion loan. The US negatively responded to this loan request, and this resulted in the IMF not approving the loan.[94] Many in the public believed that the Iranian government had mishandled the pandemic and this caused a substantial public backlash in Iran.[95] Part of the reason for the government's poor initial response was their concern about public backlash if they provided accurate and transparent communications about the impact of the pandemic.[92,95]

The severity of the pandemic worsened, forcing the government to impose a second lockdown in November in many parts of the country, which made the economic situation dire.[96] Stringent new measures, including prohibiting travel between areas and the closure of most non-essential workplaces and businesses, were instituted in 150 cities and towns, including Tehran. The lockdown was expanded to the entire country when over 13,000 cases were diagnosed in one day, and almost 6,000 patients were in intensive care.[96]

In contrast to Iran, Jordan was one of the Middle Eastern countries that managed to contain COVID-19 in the first half of 2020. Jordan shut down businesses and travel during the early part of the first wave for short periods of time and was able to control the number of cases through the summer (Chapter 2, Figure 2.23). This occurred with the help of over US$700 million in loans from the IMF.[97] The IMF noted that one of the major reasons for Jordan receiving these loans was the government prioritizing the safety of its citizens and supporting businesses impacted by the pandemic.

While the IMF loan to Jordan helped with the government's pandemic response and the economy,[98] Jordan started to experience a large increase of COVID-19 cases in September, and by November the cases per capita was approximately a third higher in Jordan than in Iran (Chapter 2, Figure 2.23), but the deaths per capita through 2020 were about a third lower than in Iran (Chapter 2, Figure 2.24). The economies of both Iran and Jordan were substantially impacted during the first year of the pandemic, each decreasing by approximately 5% in 2020 (Figures 3.46 and 3.47, respectively).[99,100] However, Jordan's economy is predicted to do better in 2024–2025.

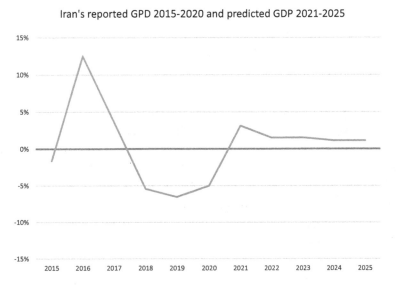

Figure 3.46. Iran's reported GDP from 2015 to 2020 and predicted GDP from 2021 to 2025. Figure modified from reference 99.

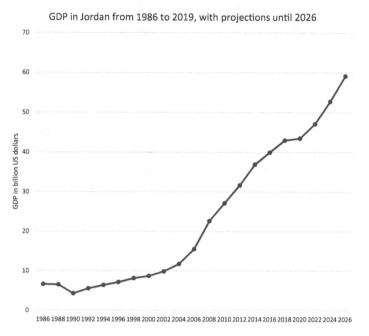

GDP in Jordan from 1986 to 2019, with projections until 2026

Figure 3.47. The GDP in Jordan from 1986 to 2019, with projections up until 2026. Modified from reference 100.

Key Point: Iran was the country in the Middle East region most impacted by the COVID-19 pandemic and had the greatest number of deaths per capita. Some of the reasons for this were also present in other countries that initially tried to downplay the impact of the pandemic to the public. However, a unique factor was that the US government reinstated economic sanctions against Iran towards the end of 2018. These sanctions were already having a deleterious impact on Iran's economy before the pandemic, and the negative impact of the sanctions further increased during the pandemic. Furthermore, the US blocked a US$5-billion loan requested by the Iran government from the IMF. In contrast, Jordan was able to obtain over US$700 million in IMF loans that helped mitigate its first wave of the pandemic. Both countries had a similar decrease in their GDP in 2020, but the economy of Jordan is expected to fare better than Iran going forward.

3. Conclusions

The WHO had a major role in helping countries respond to the pandemic. In a number of areas, the WHO did a remarkable job, particularly in coordinating research programs needed to examine the utility of tests, treatments and vaccines being developed and helping to make them available to countries across the globe (see Chapter 5 for further information). The WHO also helped low and middle-income countries obtain PPE and other supplies needed by healthcare workers and those who became ill. During the first year of the pandemic, the WHO also formed many advisory groups and published various guidelines to provide needed advice to countries.

However, the WHO also struggled in several areas. The WHO declared the SARS-CoV-2 outbreak a PHEIC on January 29, 2020, but delayed declaring it a pandemic. Initially, many countries ignored the threat and therefore delayed the needed planning to better cope with the pandemic. Additionally, the WHO early on suggested that the general public did not need to wear masks, indicating that more rigorous data was needed to prove the benefit of masks outside certain settings such as hospitals. While more data was forthcoming and the WHO did eventually recommend that everyone wear masks when in contact with other people, there already was a substantial amount of observational data to suggest that masks would help protect people from transmitting and developing the disease. Another major problem was created by the inability of the WHO Director-General to get the Chinese government to allow a WHO-appointed group to enter the country to investigate the origins of the SARS-CoV-2. While this access was finally granted, the delay and limitations of the visit made it much more difficult to determine what had happened and what could be done to prevent future outbreaks due to SARS-CoV-2 and other viruses.

Remarkably, in 2020, many of the low and middle-income countries had fewer deaths per capita than high-income countries within a region and across the globe (Figure 3.42). Indeed, the countries with the highest number of case fatality rates (CFRs) were mainly in the Americas and Europe (see Chapter 1 for further explanation of what CFR measures.)

No single reason explains this unexpected finding. Figure 3.48 examines the CFR per capita for the nine countries highlighted in this chapter, as well as the entire African region and the world.[101] The CFR for these nine countries during the first wave of the pandemic varied between 1 and 12%,

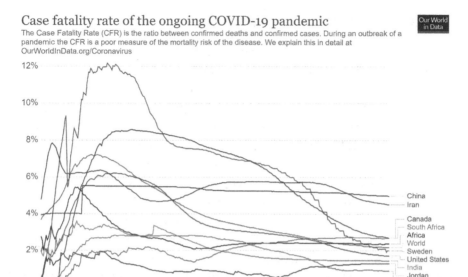

Case fatality rate of the ongoing COVID-19 pandemic

The Case Fatality Rate (CFR) is the ratio between confirmed deaths and confirmed cases. During an outbreak of a pandemic the CFR is a poor measure of the mortality risk of the disease. We explain this in detail at OurWorldInData.org/Coronavirus

Source: Johns Hopkins University CSSE COVID-19 Data – Last updated 4 February, 15:00 (London time)   CC BY

Figure 3.48. The case fatality rate in the World, Africa, Canada, China, India, Jordan, Norway, South Africa, Sweden, and the US, March 14 to December 31, 2020.[101]

but by the second wave, the CFR range for most of these countries was between 1 and 3.5%. Figure 3.48 is updated through June 30, 2022 in the Epilogue (Chapter 10- Figure 10.84) and shows the impact of subsequent COVID waves on the world, the African region and the other nine countries shown in Figure 3.48. The ability of countries to detect cases and care for their patients likely led to an improvement in the CFR during 2020. The CFR per capita was about 2% higher for China and Iran than in the other countries. In the case of China, this is due to the great majority of the cases and deaths occurring in the first few months of the pandemic when little was known about how to treat the COVID-19 disease. The higher CFR in Iran relates mostly to their initial lack of response to the pandemic, public distrust of the government advice about the pandemic, and the country's economic problems. For the other countries, the small differences in CFR do not explain why some high-income countries did poorly.

The US had a high number of deaths per capita compared to most other high, middle and low-income countries. One of the biggest reasons why various high-income countries fared poorly during the pandemic relates to the response of their governments and/or the advice of their public health sector. In the US, the government leadership downplayed the severity of the pandemic and often ignored public health advice and scientific information. The downplaying of the severity of the pandemic led to a lack of coordinated public health response and a disjointed approach to securing PPE and the testing needed to protect people.

This was also the common denominator in some other countries where the political leadership was much more concerned about the impact of the pandemic on the economy than on the health of the population. Brazil was the first South American nation to report a case of COVID-19 in February 2020, but by May, it was second only to the US for the highest number of COVID-19 cases worldwide. Similar to President Trump, President Jair Bolsonaro of Brazil downplayed the seriousness of the pandemic, had a low regard for science, and denigrated those who expressed an opposing view.[102] This turned out to have grave consequences, with some cities running out of vital supplies, including oxygen and ICU beds for those with severe disease.[103]

Some countries in Europe also experienced this type of problem. Both Sweden and the United Kingdom (UK) initially tried the approach of letting the virus spread rapidly in the hope of quickly building up herd immunity. As described earlier in this chapter, the Swedish government took this approach based on the advice of their public health leadership. In contrast, many public health experts in the UK argued against this approach, but Prime Minister Boris Johnson initially ignored their recommendations. England's healthcare system was overwhelmed, and Johnson himself developed severe COVID-19 disease requiring admission to the ICU. Unlike Trump and Bolsonaro, who also developed COVID-19 disease, Johnson became more amenable to the public health recommendations after requiring ICU care due to the COVID-19 disease.[104]

In other countries, the inability to mitigate the pandemic related more to the stringency of their mitigation policies and/or how well they enforced these policies. China's authoritarian government is the most obvious example of a country where the government used very stringent containment and mitigation policies that were tightly enforced. However, there are also multiple examples of democratic governments that were able to contain the pandemic. New Zealand all but eliminated the local transmission of COVID-19 by closing its borders to all foreigners in March 2020 and they plan to keep the country closed to visitors until their population is vaccinated, likely by mid-2021.[105] The government clearly decided to prioritize the saving of lives over the economy despite tourism being a major part of the country's economy. The impact on the economy was substantial, but except for a few short lockdowns in specific areas of the country, the public was able to move around the country freely. Overall, the government had strong support for their pandemic containment program. Australia took a similar approach with COVID-19, and the two countries along with Hong Kong, South Korea, and Japan are considering creating a "travel bubble" in 2021 to allow their citizens to travel between these countries due to their low levels of COVID-19.[106]

The lower prevalence of obesity in Asia and Africa may be another reason for the lower COVID-19 mortality rate.[107] Another possibility is that other coronavirus species may cause more frequent disease in poorer countries, particularly in those with higher rates of overcrowded living conditions, and this might result in partial immunity to SARS-CoV-2.[108]

The economies of all countries have been hurt by the pandemic, but a combination of quick lockdowns in affected areas along with reopenings based on decreasing transmission may be the best way to minimize the impact of pandemics on both health and the economy. Based on predicative modeling by the World Bank, IMF and some other groups, it seems that countries that use strong mitigation policies in conjunction with government interventions to help businesses that are forced to close and people who lose their jobs will recover faster than those that use less stringent policies.[109,110] Data from the 1918 influenza pandemic also suggests that strong mitigations policies help the economy recover faster.[111] More recently, the Independent Panel for Pandemic Preparedness and Response, in their second report to the WHO, indicated that sufficient evidence now exists that decisions to implement strict public health control measures will leave economies at least no worse off than those that do not implement these measures while averting significantly more deaths and illness.[112] This is a powerful conclusion that should help inform the approach that countries take now in dealing with COVID-19 waves and in future pandemics.

Key Point: The global impact of the first year of the Covid-19 pandemic was severe both in terms of health and the economy. The response of the WHO resulted in some remarkable achievements and also some struggles. The same can be said for the governments of most countries. The lessons already learned, those to be learned, and our ability to properly implement these lessons in the future will help determine whether pandemics become more frequent and whether we will be better able to handle them.

References

1. WHO. (2020) A guide to WHO's guidance on COVID-19. World Health Organization, July 17. https://www.who.int/news-room/feature-stories/detail/a-guide-to-who-s-guidance

2. WHO. (nd) WHO country & technical guidance — Coronavirus disease (COVID-19). World Health Organization. https://www.who.int/emergencies/diseases/novel-coronavirus-2019/technical-guidance-publications

3. WHO. (2020) WHO Director-General's opening remarks at the media briefing on COVID-19, April 13. World Health Organization. https://www.who.int/dg/speeches/detail/who-director-general-s-opening-remarks-at-the-media-briefing-on-covid-19--13-april-2020

4. Richie H, Ortiz-Opsina E, Bellekian D, et al. (nd) Policy responses to the coronavirus pandemic. https://ourworldindata.org/policy-responses-covid

5. Petherick A, Kira B, Angrist N, et al. (2021) Variations in governments responses to COVID-19. Blavatnik School Working Paper. University of Oxford. https://www.bsg.ox.ac.uk/research/publications/variation-government-responses-covid-19

6. OxCGRT/Covid-policy tracker. (2021) Methodology for calculating indices. https://github.com/OxCGRT/covid-policy-tracker/blob/master/documentation/index_methodology.md

7. Khullar D. (2021) Five countries, five experiences of the pandemic. New Yorker, January 17. https://www.newyorker.com/science/medical-dispatch/five-countries-five-experiences-of-the-pandemic

8. Han E, Tan MJ, Turk E. (2020) Lessons learnt from easing COVID-19 restrictions: An analysis of countries and regions in Asia Pacific and Europe. Lancet 396(10261):1525–1534. https://doi.org/10.1016/S0140-6736(20)32007-9

9. Pan A, Liu L, Wang C, et al. (2020) Association of public health interventions with the epidemiology of the COVID-19 outbreak in Wuhan, China. JAMA 323(19):1915–1923. DOI:10.1001/jama.2020.6130

10. Statista (nd) Number of novel coronavirus COVID-19 cumulative confirmed and death cases in China from January 20, 2020 to January 23, 2022. StatIsta. https://www.statista.com/statistics/1092918/china-wuhan-coronavirus-2019ncov-confirmed-and-deceased-number/

11. Wu A, Wang Q, Zhao J, et al. (2020) Time course of second outbreak of COVID-19 in Beijing, China, June–July 2020. JAMA 324:1458–1459.

12. The New York Times (2010) A Chinese city will test all 9.5 million of its residents. NY Times Coronavirus Briefing, October 12. https://www.nytimes.com/2020/10/12/briefing/china-vaccine-race-myanmar-soldiers.html

13. Feng E, Feng A. (2020) Critics say China has suppressed and censored information in coronavirus outbreak. Goats and Soda, National Pub-

lic Radio, Inc., February 8. https://www.npr.org/sections/goatsand-soda/2020/02/08/803766743/critics-say-china-has-suppressed-and-censored-information-in-coronavirus-outbreak.

14. Zhang R, Mozur P, Kuo J, Krulik A. (2020) 'Be sleek and silent': How China censored bad news about Covid. *NY Times*, December 20. https://www.nytimes.com/2020/12/19/technology/china-coronavirus-censorship.html

15. Mehanty P. (2009) Labour reforms: No one knows the size of India's economy. *Business Today*, July 15. https://www.businesstoday.in/sectors/jobs/labour-law-reforms-no-one-knows-actual-size-india-informal-workforce-not-even-govt/story/364361.html

16. JHU. (nd) COVID-19 dashboard by the Center for Systems Science and Engineering (CCSE) at Johns Hopkins University. https://www.arcgis.com/apps/opsdashboard/index.html#/bda7594740fd40299423467b48e9ecf6

17. Bharali I, Kumar P, and Selvaraj S (2020). How well is India responding to COVID-19? Brookings. https://www.brookings.edu/blog/future-development/2020/07/02/how-well-is-india-responding-to-covid-19/

18. Laxminarayan R, Wahl B, Dudala SR. (2020) Epidemiology and transmission dynamics of COVID-19 in two Indian states. *Science* **370**(6517):691–697. DOI:10.1126/science.abd7672

19. Yao K, Crossley G. (2020) China's economy has rebounded after a steep slump — but challenges lie ahead. *Reuters*. https://www.weforum.org/agenda/2020/07/chinas-economy-rebounds-after-steep-slump-u-s-tensions-weak-consumption-raise-challenges/

20. Statista Dossier. (2020) Coronavirus: Economic impact in India. *Statista*, Slide 7. https://www.statista.com/study/72133/coronavirus-economic-impact-in-india/

21. The New York Times. (2020) Europe scrambles to halt a rising wave of virus cases with more refined travel restrictions and closures. NY Times Coronavirus Briefing, October 13. https://www.nytimes.com/2020/10/13/briefing/amy-coney-barrett-coronavirus-nagorno-karabakh.html

22. Delussu F, Tizzoni M, Gauvin L. (2020) Evidence of pandemic fatigue associated with stricter tiered COVID-19 restrictions. *PLOS Digital Health*. https://doi.org/10.1371/journal.pdig.0000035

23. European Parliament. (2020) Public opinion monitoring at a glance in the time of COVID-19. June 3. https://www.europarl.europa.eu/at-your-service/files/be-heard/eurobarometer/2020/covid19/en-public-opinion-in-the-time-of-COVID19-03062020.pdf

24. Santora M, Kwai I. (2020) As virus surges in Europe, resistance to new restrictions also grows. *The New York Times*, October 9. https://www.nytimes.com/2020/10/09/world/europe/coronavirus-europe-fatigue.html

25. European Commission. (2020) A common approach to travel measures in the EU. October 1. https://ec.europa.eu/info/live-work-travel-eu/corona-virus-response/travel-during-coronavirus-pandemic/common-approach-travel-measures-eu_en

26. World Health Organization. (2020) Pandemic fatigue: Reinvigorating the public to prevent COVID-19. WHO European Region, October. https://apps.who.int/iris/bitstream/handle/10665/335820/WHO-EURO-2020-1160-40906-55390-eng.pdf

27. Ahrendt D, Cabrita J, Clerici EH, et al. (2020) Eurofound: Living, working and COVID-19. September 28. https://www.eurofound.europa.eu/sites/default/files/ef_publication/field_ef_document/ef20059en.pdfCOVID-19

28. Habib H. (2020) Has Sweden's controversial covid-19 strategy been success-ful? *BMJ* **369**:m2407.

29. Vogel G. (2020) "It's been so, so surreal." Critics of Sweden's lax pan-demic policies face fierce backlash. *Science*. https://www.sciencemag.org/news/2020/10/it-s-been-so-so-surreal-critics-sweden-s-lax-pandemic-policies-face-fierce-backlash

30. Ellyatt H. (2020) Sweden resisted a lockdown, and its capital Stockholm is expected to reach 'herd immunity' in weeks. CNBC, April 28. https://www.cnbc.com/2020/04/22/no-lockdown-in-sweden-but-stockholm-could-see-herd-immunity-in-weeks.html

31. Richie H, Ortiz-Opsina E, Bellekian D, et al. (nd) Cumulative confirmed COVID-19 deaths per million people. https://ourworldindata.org/covid-deaths#world-maps-confirmed-deaths-relative-to-the-size-of-the-population

32. Henley J. (2020) We should have done more, admits architect of Swe-den's Covid-19 strategy. *The Guardian*, June 3. https://www.theguard-ian.com/world/2020/jun/03/architect-of-sweden-coronavirus-strategy-admits-too-many-died-anders-tegnell

33. Ahlander J, Pollard N. (2020) Swedish antibody study shows long road to immunity as COVID-19 toll mounts *Reuters*, May 20. https://www.reuters.com/article/us-health-coronavirus-sweden-strategy/swedish-antibody-study-shows-long-road-to-immunity-as-covid-19-toll-mounts-idUSKBN22W2YC

34. Boseley S. (2020) WHO warns that few have developed antibodies to Covid-19. *The Guardian*, April 20. https://www.theguardian.com/society/2020/apr/20/studies-suggest-very-few-have-had-covid-19-without-symptoms

35. Johan-Karlsson C. (2020) Sweden's coronavirus failure started long before the pandemic. *Foreign Policy*, June 23. https://foreignpolicy.com/2020/06/23/sweden-coronavirus-failure-anders-tegnell-started-long-before-the-pandemic/

36. Richie H, Ortiz-Opsina E, Bellekian D, *et al.* (nd) What is the total number of COVID tests done per 1,000 population?

37. Savage J. (2020) How Sweden is being forced to abandon its sailing Covid-19 strategy. *The New Statesman*, December 14. https://www.newstatesman.com/world/europe/2020/12/how-sweden-being-forced-abandon-its-failing-covid-19-strategy

38. International Long Term Care Policy Network. (2020) Report of the Swedish Corona Commission on care of older people during the pandemic. International Long Term Care Policy Network, December 16. https://ltccovid.org/2020/12/16/report-of-the-swedish-corona-commission-on-care-of-older-people-during-the-pandemic/

39. Anderson C. (2020) The King of Sweden denounces his country's response to the virus. NY Times Coronavirus Briefing, December 17. https://www.nytimes.com/video/world/europe/100000007509830/sweden-king-coronavirus-failed.html

40. Kulldorf M, Guppta S, Bhattacharya J. (2020) The Great Barrington Declaration, October 4. https://gbdeclaration.org/

41. Malmo RO. (2020) Coronavirus: Norway wonders if it should have been more like Sweden. *The Telegraph*, May 30. https://www.telegraph.co.uk/news/2020/05/30/coronavirus-norway-wonders-should-have-like-sweden/

42. Statista. (2021) Norway and Sweden. https://www.statista.com/statistics/1109576/gdp-growth-forecast-in-norway/ and https://www.statista.com/statistics/1109576/gdp-growth-forecast-in-sweden/

43. International Monetary Funds. (2021) Policy Support and vaccines expected to lift activity. January. https://www.imf.org/en/Publications/WEO/Issues/2021/01/26/2021-world-economic-outlook-update

44. Fuller JA, Hakim A, Victory KR, *et al.* (2021) Mitigation policies and COVID-19-associated morality — 37 European countries, January 23 – June 30, 2020. *Morbidity and Mortality Weekly Report* **70**(2):58–62. https://www.cdc.gov/mmwr/volumes/70/wr/mm7002e4.htm.

45. Richie H, Ortiz-Opsina E, Bellekian D, *et al.* (nd) What is the total number of confirmed deaths per million population? https://ourworldindata.org/coronavirus-data-explorer?

46. Wallach PA, Myers J. (2020) The federal government's response — Public health timeline. Brookings Report, March 31. https://www.brookings.edu/research/the-federal-governments-coronavirus-actions-and-failures-timeline-and-themes/.

47. Whyte LE. (2020) Newly released COVID-19 data show most US cities are sustained hotspots. National Public Radio, Inc. https://www.npr.org/

sections/health-shots/2020/12/18/948181472/new-federal-covid-19-data-release-flags-most-u-s-cities-as-sustained-hotspots.

48. Garcia-Roberts G, Mansfield E, Anders C. (2020) It may not have started here, but the novel coronavirus became a US tragedy. *USA Today*, December 10. https://www.usatoday.com/in-depth/news/2020/12/10/how-u-s-failed-meet-coronavirus-pandemic-challenge/3507121001/

49. Shear MD, Weiland N, Lipton E, *et al.* (2020) Trump's failure: The rush to abandon leadership role on the virus. *NY Times*, July 18. https://www.nytimes.com/2020/07/18/us/politics/trump-coronavirus-response-failure-leadership.html

50. World Health Organization and World Bank. (2019) Global Preparedness Monitoring Board. Annual report on global preparedness for health emergencies. https://www.gpmb.org/annual-reports/annual-report-2019

51. Council on Foreign Relations. (2020) Improving pandemic preparedness: Lessons from COVID-19. Independent Task Force Report No. 78. https://www.cfr.org/report/pandemic-preparedness-lessons-covid-19

52. Wright L. (2020) The Plague Year. *The New Yorker*, December 28. https://www.newyorker.com/magazine/2021/01/04/the-plague-year.

53. University of Washington Institute for Health Metrics and Evaluation. (nd) COVID-19 projections. https://covid19.healthdata.org/united-states-of-america?view=total-deaths&tab=trend

54. Covidstim COVID-19 nowcasting. (nd) https://www.covidestim.org/. Accessed: April 26, 2020.

55. Sun LH, Achenback J. (2020) CDC chief says that coronavirus cases may be 10 times higher than reported. *Washington Post*, June 25. https://www.washingtonpost.com/health/2020/06/25/coronavirus-cases-10-times-larger/

56. Sheridan K. (2021) I'm not looking to be vindicated, Dr. Brix says in televised interview. *STAT*, January 24. https://www.statnews.com/2021/01/24/im-not-looking-to-be-vindicated-deborah-birx-says-in-televised-interview/

56a. Bump P. (2021) A better pandemic response might have saved hundreds of thousands of lives — and Trump's presidency. *Washington Post*, March 25. https://www.washingtonpost.com/politics/2021/03/25/better-pandemic-response-might-have-saved-hundreds-thousands-lives-trumps-presidency/

57. Dearen J, Strobe M. (2020) Trump Administration buries detailed advise on reopening. *AP News*, May 7. https://apnews.com/article/7a00d5fba3249e-573d2ead4bd323a4d4

58. Stein R. (2020) Fauci reveals he has received death threats and his daughters have been harassed. National Public Radio Inc., August 5. https://www.npr.org/sections/coronavirus-live-updates/2020/08/05/899415906/fauci-reveals-he-has-received-death-threats-and-his-daughters-have-been-harasse

59. Stolberg SG. (2020) White House embraces a declaration from scientists that opposes lockdowns and relies on herd immunity. *NY Times*, October 13. https://www.nytimes.com/2020/10/13/world/white-house-embraces-a-declaration-from-scientists-that-opposes-lockdowns-and-relies-on-herd-immunity.html

60. VOA News (2020) Trump events leave trail of COVID-19 infections. *VOA News*, October 3. https://www.voanews.com/covid-19-pandemic/trump-events-leave-trail-covid-19-infections

61. Bulfone TC, Malekinejad M, Rutherford GW, Razani N. (2021) Outdoor transmission of SARS-CoV-2 and other respiratory viruses: A systematic review. *Journal of Infectious Diseases* **223**(4):550–556. DOI:10.1093/infdis/jiaa742

62. The New York Times. (2020) A letter from more than 1,000 current and former "disease detectives" decries the politicization of the CDC. NY Times Coronavirus Briefing, October 16. https://www.nytimes.com/2020/10/16/us/coronavirus-today.html

63. Allassan F. (2020) 7 former FDA commissioners say Trump is undermining the agency's credibility. *Axios*, September 29. https://www.axios.com/fda-commissioners-trump-credibility-coronavirus-vaccine-81da52d1-8c88-4b3b-a305-e17e669d4fc3.html

64. Taylor M, Roston A. (2020) Exclusive: Pressed by Trump, US pushed unproven coronavirus treatment guidance. *Reuters*, April 4. https://www.reuters.com/article/us-health-coronavirus-usa-guidance-exclu/exclusive-pressed-by-trump-u-s-pushed-unproven-coronavirus-treatment-guidance-idUSKBN21M0R2

65. Eaton M, King AB, Dalmayne E, Seigler A. (2020) Trump suggested "injecting" disinfectant to cure coronavirus? We're not surprised. *NY Times*, April 26. https://www.nytimes.com/2020/04/26/opinion/coronavirus-bleach-trump-autism.html

66. Joseph A. (2020) CDC: Some Americans are misusing cleaning products — including drinking them — in effort to kill coronavirus. June 5. https://www.statnews.com/2020/06/05/cdc-misusing-bleach-try-kill-coronavirus/

67. The Editors. (2020) Dying in a leadership vacuum. *New England Journal of Medicine* **383**:1479–1480. https://www.nejm.org/doi/full/10.1056/NEJMe2029812

68. Crabtree S. (2020) Americans' social distancing habits have tapered since July. *Gallup*, October 19. https://news.gallup.com/poll/322064/americans-social-distancing-habits-tapered-july.aspx

69. WHO. (2020) Pandemic fatigue Reinvigorating the public to prevent COVID-19 Policy framework for supporting pandemic prevention and management. https://www.aarp.org/health/conditions-treatments/info-2020/cdc-coronavirus-bleach.html

70. Jones S, Waldrop T. (2020) 14th person charged in alleged plot to kidnap Michigan governor. CNN. https://www.cnn.com/2020/10/15/us/michigan-governor-plot-charge/index.html

71. Baker M. (2020) Armed protesters angry over virus restrictions try to force their way into the Oregon Statehouse. NY Times Coronavirus Briefing, December 21. https://www.nytimes.com/2020/12/21/world/oregon-coronavirus-protests.html

72. Bokat-Lindell S. (2020) Pandemic fatigue, meet pandemic anger. NY Times, December 8. https://www.nytimes.com/2020/12/08/opinion/pandemic-anger-shaming.html

73. Poon L, Patino M. (2020) Tens of millions of Americans projected to travel for Thanksgiving despite Covid surge. Bloomberg Citylab, November 25. https://www.bloomberg.com/news/articles/2020-11-25/u-s-travel-is-up-during-the-thanksgiving-holiday

74. Waller A, McCarthy L, Levin D. (2020) Air Travel is down 60% from last Christmas, but many still traveling. NY Times Coronavirus Briefing, December 24. https://www.nytimes.com/live/2020/12/24/world/covid--updates-coronavirus#air-travel-is-down-60-percent-from-last-christmas-but-many-people-are-still-flying

75. Hess DB, Bitterman A. (2020) The conversation. COVID-19 response highlights major differences between US and Canada: US Profs. Canadian Broadcasting Company — Hamilton Point of View. CBC News, June 3. https://www.cbc.ca/news/canada/hamilton/american-canadian-covid-1.5596226.

76. Detsky AS, Bogooch II. (2020) COVID-19 in Canada: Experience and response. JAMA 324(8):743–744. DOI:10.1001/jama.2020.14033

77. Statista. (2020) Percentage of Canadians concerned about friends and family contracting COVID-19 from February to September 2020. https://www.statista.com/statistics/1133772/concern-family-and-friends-covid19-canada

78. Statista. (2021) North America: Gross domestic product (GDP) of Canada and the United States from 2009 to 2021. https://www.statista.com/statistics/527955/north-america-gross-domestic-product-forecast/. Accessed: January 29, 2021.

79. Pirlea F. (2019) Birth registration is less than 50% in many African countries. World Bank... Blogs, July 26. https://blogs.worldbank.org/opendata/birth-registration-less-50-many-african-countries

80. WHO. (nd) WHO coronavirus disease (COVID-19) dashboard. World Health Organization. https://covid19.who.int/?gclid=CjwKCAiArbv_BRA8EiwAYG-s23PaGIsx-9elreBB93Mo6TmA0bd6vRg8ACon-1pKxHxN5zZ8no0Sx8Ro-CrqgQAvD_BwE. Accessed: January 1, 2021.

81. Africa CDC. (nd) Coronavirus Disease 2019 (COVID-19). https://africacdc. org/covid-19/. Accessed: January 1, 2021.

82. Mwai P. (2020) Coronavirus: What's happening to the numbers in Africa? *BBC News*, December 21. https://www.bbc.com/news/world-africa-53181555

83. WHO. (2020) Emergency preparedness response — SARS-CoV-2 Variants. World Health Organization, December 31. https://www.who.int/csr/don/31-december-2020-sars-cov2-variants/en/

84. Munyaradz M. (2021) South Africa responds to new SARS-CoV-2 variant. *Lancet* **397**(10271):267. doi.org/10.1016/S0140-6736(21)00144-6

85. Desjerdine J. (2019) Mapped: The median age of the population on every continent. *World Economic Forum*, February 15. https://www.weforum.org/agenda/2019/02/mapped-the-median-age-of-the-population-on-every-continent/

86. CDC. (nd) COVID-19 hospitalization and death by age. Centers for Disease Control and Prevention. https://www.cdc.gov/coronavirus/2019-ncov/covid-data/investigations-discovery/hospitalization-death-by-age.html. Updated: August 18, 2020.

87. Kuhen BM. (2021) Africa succeeded against COVID-19's first wave, but the second wave brings new changes. *JAMA* **325**(4):327–328. DOI:10.1001/jama.2020.24288

88. WHO. (2020) WHO issues its first emergency use validation for a COVID-19 vaccine and emphasizes need for equitable global access. World Health Organization, December 31. https://www.who.int/news/item/31-12-2020-who-issues-its-first-emergency-use-validation-for-a-covid-19-vaccine-and-emphasizes-need-for-equitable-global-access

89. Science X. (2021) One third of Africa will be vaccinated this year. *MedicalXPress*, January 28. https://medicalxpress.com/news/2021-01-africa-vaccinated-year.html

90. Dyer P, Schaider I, Letzkus A. (2021) Infographic: The stringency of Middle East and North Africa's COVID-19 response. Booking Institute, January 5. https://www.brookings.edu/interactives/infographic-the-stringency-of-middle-east-and-north-africas-covid-19-response/

91. World Bank. (nd) GDP of Middle East & North Africa. https://data.world-bank.org/indicator/NY.GDP.MKTP.CD?locations=ZQ. Accessed: February 3, 2021.

92. WHO Eastern Mediterranean Region. (2020) WHO and public health experts conclude COVID-19 mission to Islamic Republic of Iran. March 12. http://www.emro.who.int/irn/iran-news/delegation-of-who-and-public-health-experts-concludes-covid-19-mission-to-iran.html

93. Nephew R. (2020) The "chilling effect" of US sanctions on Iran. The Iran Primer, US Institute of Peace, October 11. https://iranprimer.usip.org/blog/2020/oct/11/chilling-effect-us-sanctions-iran

94. Williams N. (2020) US will block Iran's $5 billion IMF loan to fight virus. *Bloomberg*, April 8. https://www.bloomberg.com/news/articles/2020-04-08/trump-administration-will-block-iran-s-5-billion-imf-loan-bid

95. Schneider C, Kowsar N. (2020) Iran's mishandled coronavirus response is triggering a backlash against the regime. *Business Insider*, May 11. https://www.businessinsider.com/iran-mishandled-coronavirus-response-is-triggering-anti-regime-backlash-2020-5

96. Hadian-Jazy T. (2020) Iran tries another lockdown as coronavirus cases soar. Atlantic Council, November 20. https://www.atlanticcouncil.org/blogs/iransource/iran-tries-another-lockdown-as-coronavirus-cases-soar/

97. IMF. (2020) IMF Executive Board approves US$ 396 Million in emergency assistance to Jordan to address the COVID-19 pandemic. International Money Fund, May 12. https://www.imf.org/en/News/Articles/2020/05/21/pr20222-jordan-imf-executive-board-approves-emergency-assistance-to-address-the-covid-19-pandemic

98. Thorpe I. (2020) IMF financing soften blow of the pandemic. *The Borgen Project*, October 2. https://borgenproject.org/imf-in-jordan/

99. Statista. (nd) Iran: Real gross domestic product (GDP) growth from 2015 to 2025. https://www.statista.com/statistics/294301/iran-gross-domestic-product-gdp-growth/. Accessed: February 3, 2021.

100. O'Neill A. (2021) Jordan: Gross domestic product (GDP) in current prices from 1986 to 2026. *Statista*, November 2. https://www.statista.com/statistics/385576/gross-domestic-product-gdp-in-jordan/

101. Richie H, Ortiz-Opsina E, Bellekian D, *et al.* (nd) What is the case fatality rate of the COVID-19 pandemic? https://ourworldindata.org/mortality-risk-covid

102. Savarese M. (2020) Brazil's Bolsonaro rejects COVID-19 shot, calls masks taboo. *AP News*, November 27. https://abcnews.go.com/International/wireStory/brazils-bolsonaro-rejects-covid-19-shot-calls-masks-74428885

103. Daniels JP. (2021) Health experts slam Bolsonaro's vaccine. *Lancet* **397**(10272):P361. https://doi.org/10.1016/S0140-6736(21)00181-10

104. VOA. (2020) British Prime Minister takes responsibility for COVID-19 response. *VOA News*, July 8. https://www.voanews.com/covid-19-pandemic/british-prime-minister-takes-responsibility-covid-19-response

105. Frost N. (2021) Tourism down, New Zealand dares locals to step up. *NY Times*, February 7. https://www.nytimes.com/2021/02/05/world/asia/new-zealand-ad-tourists-photos.html

106. Manning J. (2021) Travel to Australia might not restart until the end of 2021. *TimeOut*, January 18. https://www.timeout.com/news/australia-travel-restrictions-border-closures-latest-news-010621

107. The World Fact Book. (nd) Country comparisons: Obesity — Adult prevalence rate. https://www.cia.gov/the-world-factbook/field/obesity-adult-prevalence-rate/country-comparison?campaign_id=9&emc=edit_nn_20210311&instance_id=27987&nl=the-morning&regi_id=93312921&segment_id=53295&te=1&user_id=51e87c97eff6fb3416b9ab2e64d1a65a. Accessed: March 12, 2021.

108. Leonhardt D. (2021) An epidemiologic whodunit. *NY Times — The Morning Newsletter*, March 8. https://www.nytimes.com/series/us-morning-briefing

109. Deb P, Furceri D, Ostry JD, Tawk N. (2020) The economic effects of COVID-19 containment measures. *VOX*, June 17. https://voxeu.org/article/economic-effects-covid-19-containment-measures

110. Cantore N, Jartwich F, Laplane A, *et al.* (2020) Recovery or protracted economic downturn? The role of policies based on evidence. United Nations Industrial Development Organization, October 21. https://www.unido.org/stories/coronavirus-economic-impact-21-october-2020#story-start.

111. Dizikes P. (2020) The data speak: Stronger pandemic response yields better economic recovery. *MIT News*, March 31. https://news.mit.edu/2020/pandemic-health-response-economic-recovery-0401.

112. The Independent Panal. (2021) Second report on progress: Prepared by the Independent Panel for Pandemic Preparedness and Response for the WHO Executive Board, January 2021. https://theindependentpanel.org/wp-content/uploads/2021/01/Independent-Panel_Second-Report-on-Progress_Final-15-Jan-2021.pdf

4   Airborne Assassin

"We will get you home."

Written by one of Nic Brown's nurses on the window to his ICU room, to which he later responded by asking a nurse to write his letter of gratitude on the same window. An excerpt from that letter follows…

"I watched you work hard to keep me and the others alive, unable to thank you for the time that you poured into me — and although I will probably never get the chance to pour that same love and support into you, I want you to know that I think you all are rockstars."

Nic Brown, a patient hospitalized with COVID-19. With permission. https://my.clevelandclinic.org/patient-stories/375-covid-19-patient-writes-inspiring-message-on-glass-to-caregivers

Contents

1. Clinical Presentations
   a. Case #1 — Risk of transmission
      i. No symptoms vs. symptoms
      ii. Superspreaders
      iii. Risk of transmission to healthcare workers
      iv. How well do personal protective equipment work?
      v. SARS-CoV-2 survival on surfaces
   b. Case #2 — Mild COVID-19 pneumonia
      i. COVID-19 presentations at Emergency Departments
      ii. Laboratory abnormalities
      iii. Imaging: Chest computerized tomography vs. chest X-rays
      iv. Diagnostic testing: PCR vs. antigen vs. antibodies
      v. Risk factors for COVID-19 admissions

     c. Case #3 — COVID-19 with embolic and thrombotic events
        i. Deep venous thrombosis
        ii. Pulmonary emboli
        iii. Myocardial infarctions and strokes
     d. Case #4 — COVID-19 reinfection with fatal outcome
        i. Reinfection vs. persistent infection
        ii. Treatment effectiveness
        iii. Overall impact of treatment on mortality
        iv. Ethics
     e. Case #5 — MIS-C in children
     f. Case #6 — Pregnant females with COVID-19
     g. Case #7 — Immunocompromised patients
     h. Case #8 — Central nervous system manifestations
     i. Case #9 — "Long Haulers" or "Long COVID"
2. Pathogenesis of COVID-19
     a. ACE2 receptor
        i. Role of binding to ACE2 receptor (angiotensin-converting enzyme 2 receptor)
     b. Lung disease
     c. Heart disease
     d. Immune response
        i. Are asymptomatic COVID-19 infections due to persistent immunity from prior nonSARS-CoV-2 coronavirus infections?
        ii. Are the most severe COVID-19 pneumonias a consequence of cytokine storm?
     e. Coagulopathy
     f. Sars-CoV-2 mutation

1. Clinical Presentations

Although SARS-CoV-2 initially infects the respiratory tract, subsequently, almost all organs and organ systems can be involved. The clinical consequence is that while the most common clinical presentation of COVID-19 involves respiratory symptoms, it may otherwise be quite diverse with protean symptoms and signs. It is that diversity of clinical presentations that may make the diagnosis of COVID-19 quite challenging. The following nine clinical cases, hospitalized during 2020, illustrate the broad range of clinical manifestations of COVID-19.

a. Case #1 — Risk of transmission

A geriatric male without significant past medical history (PMH) except for mild short-term memory difficulties was brought to the Emergency Department (ED) because of confusion. He had acute kidney injury with a creatinine of 2.4 (normal ≤1.3) that resolved overnight with hydration, as did his confusion. A physical therapy evaluation determined that he would benefit from a stay at an inpatient rehabilitation facility, so he underwent COVID-19 antigen testing as part of the rehabilitation admission process. He was found to be SARS-CoV-2 positive, making him ineligible for admission to the rehabilitation center. Upon further questioning, the patient admitted that prior to admission, he had mild nausea and did not drink or eat well for several days. Although COVID-19 was not initially suspected due to incomplete clinical information, there were no secondary cases in medical personnel, likely due to the wearing of appropriate personal protective equipment (PPE), including surgical masks and eye shields.

i. *No symptoms vs. symptoms*

About 20 to 40% of COVID-19-infected individuals remain totally asymptomatic (Table 4.4).[1,2] Because asymptomatic individuals rarely get tested, this leads to COVID-19 mortality rates being calculated as case fatality rates (CFR), which exclude asymptomatic individuals and are higher, rather than infectivity fatality rates (IFR), which include asymptomatic cases and are lower (see Chapter 1 for a further discussion of the definitions of CFR and IFR and the mortality discussion under Case 4 of this chapter).

For the 60 to 80% of individuals who are symptomatic, symptoms first appear, on average, five days after infection.[3] The most common symptoms are fever, cough, shortness of breath, confusion, nausea, vomiting, diarrhea, and a loss of taste or smell (Table 4.4).[3-9] None of these symptoms are specific to COVID-19 infection.[9] Asymptomatic infected individuals can shed the virus for as long as those who are mildly symptomatic, typically 10-14 days (rarely out to 28 days), but this shedding can go on for much longer (many months) in immunocompromised patients.[10]

Table 4.4. Adult manifestations of COVID-19.

Clinical Manifestations	Percentage Range	Comments Median (range)
Asymptomatic	18–40%[1,2]	Lower if community testing low
Symptomatic	60–82%	
No admission	80%	
Admission: No ICU	15%	
Yes ICU	5%	
Time to symptom onset	5 (4–6) days	Median (range)
Active Symptoms[3-7,9]		At time of presentation
Most common		>10% incidence
Fever	43.8–68.0%	
Shortness of breath	18.7–60.9%	
Cough	29.3–74.9%	
Malaise or fatigue	38.1–42%	
Loss of taste	56%	
Loss of smell	83%	
Confusion	27.9%	
Other		<10% incidence
Sore throat	2.0–13.9%	
Runny nose	4.8–24.5%	
Muscle aches or joint aches	0.7–14.9%	
Diarrhea	3.8–21.7%	
Nausea or vomiting	5.0–20%	
Chest pain or pressure	3.0%	
Headache	2.7–16%	
Conjunctival congestion	0.8%	
Associated Complications[39,40,61-75]		
Common		>10% incidence
Deep venous thrombosis	46%	Overall
Pulmonary embolus	20.6–24%	All, higher in ICU
Admission myocardial injury	7–27.8%	Based on elevated troponins
Acute kidney injury	36.6%, 52%	Within 48h of admission, intubated
Requiring RRT	23.2%	Of those on ventilators
Liver dysfunction (liver function tests)	14.8–78%	Multifactorial
Other		<10% incidence
Stroke	0.9%	Based on imaging
Bleeding	4.8%	Higher if d-dimer elevated
Secondary bacterial infection	3.5%, 14.3%	On admission, after admission

ii. *Superspreaders*

Recent studies looking at the airborne transmission of Influenza A, the pandemic pathogen that is most similar to SARS-CoV-2 (Chapter 8), demonstrated that 25% of influenza particles detectable at a distance of 1 foot from the hospitalized patient's head were still detectable 6 feet from the patient's head, and greater than 90% of the particles detectable at 6 feet were <5 microns in size.[11] The same study further demonstrated that Influenza A airborne transmission was heterogeneic (definition: individuals had a wide range of how much virus they expelled into the air), with 19% of the patients studied being superemitters (superspreaders, Chapter 8), emitting 32 times more virus than the other 81% of the patients, which correlated with the high viral loads in nasopharyngeal samples. Others have shown that influenza A-infected persons with greater symptoms have higher viral loads and shed for longer periods of time.[12,13] Similarly, COVID-19 patients with more severe disease have higher nasopharyngeal viral loads, and theoretically are more likely to shed virus or possibly be a superspreader (Chapter 8).[14,15]

iii. *Risk of transmission to healthcare workers*

The healthcare workers (HCWs) associated with Case #1 were fortunate in not acquiring COVID-19, because it is human nature to be more careful when you have higher levels of suspicion for acquiring an infectious disease. An important question then is: How great is the risk of HCWs acquiring COVID-19 infection? In a prospective, observational study in the United States (US) and the United Kingdom (UK), it was found that HCWs working in acute care hospitals were 24 times more likely to acquire COVID-19 than the general public, 16 times more likely if they worked in a nursing home, and 11 times more likely if they worked in an outpatient clinic.[16] In UK university hospitals, Shields and colleagues found the prevalence of COVID-19 antibodies in the blood — suggesting prior infection — ranged from 34.5% in housekeeping down to 14.8% for individuals working in intensive care, with an average seroprevalence of 24.4%.[17] It has been further shown that the reuse of masks or poor quality masks increased the risk of HCWs acquiring COVID-19.[16,18]

iv. *How well do personal protective equipment work?*

What is known and recommended about personal protective equipment (PPE) effectiveness related to preventing SARS-CoV-2 transmission? There are data that strongly supports that SARS-CoV-2 can be transmitted through the air.[19,20] Airborne transmission of infectious organisms occurs by both large and small particles (see Chapter 8 for more details).[21,22] Large airborne particles (>5 microns), so-called droplet nuclei, are thought to be transmissible only a short distance (less than 6 feet). Small airborne particles (<5 microns) can be transmitted a greater distance (>6 feet) and remain suspended in the air for longer periods of time (greater than one hour), depending upon ventilation in the room.[22] Large airborne particles are thought to mainly impact on the upper respiratory tract (nose, nasopharynx or throat). Small airborne particles are thought to go into the lungs, as well as impacting the upper respiratory tract.

Surgical masks or ASTM (American Society of Testing and Materials) level three masks or EN (Europe) Type IIR are designed to prevent the transmission of large airborne particles (>5 microns). NIOSH (National Institute for Occupational Safety and Health) N95 masks or European FFP (filtering facepiece) P2 masks are certified to filter 95% of airborne particles and designed to prevent the airborne transmission of both large and small airborne particles (>5 microns, <5 microns). Since a significant percentage of influenza virus particles in the air are smaller than 5 microns, it is logical to assume that N95 masks and European FFP P2 masks would be more effective at preventing transmission of the Influenza virus than standard surgical masks; however, existing studies do not support this contention.[23,24] The reason for this is likely multifactorial and may include poor study design, lack of mask fit testing, substantial variation in the effectiveness of surgical masks, and the fact that inhaling the organism may not be the only route of transmission.[23–25] For example, using the live attenuated influenza vaccine, it has been demonstrated that for individuals wearing an N95 mask, 60% of individuals exposed to the vaccine virus aerosol became infected if their eyes are not protected.[26] There are a few studies that suggest eye protection, in addition to masks, can decrease the overall risk of transmitting an airborne infectious disease.[26,27] Many other kinds of masks exist (including homemade bandanas and neck gaiters), made from a wide variety of materials, and virtually all of them are less effective at filtering airborne particles than surgical or N95 masks.[28,29] One new important finding is that masking the patient may turn out to be as important, or more important, at preventing the transmission of airborne infectious diseases.[30]

One must be cautious of popularized methodologies of mask effectiveness, such as seeing if you can blow out a candle while wearing a mask, i.e., failure equaling an effective mask; such methods have not been rigorously tested.

Limited data are available about whether gowns and gloves have added efficacy at preventing transmission versus wearing masks and using eye protection.[31,32]

v. *SARS-CoV-2 survival on surfaces*

Surfaces may be important related to transmission, as SARS-CoV-2 can survive and remain infectious on surfaces that are not disinfected.[33,34] Surfaces studied have included stainless steel, plastic and cardboard.[33,34] The US CDC recommends that usual hospital or home surface disinfection is adequate for reducing the risk of surface transmission.[35] This suggests that great care must be taken in rooms where COVID-19-infected patients reside, and special care must be taken with room disinfection after they depart the room. The CDC currently recommends either alcohol hand disinfection or soap and water for at least 20 seconds after interaction with COVID-19 patients or surfaces.[36]

Key Points: Approximately 60% of COVID-19 infected people have symptoms, and up to 80% of symptomatic COVID-19 infections have nonspecific, mild symptoms that may or may not result in seeking medical care, including confusion, nausea, runny nose, and a headache (Table 4.4). Asymptomatic and mild COVID-19 illnesses appear to be equally infectious, but severe infections are likely more infectious. Transmission can be reduced by wearing masks and eye protection. Handwashing and environmental disinfection are also likely important at minimizing transmission.

b. Case #2 — Mild COVID-19 pneumonia

A young adult Hispanic male with PMH (past medical history) significant only for obesity (Body Mass Index: 38), was admitted due to an 8-day history of shortness of breath, intermittent diarrhea, mild chest tightness, fevers greater than 104°F, hypoxia (less than 88% hemoglobin oxygen saturation; his was in the low 80s), and outpatient testing three days prior to admission that was positive for SARS-CoV-2. Of additional note, multiple family members had already tested positive for SARS-CoV-2. He required 5 liters/minute oxygen in the ED (emergency department) to maintain oxygen saturation greater than 90%. His chest X-ray was suggestive of possible pneumonia, and chest CT (computerized tomography) showed infiltrates typical of COVID-19 pneumonia (Figure 4.49). He was admitted and started on dexamethasone (a steroid medication) and antibiotics. The next day, his oxygen needs increased and remdesivir (an antiviral medication) and convalescent plasma (contains antibodies against SARS-CoV-2) were added. He improved and was discharged on his 8th hospital day.

i. *COVID-19 presentations at Emergency Departments*

Early on in the coronavirus pandemic, 20% of symptomatic patients were admitted and 25% of the admitted patients ended up in the ICU (less now since proven treatments and vaccines are available). The most common reason for admission to the hospital is pneumonia, with or without fever and hypoxia, and with or without an abnormal chest X-ray or chest CT scan (Table 4.4, Table 4.5, Table 4.7).[8] Upon examination in the ED, a significant proportion of patients have fever (26% to nearly 70% depending upon the study, see Tables 4.4 and 4.5) but few other exam abnormalities. Most patients have minimal initial O_2 needs in the ED (none, 62%; nasal cannula O_2, 25%; higher O_2 needs, 13%; see Table 4.5).[8]

ii. *Laboratory abnormalities*

Laboratory abnormalities (Table 4.6) that help distinguish COVID-19 infection from other diseases include lymphocytopenia (lymphocyte: type of white blood cell; penia = low number; frequency: 63%), elevated LDH (lactate dehydrogenase; frequency: 41–73%), elevated d-dimer (elevated when

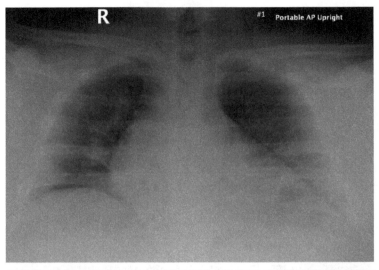

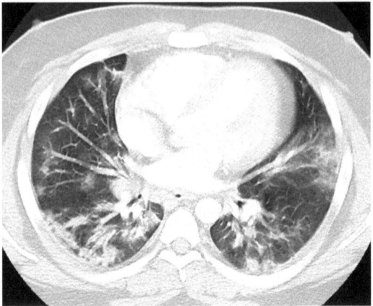

Figure 4.49. Case #2. Top figure. Chest X-ray showing possible interstitial edema (fluid), cardiomegaly (heart enlargement). Bottom figure. Chest CT from the same day showing bilateral, peripheral (near the ribs) ground glass infiltrates (grey-white areas) compatible with COVID-19 pneumonia.

Table 4.5. Emergency Department vital signs, O_2 requirements.

Exam Findings in ED[8]	Percent
Fever > 38°C	25.5%
Heart rate ≥ 125	5.6%
Systolic BP < 90 mm Hg	1.5%
Respiratory rate > 24/min	9.9%
Supplemental O_2 needs first three hours	
None	62.1%
Nasal cannula	25.4%
Non-rebreather	4.8%
High flow O_2	1.3%
Mechanical ventilation	4.8%
Other (venti mask, BIPAP)	1.6%

BIPAP = a form of noninvasive, positive pressure ventilation therapy

Table 4.6. Laboratory abnormalities in COVID-19 patients admitted to the hospital.

Laboratory Studies[3–8]	Percent Abnormal
Bacteremia	4.8%
CK elevation (>200 U/l)	13.7%
Creatinine (≥133 umol/l)	1.6–36.6%
CRP elevation (≥10 mg/l)	60.7%
D-dimer elevation (≥0.5 mg/l)	36–46%
ESR elevation (>26 mm/h)	67%
Ferritin (>300 ug/ml)	66.2%
LDH elevation (>250 U/l)	41–73%
Platelet count (<100)	5%
Procalcitonin (≥0.5 ng/ml)	5.5–16.9%
Transaminase elevation (>40 U/l)	21–22%
Total bilirubin (>17.1 umol/l)	10.5%
Troponin elevation (>0.5 ng/ml)	5–27.8%
WBC	
Leukocytosis (>10,000)	5.9–30%
Leukopenia (<4,000)	25–33.7%
Lymphocytopenia (<1,000/mm³)	63%

CK = creatinine kinase, CRP = C-reactive protein, ESR = erythrocyte sedimentation rate, LDH = lactate dehydrogenase, WBC = white blood cell count.

blood is actively clotting; frequency: 36–46%), and elevated inflammatory parameters: ferritin (carries iron in the blood; frequency: 66%), CRP (C-reactive protein — elevated with infection and other inflammatory states; frequency: 61%) or ESR (erythrocyte sedimentation rate — elevated with infection and other inflammatory states; frequency: 67%).[3–8]

iii. *Imaging: Chest computerized tomography vs. chest X-rays*

Perhaps the most sensitive indicator of COVID-19 lung infection is the chest CT (Table 4.7). Chest CTs are 50% more sensitive than routine chest X-rays for detecting pneumonia (90% vs. 60%, Table 4.7) and may have the added benefit of detecting pulmonary emboli, if an intravenous contrast agent is also given (CTA, where A = angiogram; see below and Table 4.7).[3–8,37–40] One recent study showed that of those patients with COVID-19 with pulmonary emboli diagnosed in the hospital, half were diagnosed in the ED. This suggests that any patient with suspected COVID-19 pneumonia and an elevated d-dimer in the ED should have a chest CTA, rather than just a chest CT (Table 4.7).[39,40]

Although many studies have been done comparing various diagnostic and imaging parameters using multivariate analysis approaches, almost

Table 4.7. Chest imaging abnormalities in COVID-19 adult patients admitted to the hospital.

Imaging[8,48,49,54–56]		
Chest X-ray abnormalities		Admission
Bilateral infiltrates	60%	
Unilateral infiltrates	16%	
Pleural effusion	6%	
Chest CT abnormalities		Admission
Bilateral infiltrates	81.5–92.9%	
Ground glass	21.8%	
Consolidation	35.5%	
Crazy-paving pattern	42.7	Higher association with mortality
Unilateral infiltrates	7.1–16.1%	
Pleural effusion	0%	
Chest CTA showing PE	22%	RF: Elevated d-dimer, CRP; obesity

all of these studies are small and/or not designed to answer the question of which parameters are the most sensitive and specific for making the diagnosis of COVID-19. In particular, since the most common abnormal studies (LDH, d-dimer, ferritin, CRP, ESR, chest CT) for patients admitted with suspected COVID-19 infection are not commonly ordered for patients with community-acquired pneumonia, it is difficult understanding how well they discriminate COVID-19 from other diseases.

iv. *Diagnostic testing: PCR vs. antigen vs. antibodies*

Developing diagnostic testing was an immediate need right from the beginning of the COVID-19 pandemic. To understand the tests that became available, one must first understand a little about the natural history of the infection. As shown in Figure 4.50, within a few days after exposure to SARS-CoV-2, the infected person begins having detectable RNA and viral antigens (mainly proteins) in the respiratory tract, that are produced as part of viral replication.[41] Within two weeks of the onset of detecting viral RNA and viral proteins, the body is producing IgG, IgM and IgA antibodies (Figure 4.50, IgA not shown). IgA antibodies appear in nasal secretions and help decrease the attachment of SARS-CoV-2 to mucosal surfaces (e.g., nose). All three of these biologic processes occur whether the person is symptomatic or asymptomatic.

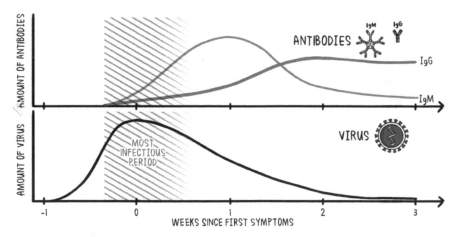

Figure 4.50. Time course for the detection of SARS-CoV-2 RNA (grey line), viral antigens (red line), and antibodies (blue lines).[1]

The natural history of SARS-CoV-2 viral infection has led to the development of three types of diagnostic tests: (1) PCR tests for detecting SARS-CoV-2 RNA, (2) Antigen tests that detect SARS-CoV-2 proteins, and (3) Antibody tests that detect IgG and/or IgM antibodies in the blood directed against the SARS-CoV-2 virus (Figure 4.51).[42] PCR tests are performed to detect the presence of RNA from the SARS-CoV-2 virus by first swabbing

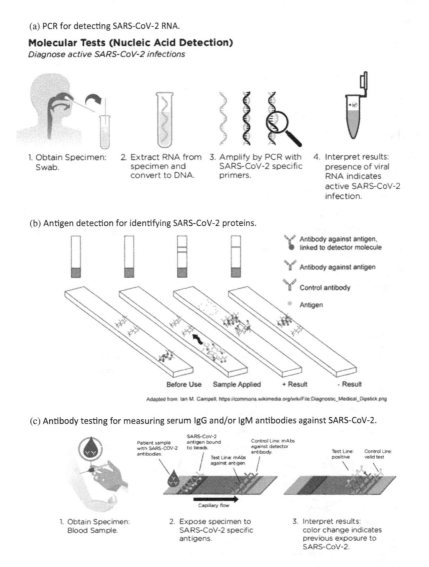

(a) PCR for detecting SARS-CoV-2 RNA.

Molecular Tests (Nucleic Acid Detection)
Diagnose active SARS-CoV-2 infections

1. Obtain Specimen: Swab.

2. Extract RNA from specimen and convert to DNA.

3. Amplify by PCR with SARS-CoV-2 specific primers.

4. Interpret results: presence of viral RNA indicates active SARS-CoV-2 infection.

(b) Antigen detection for identifying SARS-CoV-2 proteins.

Antibody against antigen, linked to detector molecule

Antibody against antigen

Control antibody

Antigen

Before Use   Sample Applied   + Result   - Result

Adapted from: Ian M. Campell. https://commons.wikimedia.org/wiki/File:Diagnostic_Medical_Dipstick.png

(c) Antibody testing for measuring serum IgG and/or IgM antibodies against SARS-CoV-2.

Patient sample with SARS-COV-2 antibodies

SARS-CoV-2 antigen bound to beads

Test Line: mAbs against antigen

Control Line: mAbs against detector antibody

Test Line: positive

Control Line: valid test

Capillary flow

1. Obtain Specimen: Blood Sample.

2. Expose specimen to SARS-CoV-2 specific antigens.

3. Interpret results: color change indicates previous exposure to SARS-CoV-2.

Figure 4.51. Diagnostic testing available for SARS-CoV-2 infection: (a) PCR, (b) Antigens, (c) Antibodies.[2]

the nasopharynx, removing any attached RNA from the swab into a solution followed by purifying the RNA, converting the RNA to DNA with an enzyme, and then amplifying the DNA using PCR to increase the sensitivity (Figure 4.51a). Antigen tests typically involve removing the antigens from a nasal or oral swab into a solution, placing the antigen-containing solution onto slides containing antibodies that are specific for a SARS-CoV-2 protein(s), and then adding a reagent that leads to a visible band indicating the presence of SARS-CoV-2 (Figure 4.51b). SARS-CoV-2 antibody testing is performed on blood, similar to detecting SARS-CoV-2 proteins; only the antibodies on the slides are specific to IgG and IgM antibodies that target the SARS-CoV-2 virus (Figure 4.51c).

By January 20, ten days after the Chinese had posted the genetic sequence of SARS-CoV-2, the CDC had developed a diagnostic test that had been given Emergency Use Authorization (EUA) by the FDA on February 4, 2020.[43,44] The CDC test subsequently failed, but through the end of 2020, the US FDA issued EUAs for >150 PCR tests, 8 antigen tests, and 70 antibody tests.[44,45] Some of these tests have been excellent, and some have failed, so it is important not to assume they are equally accurate.

PCR and antigen tests were the most useful because they are positive when the patient is infectious (Figure 4.50).[46–49] PCR is 10–20% more sensitive than antigen detection (Table 4.8). In spite of the extremely large number of PCR tests approved in the US alone, most clinicians would still

Table 4.8. Sensitivity and/or specificity of PCR for SARS-CoV-2 versus antibody tests for diagnosing COVID-19 infection.

Diagnostic Test[46–49]	Percent Positive	Comments
PCR		Takes about two hours
Throat	32–50	
Nasopharynx	63–72	
Lung	93–100	Bronchoalveolar lavage
Antigen		Takes 15–20 minutes
Sensitivity vs. PCR	84–97	Less sensitive than PCR
Antibody (IgG only)		Wane rapidly, so negatives do not rule out prior infection
Sensitivity	88–99	
Specificity	95–99	

likely say that the PCR turn-around time was too slow. In the first half of 2020, it was not uncommon for a PCR test to take a week or longer before results were available, which made patient care very difficult. The reasons for the delay are multifactorial and included politics (Chapter 3).

Antibody tests are not useful for diagnosing acute infection, because they may only indicate prior infection. However, they are very useful to help estimate how long immunity may persist, either due to natural infection or to vaccination.

v. *Risk factors for COVID-19 admissions*

Early in the COVID-19 pandemic, small studies suggested risk factors for admission included older age, cardiovascular disease, obesity, chronic lung disease, diabetes, and belonging to a nonwhite race.[3-8] One year into the pandemic, larger studies were available that confirmed these risk factors and demonstrated that they were essentially identical to the risk factors for dying from COVID-19.[50-59]

The risk factor that confers the highest risk of dying is advanced age. A metaanalysis using international data from 27 studies found that the risk of dying with COVID-19 infection increased from 0.002% at age 10, to 0.01% at age 25, 0.4% at age 55, 1.4% at age 65, 4.6% at age 75, 15% at age 85 and exceeded 25% for ages 90 and above.[51] Another large meta-analysis published in December 2020 confirmed the age of >60 as being the most highly correlated with mortality (odds ratio [OR]: 6.09) (when the OR is greater than 1, it indicates a higher likelihood of the outcome occurring), followed by cardiovascular disease (OR: 5.16), cerebrovascular disease (OR: 5.14), chronic respiratory disease (OR: 2.83), hypertension (OR: 2.6), diabetes (OR: 2.11), and being male (OR: 1.34).[52] Other studies have looked at modifiers to the above risk factors. In one large study of 66,646 COVID-19 patients, diabetes was not a risk factor unless it was accompanied by chronic diabetes complications, and hypertension was only minimally a risk factor unless accompanied by chronic hypertension complications.[53] In a December 2020 publication, obesity (Body Mass Index >35) increased the risk of mortality in a large meta-analysis of 45,650 patients (OR: 1.49).[54]

One of the most striking and controversial risk factors for COVID-19 deaths is race. One large meta-analysis looking at greater than 18 million COVID-19 patients by race found that black and Asian races had a greater likelihood of death than those designated white (OR: 2.02, 1.5, respectively).[55] The increased risk of death associated with black and Asian races has been confirmed by others and expanded to show a greater risk of dying among those of Hispanic ethnicity (OR: 2.56).[56] A similar meta-analysis of COVID-19 infections in American Indians/Alaska Native Persons showed an increased death rate when compared with white patients (OR: 1.8).[57] At this point, the mechanism for the increased risk of COVID-19 death associated with nonwhite ethnicities is unknown but could be due to a higher prevalence of the risk factors cited above, socioeconomic factors, a greater representation of these groups in certain high-risk jobs (meatpacking, for example; see Chapter 8), or less access to medical care.[58] See Chapter 6's section on racial disparity for further discussion.

So far, only a few studies are demonstrating that genetic factors can increase the risk for severe COVID-19 infection. One Spanish study of 1,980 patients with COVID-19 infection compared with controls found that COVID-19 patients with severe infection were more likely to have a unique gene cluster and type A blood group than those without severe infection. A UK study of 2,244 critically ill COVID-19 patients identified four gene clusters that correlated with worse outcomes that may ultimately provide targets for new or existing drugs.[59,60] It is highly likely that ongoing research will identify additional genetic loci and ultimately, the mechanisms of how our genes contribute to mortality.

Key Points: The most common reason for COVID-19 admission is pneumonia with or without hypoxia. Patients requiring admission have risk factors that include obesity, hypertension, heart failure, diabetes, chronic obstructive pulmonary disease, and advanced age (>80). Asian Americans, Native Americans, Hispanics and African Americans have had greater mortality rates, but for as yet explained reasons.

---

c. Case #3 — COVID-19 with embolic and thrombotic events

A middle aged adult with PMH significant for diabetes mellitus came to the ED with fever, chills, and normal oxygen saturation (94–96% saturation on room air). His exam was remarkable for a fever of 100.4°F and abnormal lung sounds by stethoscope exam posteriorly on the left side of his chest. His white blood cell count was within normal limits without lymphocytopenia. A chest X-ray showed bilateral increased interstitial markings. He was diagnosed with community-acquired pneumonia versus COVID-19 pneumonia and placed on azithromycin (an antibiotic) and steroids, and sent home. Nasopharyngeal SARS-CoV-2 PCR testing was negative. Six days later, he returned to the ED with diffuse, severe back and abdominal pain. His exam was remarkable for hypoxia requiring supplemental oxygen. Laboratory evaluation demonstrated an elevated white blood cell count (15.2, normal ≤10.0), elevated glucose (378, normal <140), and serum acetone elevation consistent with mild diabetic ketoacidosis, d-dimer elevation consistent with possible clots in the vascular system (5,900, normal ≤500), and elevated LDH, CRP and ferritin consistent with COVID-19 infection; his nasopharyngeal SARS-CoV-2 PCR was positive. Chest CTA showed bilateral lung infiltrates consistent with COVID-19 pneumonia (Figure 4.52a), a 2x1 cm

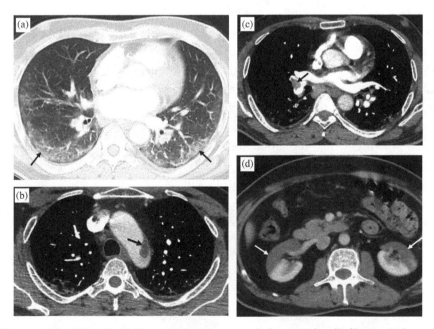

Figure 4.52. Case #3. (a) Chest CT showing ground glass peripheral infiltrates at the periphery of both lungs (see arrows). (b) Chest CT angiogram showing clot in the aortic arch (see arrow). (c) Chest CT angiogram showing pulmonary embolus in R pulmonary artery (see arrow). (d) Abdominal CT showing bilateral kidney infarcts (dark gray areas, see arrows).

thrombus on the internal wall of the aortic arch (Figure 4.52b), and bilateral pulmonary emboli (Figure 4.52c). Abdominal CTA showed bilateral kidney infarcts suggestive of emboli (Figure 4.52d). He was treated with antibiotics, heparin (blood thinner), dexamethasone, and insulin with improvement of all his laboratory and clinical parameters (Figure 4.53). The patient was discharged on his sixth day of hospitalization, after steady improvement on a blood thinner (rivaroxaban) and insulin.

Complications of COVID-19 usually occur in conjunction with pneumonia and may be the presenting problem in the ED. Complications include thrombotic events (clots in blood vessels causing heart attacks, strokes, deep venous thrombosis / pulmonary emboli, or arterial clots), renal failure, elevated liver function tests and secondary bacterial infection (Table 4.4).[39,40,61–75]

i. *Deep venous thrombosis*

The highest frequency complication of COVID-19 is deep venous thrombosis (DVT) with or without pulmonary emboli.[65–67] A Wuhan China study evaluated 143 consecutive patients admitted to a hospital with COVID-19 and found that 66 patients had lower extremity DVTs — 46% proximal (above the knee) and 65% distal (below the knee).[65] The median time after admission to the diagnosis of DVT was ten days. Multivariate analysis predictors of DVT included an elevated CURB-65 score (used to assess the risk of community-acquired pneumonia), an elevated Padua score ≥4 (used to assess the risk of DVT), and an elevated d-dimer. A New York City hospital performed a retrospective analysis of 158 COVID-19 patients admitted to a hospital in New York City and also had d-dimer testing and lower extremity ultrasound looking for DVT.[66] Patients with DVT upon admission were excluded. Wells criteria for DVT (predictive criteria for DVT in other patient populations) were not a good predictor in this study, but a d-dimer value of ≤6,494 had an 88% negative predictive value for diagnosing DVT, i.e., ruling out DVT.

In COVID-19 patients admitted to the ICU, the risk of DVT is even higher. A French study examined 34 consecutive COVID-19 patients

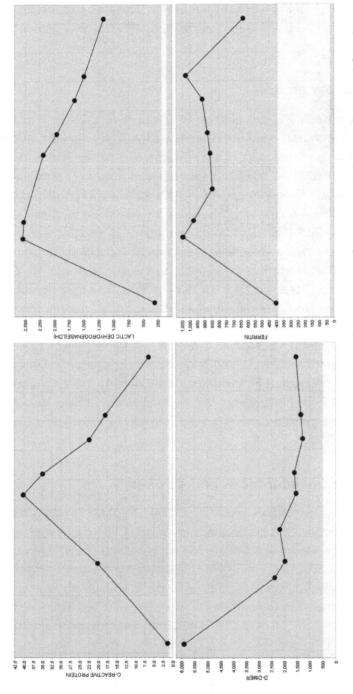

Figure 4.53. Case #3. COVID-consistent laboratory abnormalities with improvement after treatment (6-day period). Bottom left, D-dimer; top left, C-reactive protein; top right, lactate dehydrogenase; bottom right, ferritin. Green equals normal range.

admitted to an ICU in France. At the time of admission to the ICU, 65% of the patients had DVT.[67] Two days later, the DVT prevalence had risen to 76%.

ii. *Pulmonary emboli*

Pulmonary emboli (PE) are also quite frequent in COVID-19 patients. Spanish investigators studied 30 consecutive patients admitted with COVID-19 pneumonia who had an elevated d-dimer and found that 50% of them had PE — 60% were bilateral and 86% were mainly in segmental arteries.[39] Given an approximately 40% elevation of d-dimer at admission (Table 4.6), this would suggest an admission PE prevalence of approximately 20% (15/70). A European group studied 107 consecutive patients with chest CTA at the time of admission and found the prevalence of PE was 15%.[68] Together, these two studies suggest that 15–20% of the patients admitted with COVID-19 have PE at the time of admission to the hospital. No similar studies have been done for patients in ICUs because many of these patients are intubated and CTAs are relatively or absolutely contraindicated. In a recent meta-analysis comparing the risk of pulmonary emboli in COVID-19 patients housed in general wards versus ICUs, the pooled PE incidence rates were 14.7% on the general wards and 23.4% in ICU patients.[40] If the relative risk of PE is indeed 50% greater in ICUs than on general wards, than ICU PE rates could easily be greater than 30%.

iii. *Myocardial infarctions and strokes*

The high frequency of DVT and PE in COVID-19 patients raised the possibility that there might be frequent myocardial infarctions and strokes. However, the opposite was actually found. In many medical communities, there was a sudden and significant decline in the number of myocardial infarctions, as well as strokes admitted to the hospital, with an associated significant increase in the number of out-of-hospital cardiac arrests and resuscitations.[62–64,76–79] It was speculated that patients were afraid to go to the hospital for fear of acquiring COVID-19. They, therefore, may have stayed home with their cardiovascular events without treatment.

Key Points: An unexpected finding in COVID-19 patients was an increased frequency of thrombotic events involving both arteries and veins. In prospective studies, the frequency of deep venous thrombosis (DVT) and pulmonary emboli (PE) was very high in patients admitted with COVID-19 (DVT: 46–65%; PE: 15–20%). DVT rates in ICU patients approached 75%, and PE rates in ICU patients were likely to be significantly higher than at the time of admission. During the same time period, heart attacks and strokes seemed to decrease in frequency, but this was likely an artifact of people being afraid to come to the hospital for fear of catching COVID-19.

d. Case #4 — COVID-19 reinfection with fatal outcome

A geriatric male with PMH significant for hypertension, elevated cholesterol, coronary artery disease requiring placement of a stent in his coronary artery, type 2 diabetes, and remote smoking history was initially evaluated in the ED due to a 4-day history of fever. His chest X-ray was negative, but his SARS-CoV-2 PCR was positive. He was sent home to self-isolate, and his fever resolved. Twenty days later, he returned to the ED with a recurrence of fever and chest pressure. Temperature was 97.4°F, respiratory rate 16, and oxygen saturation was 96% on room air. Chest CTA was negative for pulmonary emboli and showed minimal ground glass-like infiltrates in the lungs. His SARS-CoV-2 PCR was negative. He was admitted for a cardiac stress test and discharged when negative. Twenty-one days later (now 45 days since his first fever appeared), he returned to the ED with a fever and cough. He remained stable for several hours in the ED and was discharged home. Three days later, he returned (48 days since his fever first appeared), complaining of persistent fever and progressive shortness of breath. Exam was significant for fever 101.7°F, RR (respiratory rate) over 20, and progressive hypoxia. Chest X-ray showed bilateral infiltrates and chest CT showed bilateral ground glass infiltrates (Figure 4.54). His SARS-CoV-2 PCR was positive. He was treated with broad-spectrum antibiotics, dexamethasone and anticoagulation but got worse. Remdesivir and convalescent plasma were added on the second day, but he progressed and required intubation. Vitamin C, zinc and thiamine were added.

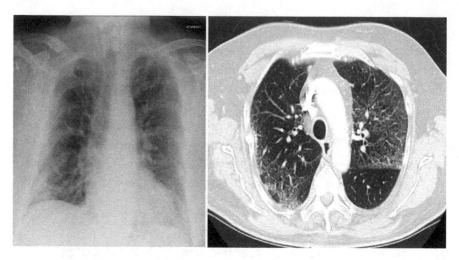

Figure 4.54.   Case #4. (a) Admission Chest X-ray showing bilateral infiltrates, (b) Admission Chest CT showing bilateral ground glass infiltrates.

He developed hemoptysis (coughing up blood) on Day 3 of his hospitalization, and his anticoagulation was stopped, followed by a steady rise in his d-dimer (Figure 4.55). Then he developed ventricular fibrillation with cardiac arrest requiring cardioversion, associated with myocardial infarction, and died on Day 8 of his hospitalization.

Case #4 brings up a number of important COVID-19 questions. First, how likely is it to develop a second SARS-CoV-2 infection? Alternatively, is persistent infection possible? Second, given the fatal outcome, what treatment modalities are most effective for COVID-19, and is there an optimal combination of these treatment modalities? Third, what ethical issues exist for treating COVID-19?

i. *Reinfection vs. persistent infection*

Reinfection (due to a new viral strain) versus persistent SARS-CoV-2 infection (by the same strain) is a rapidly evolving area of research. In a study of HCWs in the UK between June 2020 and November 2020, it was shown that HCWs with antibodies against SARS-CoV-2 had a roughly 6.7/1000 risk of developing a second SARS-CoV-2 infection, in comparison to a roughly 22.4/1000 in the absence of pre-existing antibodies.[80] There was no data from the reinfection group as to whether the first SARS-CoV-2 strain was

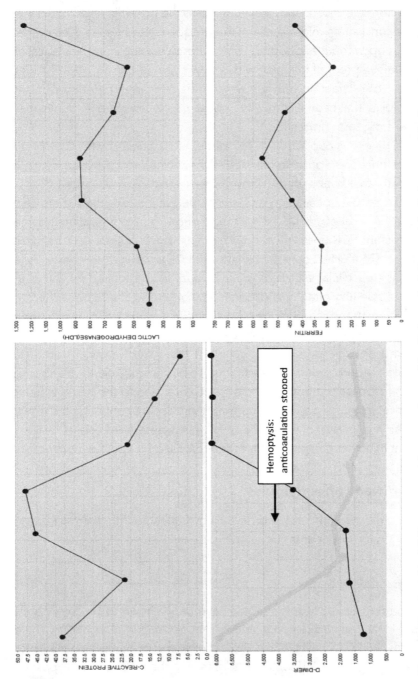

Figure 4.55. Case #4. COVID-consistent laboratory abnormalities (8-day period). Bottom left, D-dimer; top left, C-reactive protein; top right, lactate dehydrogenase; bottom right, ferritin. Green equals normal range.

different from the second, but the study raises the possibility that reinfection with a second strain might occur with a frequency as high as 30% of that of the group without antibodies. There are increasing numbers of cases with definitive proof of infection with a new strain of SARS-CoV-2.[81–84] The possibility of reinfection with a new strain is concerning, in that it raises the possibility that natural immunity or even vaccine-derived immunity may not offer long term protection.[85]

A Chinese group studied 289 patients diagnosed with COVID-19 by pharyngeal swab positive for SARS-CoV-2 RNA, who additionally were tested with anal swabs, both at the time of their initial diagnosis (53.8% tested SARS-CoV-2 positive by anal swab), and at intervals thereafter up to 8 weeks.[86] A total of 7% (21/289) of this cohort required readmission and had persistent PCR positivity in their pharynx; simultaneously, 15 of these 21 patients (71.4%) had persistent anal swab PCR positivity.[86] Further analysis looking at intracellular subgenomic messenger RNA (required for a virus to express its assembly proteins and more commonly present in actively infected cells) demonstrated that 3 of the 16 patients in the readmission subgroup had active viral replication in the GI tract, but not in their respiratory tracts, suggesting possible persistent infection in the gastrointestinal tract. The persistent infection group was also found to be half as likely to develop an antibody response to the spike protein in comparison to the group without persistence, suggesting an inadequate immune response might be the explanation for viral persistence. See Case #9, this chapter, and Long-COVID = Persistent infection, Chapter 10 for further discussion of persistent infection.

ii. *Treatment effectiveness*

What treatments work has become a crucial question for clinicians taking care of COVID-19 patients (Table 4.9).

Decreased mortality

Through midyear 2021, only steroids have been shown to be consistently effective in randomized clinical trials (RCTs) at decreasing mortality.[87–90] There are at least 16 RCTs available that show clinical and/or mortality benefits for steroids used in COVID-19 patients admitted to the hospital with hypoxia.[88] The first report demonstrating effectiveness was the RECOVERY study from

Table 4.9. COVID-19 treatments tried globally through midyear 2021. RCT = randomized controlled trial. Anticoagulation is therapeutic dosing.

COVID-19 Treatment	Study	Comment[91,92]
Most Effective		
Steroids	RCT	>30% mortality reduction, intubated patients
Possibly Effective		
Anticoagulation	RCT	No value in ICUs, trials continue in less ill patients
Convalescent Plasma	RCT	High titer given early decreased severe disease by 50%
Remdesivir	RCT	No mortality benefit, decreased hospitalization 5 days
Monoclonal Ab	RCT	No mortality benefit, but decrease respiratory viral load
Tocilizumab Ab	RCT	No mortality benefit, but decreased risk of clinical decline
Ineffective		
Hydroxychloroquine	RCT	No benefit, not recommended
Ivermectin	RCT	No benefit, not recommended
Lopinavir-ritonavir	RCT	No benefit, not recommended

Oxford England, which randomized 6,425 patients to either dexamethasone or usual therapy.[89] It used 6 mg dexamethasone daily for up to 10 days and found, in comparison to usual care, a 12% reduction in mortality for ventilated patients, a 3% reduction in mortality for those requiring oxygen without ventilation, and no benefit for patients receiving no respiratory support at the time of randomization. The WHO recently reported a meta-analysis of 1,703 ventilated patients collected from 7 RCTs.[90] They found a 32% mortality reduction in the steroid group that was consistent across all seven clinical trials. As in the RECOVERY study, other studies have found minimal to no mortality benefit in patients not requiring mechanical ventilation or supplemental oxygen. Of additional note, the benefit in ventilated patients occurred even if steroids were not started prior to ICU admission.[90] Finally, there is now a small study that demonstrated that methylprednisolone was significantly more effective than dexamethasone (both are steroid drugs), so there may turn out to be efficacy differences between different steroid drugs.[91]

Possibly effective

Many other treatments have been investigated, but through midyear 2021, no other medication has clearly led to reduced mortality.[92–94] Remdesivir, an antiviral drug that causes termination of viral RNA transcription, has demonstrated efficacy in the treatment of Ebola (another RNA virus), so it was one of the earliest treatments studied for COVID-19. It was studied in a multicenter, double blind, randomized trial in 1,062 patients. It did not show a benefit in mortality but did show a benefit in reduced duration of hospitalization (5 days less, see Table 4.9). It is currently not recommended for mild COVID-19 but is recommended for the treatment of severe COVID-19 with oxygen saturations ≤94%.[93,95]

Monoclonal antibodies directed at the receptor-binding domain of the SARS-CoV-2 spike protein have been studied for clinical efficacy. Neither bamlanivimab and etesevimab, bamlanivimab alone, nor casirivimab and imdevimab demonstrated mortality benefit but all showed a reduction in the duration of hospitalization.[96] The latter combination gained brief notoriety when it was used in October, 2020 to treat President Donald Trump.[96A] Guideline documents have recommended their use be considered in individuals with mild to moderate COVID-19 at high risk of developing severe disease and that they not be used alone due to poor activity against emerging SARS-CoV-2 variants.[93,96]

Tocilizumab and Sarilumab, monoclonal antibodies that block the inter-leukin-6 receptor (IL-6), an important mediator of inflammation in processes such as cytokine storms, have been studied as treatments for COVID-19.[92,93] Multiple studies have shown a reduced risk of clinical deterioration as measured by a combined index consisting of death, need for mechanical ventilation, ECMO, and ICU admission. One study has shown a reduction in ICU time off organ support and in mortality.[92,93,97] It is recommended for recently hospitalized patients showing rapid respiratory decline.[92,93]

Given the high frequency of DVT and PE discussed above, in Case #3, and one large retrospective study that suggested a therapeutic benefit to anticoagulation, a significant question during the first year of the pandemic was whether there is any mortality benefit to therapeutic anticoagulation.[98] Although there are at least 20 RCTs ongoing globally, there is only one small completed study at this point.[99,100] In a study of 20 COVID-19 patients requiring ventilation in an ICU that were randomized to either prophylactic versus therapeutic anticoagulation, the latter group was found to have more ventilator-free days.[99] Unfortunately, a much larger NIH trial also looking at prophylactic versus therapeutic anticoagulation recently paused the enrollment of ICU patients because an interim analysis found that therapeutic anticoagulation did not reduce the need for organ support, such as the use of ventilators.[101] The trial will continue to enroll moderately ill, non-ICU patients. We will have to wait for the results of ongoing trials to answer the question of what is optimal anticoagulation for hospitalized COVID-19 patients.

A related question is whether anticoagulation of patients at the time of discharge should occur. In a prospective study of 163 patients not placed on anticoagulation at the time of discharge, the risk of thrombosis during the next 30 days was 2.5%.[102] A second study looked retrospectively at 1,877 patients hospitalized with COVID-19, more specifically, at their rate of venous thromboembolism in hospital (4.0%) and post-discharge rate (0.3%).[103] It appears that the overall risk after discharge is low, and anticoagulation is not warranted unless a prehospitalization or in-hospital thrombotic event warranted continued anticoagulation.

Convalescent plasma obtained from persons who recovered from COVID-19 was initially thought to hold great promise, given its successful historical use to treat important infections like pneumococcal pneumonia and diphtheria. Early RCT results looked promising but finished randomized trials showed no mortality benefit, and NIH and IDSA guideline documents no longer recommend its use.[92,104] A possible explanation for the convalescent plasma's lack of mortality benefit was offered by a Dutch randomized trial.[105] The study was halted after 86 patients were enrolled because there was (1) no difference in mortality or Day 15 disease severity, and (2) they found that prior to convalescent plasma administration, 79% of the patients in the study already had SARS-CoV-2 virus neutralization titers of 1:160 (dilution that effectively neutralizes the virus), which was identical to the titers in the convalescent plasma that was administered.[105] In another randomized trial looking at 160 patients randomized to receive either high titer convalescent plasma (>1:1,000 neutralization titer against spike protein) or a placebo within 72 hours of the onset of mild symptoms, convalescent plasma reduced the progression of COVID-19 by 48%.[106] The latter study suggests that convalescent plasma with high titer antibodies against COVID-19 is necessary to be efficacious, and this has recently been confirmed by another study that looked retrospectively at the efficacy of both low and high titer convalescent plasma in 3,082 patients.[107]

Some questions that still need to be addressed:

1. Steroids, drugs with wide-ranging anti-inflammatory effects, have increased the mortality associated with influenza, SARS and MERS but decreased the mortality with COVID-19. Why?[108–116]

2. Is methylprednisolone clearly superior to dexamethasone, as the one study cited above suggests?[91]

3. Two other anti-inflammatory agents, Tocilizumab and Sarilumab (IL-6 receptor antagonists), have been shown to shorten the course of COVID-19 and in ICU patients, to reduce organ support days and mortality, but not as effectively as dexamethasone.[117] This is despite 93% of the control group having received dexamethasone. Should an IL-6 receptor antagonist be given to all COVID patients requiring ICU care?

4. Remdesivir, monoclonal antibodies (bamlanivimab and etesevimab, bamlanivimab, casirivimab and imdevimab in combination; directed at the SARS-CoV-2 receptor binding domain), and high titer convalescent plasma given early in the course of COVID-19 have all been shown to reduce the progression of COVID-19, but not mortality.[96,118] Under what circumstances should one or more of the other agents be added to dexamethasone ± IL-6 receptor inhibitors?

5. Multiple ongoing, randomized clinical trials are looking at whether treating COVID-19 patients with anticoagulation will improve outcomes.[119] If the trials show efficacy, what do they tell us about the pathogenesis of the COVID-19?

6. Can we use the SARS-CoV-2 genome sequences to determine which patients will benefit from which treatment or combinations of treatment?

Possible solutions: The US has just approved US$3 billion for further research into drugs to treat COVID-19.[120]

Ineffective

A number of other agents, such as hydroxychloroquine (anti-inflammatory, antimalarial medication), ivermectin (anti-parasite medication), and lopinavir-ritonavir (HIV medication), received a lot of attention as treatment for COVID-19, but large RCTs have not shown efficacy, and they are not recommended by guideline documents.[92,93] Massive early interest in hydroxychloroquine occurred when it was promoted by President Trump, resulting in great difficulty obtaining the drug for patients needing it for other medical indications.[120A]

iii. *Overall impact of treatment on mortality*

At this point, it is worth asking the question of whether our overall approach to COVID-19 treatment is having an impact on mortality. The Centre for Evidence-Based Medicine at the University of Oxford in England published an analysis of German data spanning the third week of March 2020 through the end of August 2020[121] — the CFR in those aged over 80, 60–79, and 35–59 declined from 28% to 12%, 8% to 2%, and 1% to almost 0, respectively. It should be pointed out here that the infection fatality ratio (IFR), because it includes asymptomatic cases in the denominator, will be lower in all of the categories discussed above.

A similar study from 955 US hospitals found a reduction in risk-adjusted mortality rates comparing the months of January to April with May to June 2020, with the added finding that mortality was lower in hospitalized patients when the prevalence in the community was lower.[122] While it is difficult to attribute this decline in mortality to any particular intervention, or even to say how much of the decline is an artifact of greater COVID-19 testing, it is likely that some of this decline represents better care being provided from lessons learned.

iv. *Ethics*

During the coronavirus pandemic, the number of cases of COVID-19 in various areas of the world (for example, Italy, New York City, Brazil, India) exceeded local hospital capacity, requiring ethical decisions related to rationing of hospital beds, especially in ICUs.[123] Rationing also occurred with ventilators and dialysis machines. This led to doctors having to make decisions about who lived and who died. Many hospitals adopted policies that restricted access of family and friends to see hospitalized patients in order to minimize the spread of COVID-19. This meant that many patients died alone without family or friends (see Prologue). For a more detailed discussion of ethical issues, see Chapter 6.

Key Points: Dexamethasone has decreased the mortality associated with COVID-19 infection. Other treatments, such as remdesivir, actemra, and monoclonal antibodies, reduce hospital stays but so far have not shown mortality benefits. Anticoagulation may have additional mortality benefits, but confirmation of this awaits ongoing randomized trials. Low titer convalescent plasma is not beneficial, but high titer may be, if available. Overall mortality has declined, especially in those over age 80, with better care following lessons learned.

---

e. Case #5 — MIS-C in children

A teenaged female without significant PMH presented to the ED in April 2020 with a 7-day history of fever, malaise, myalgia, headache, sore throat and painful swallowing, painful lumps in her neck, nausea, vomiting, and abdominal pain. One month prior to admission, she had several days of febrile upper respiratory illness that resolved totally. At that time, her mother was COVID-19 positive. The patient was presumed to have mild COVID-19 disease, but she was not tested. In the ED, her physical examination was significant for fever, elevated respiratory rate, tachycardia (elevated heart rate), hypotension, bilateral conjunctivitis, bilateral cervical lymphadenopathy, distended abdomen, red palms, and a variable rash. Labs were significant for leukocytosis with lymphocytopenia, thrombocytopenia (low platelet count), and marked systemic inflammation with elevated ESR, CRP, ferritin, and d-dimer. She also had elevated troponin and brain natriuretic peptide, raising the possibility of cardiac disease; her cardiac echo showed mildly depressed cardiac output. Her chest radiograph showed bilateral pulmonary edema, and a CT scan of the neck with contrast revealed mild tonsillitis with reactive lymphadenopathy. A PCR respiratory viral panel was negative for all viruses, including SARS-CoV-2. Her IgG serology for SARS-CoV-2 was positive on the day of admission.

Although other diagnoses were considered, they were ruled out, such that the physicians caring for her thought the most likely diagnosis was Multisystem Inflammatory Syndrome in Children (MIS-C). The patient was treated with antibiotics, intravenous immunoglobulin (IVIG), aspirin, methylprednisolone, and anikinra (a recombinant IL-1 receptor antagonist, which binds competitively to the Interleukin-1 type I receptor [IL-1RI]). The patient's symptoms and signs improved over the next few days, and she was discharged home with a diagnosis of MIS-C after eight days. A cardiac MRI done six weeks later was normal with no evidence of scarring.

Through October 2020, children represented 11.1% of all confirmed COVID-19 cases in the US, with a rate of 1.12 cases per 100,000 children in the population.[124] The overall risk of hospitalization and death is much lower in pediatric patients than in adults (see the discussion in Case 2 above).[125] The rate of asymptomatic infection in pediatric patients appears to be higher when compared to adults.[125A]

Most pediatric patients who develop symptoms have mild disease, with infants and adolescents more likely to have acute respiratory illness than those 1–6 years of age. Table 4.10 notes the relative frequency of various symptoms in pediatric patients who develop the disease compared to adults.[126] The most striking difference is that pediatric patients, compared to adults, less frequently have shortness of breath. Risk factors for severe disease in pediatric patients are similar to adults and include being Black or of Hispanic ethnicity, having chronic underlying diseases, and being obese.[127] However, while more than 90% of hospitalized adults have at least one reported underlying medical condition, only about half of the children have one or more underlying medical conditions.[128]

MIS-C is a new clinical syndrome (Table 4.11).[127–135] Cases of MIS-C initially were reported from England in late April 2020. Since then, additional cases from Europe, the US, and other regions have also been reported. By the end of 2020, the CDC had reported well over 1,000 MIS-C cases with >20 deaths in the US.[133] Most of the cases are of children and adolescents between the ages of 1 and 14 years, with a median age of 8 to 9 years. Over 75% of the cases have occurred in children who are Hispanic or Black. Most children developed MIS-C 2–4 weeks after infection with SARS-CoV-2 and almost all of them tested positive for SARS-CoV-2 antibodies in their blood. Males made up 56% of the reported cases. The fact that the symptoms for MIS-C appear 2–4 weeks after the onset of COVID-19 infection strongly suggests that it is mediated by the immune system,

Table 4.10.   Signs and symptoms in pediatric (<18 years old) and adult (18–64 years old) patients with laboratory-confirmed COVID-19 (United States, February 12 to April 2, 2020).*

Sign/Symptom	Sign/Symptom No. (%) Pediatric[+]	Sign/Symptom No. (%) Adult[+]
Fever, cough, or shortness of breath[%]	213 (73)	10,167 (93)
Fever[&]	163 (56)	7,794 (71)
Cough	158 (54)	8,775 (80)
Shortness of breath	39 (13)	4,674 (43)
Myalgia	66 (23)	6,713 (61)
Runny nose[$]	21 (7.2)	757 (6.9)
Sore throat	71 (24)	3,795 (35)
Headache	81 (28)	6,335 (58)
Nausea/Vomiting	31 (11)	1,746 (16)
Abdominal pain[¶]	17 (5.8)	1,329 (12)

*Table modified from CDC Covid-19 Response Team. Coronavirus Disease 2019 in children — United States. February 12 to April 2, 2020, *MMWR*, April 6, 2020.[109]

[+]Total number of patients by age group: <18 years (N = 2,572), 18–64 years (N = 113,985).

Cases were included in the denominator if they had a known symptom status for fever, cough, shortness of breath, nausea/vomiting, and diarrhea.

[%] Includes all cases with one or more of these symptoms.

[&] Patients were included if they had information for either measured or subjective fever variables and were considered to have a fever if "yes" was indicated for either variable.

[$] Runny nose and abdominal pain were less frequently completed in the survey forms than other symptoms; therefore, percentages with these symptoms are likely underestimates.

Table 4.11.   Case definition for Multisystem Inflammatory Syndrome in Children (MIS-C).[113]

- An individual aged <21 years presenting with fever*, laboratory** evidence of inflammation, and evidence of clinically severe illness requiring hospitalization, with multisystem (>2) organ involvement (cardiac, renal, respiratory, hematologic, gastrointestinal, dermatologic or neurological); AND
- No alternative plausible diagnoses; AND
- Positive for current or recent SARS-CoV-2 infection by RT-PCR, serology, or antigen test; or COVID-19 exposure within the 4 weeks prior to the onset of symptoms

*Fever >38.0°C for ≥24 hours, or report of subjective fever lasting ≥24 hours
**Laboratory results, including, but not limited to, one or more of the following: an elevated C-reactive protein (CRP), erythrocyte sedimentation rate (ESR), fibrinogen, procalcitonin, d-dimer, ferritin, lactic acid dehydrogenase (LDH), or interleukin 6 (IL-6), elevated neutrophils, reduced lymphocytes and low albumin
Additional comments
- Some individuals may fulfill full or partial criteria for Kawasaki disease but should be reported if they meet the case definition for MIS-C
- Consider MIS-C in any pediatric death with evidence of SARS-CoV-2 infection

Table 4.12. Clinical and pathologic findings that can help distinguish Kawasaki disease from MIS-C.[115,116]

Characteristic	Kawasaki disease	MIS-C
Age	Usually 0–5 years of age	Median age 9 years
Major clinical manifestations		
Cardiac shock	Rare on presentation	Common on presentation
Vascular	Coronary aneurysms	Hypercoagulability with vascular thrombosis
Respiratory tract	Inclusion bodies in ciliated bronchial epithelium have been identified	No inclusion bodies are identifiable in bronchial epithelium
Etiology	Intensely studied but remains unclear	Immune response occurring several weeks after SARS-CoV-2 infection
Clinical outcome	Aneurysms can be present for many years	Almost all children appear to completely recover

as most antibody and lymphocyte immune responses take two weeks or longer to manifest symptoms.[128] It has been reported that adults can have similar manifestations of MIS, although less frequently.[131]

MIS-C patients have symptoms resembling Kawasaki disease (Table 4.12) and Toxic Shock Syndrome with rash, conjunctivitis, abdominal pain, shock, cardiac dysfunction, and markedly elevated inflammatory parameters (CRP, ESR). The clinical aspects that differentiate MIS-C from Kawasaki disease are noted in Table 4.12.[130,132] Many of the patients are ill on presentation and can have cardiac shock. As highlighted in this case, the differential diagnosis often includes other bacterial, viral and rickettsial infections and cardiac and rheumatologic diseases, so the initial workup involves laboratory and imaging studies to help rule out other diseases. Initial treatment of patients thought to have MIS-C includes intravenous fluids and a variety of different drugs that may include antimicrobials, anti-inflammatory drugs, and/or immunomodulatory agents.[133] Although most children hospitalized with MIS-C are seriously ill on admission, the mortality rate is under 2%, and the median duration of hospitalization is seven days.[133] Studies of potential long-term consequences of MIS-C are ongoing.

Key Points: Severe, life-threatening disease due to SARS-CoV-2 infection in children is rare, and most children infected by the virus are either asymptomatic or have mild diseases. MIS-C is a unique presentation following COVID-19 disease, which can cause severe symptoms and signs, but most children are better within a few weeks. MIS-C has a number of clinical and laboratory features similar to Kawasaki disease, but there are distinct differences, including the age of those who develop MIS-C, which usually occurs in older children compared to Kawasaki disease. The etiology of Kawasaki disease has been under investigation for decades, but its cause(s) remains elusive. Thus, whether SARS-CoV-2-induced MIS-C is a unique disease or one of the multiple agents that can cause Kawasaki disease remains to be determined.

f. Case #6 — Pregnant females with COVID-19

A young adult female in her 38ᵗʰ week of pregnancy and without significant PMH came to the ED with a fever of 103. Her exam was otherwise unremarkable. SARS-CoV-2 PCR testing was positive. Labor ensued, and she delivered a healthy baby girl. After 48 hours of observation, they were both discharged and are doing well at a 2-week follow-up visit.

One of the key questions pertaining to any new or emerging infection is the impact of that infection upon pregnant females and their fetus and newborn. In a report from Wuhan, China, among 118 pregnant females with COVID-19 at the time of delivery, all survived, and no infants had any evidence of COVID-19 infection.[134] Eight newborns had their throats swabbed for COVID-19 and were negative. The largest study done to date involving 3,912 infants with known gestational age born to women with COVID-19 suggested that there is a small increase in the risk of premature births (delivery before 37 weeks — 12% versus a national estimated rate of 10.2%).[135] Among 610 mothers who tested positive for SARS-CoV-2 at the time of delivery, 2.6% of their newborn infants tested positive for SARS-CoV-2. Most of these infants were either asymptomatic or had mild disease.

In contrast, a prospective multinational study (18 countries), 706 women with COVID-19 were prospectively followed and compared to a matched group (1 COVID-19 patient to 2 non-COVID-19 patients) of 1,424 non-COVID-19 infected women. Women with COVID-19 were at higher risk of preeclampsia/eclampsia, severe infections, ICU admission, and preterm birth.[136] In a study comparing 1,062 pregnant females with 9,815 non-pregnant patients, both with COVID-19 pneumonia, the mortality rate was lower in the pregnant group.[137] However, in a much larger study comparing maternal mortality rates for all US pregnancies in 2018 and 2019 versus 2020, there was a significant increase in mortality in 2020.[137A] Subsequent studies confirmed these findings in 2021. Additionally, whether there is an increased risk of stillbirths and/or congenital abnormalities that occur in pregnant women infected in the first two trimesters needs to be determined.

> Key Points: COVID-19 infection increases the risk of maternal mortality and other complications associated with pregnancy. It only infrequently infects newborn children.

g. Case #7 — Immunocompromised patients

A young adult male with PMH significant for treated primary syphilis, newly diagnosed HIV infection (4 days prior to admission; CD4 count 126, viral load 857,000, meeting AIDS definitions), and remote methamphetamine use, was admitted due to headache, fever 102.3°F, and meningeal irritation (neck stiffness). Meningitis was suspected, so a lumbar puncture was performed; cerebrospinal fluid showed three white blood cells (abnormal) and was otherwise negative. His serum VDRL was positive at a titer of 1:128, diagnostic of secondary syphilis, but it was unclear whether he had been inadequately treated previously or reinfected. He was thought to have possible central nervous system involvement and was treated with intravenous ceftriaxone and benzathine penicillin. Because of his admission fever, SARS-CoV-2 PCR was ordered and positive; his chest X-ray was negative for pneumonia, and he was not hypoxic. He was discharged on anti-retroviral treatment with outpatient follow-up for his syphilis, AIDS, and COVID-19.

A concern with any new infectious agent is how it will behave in immunocompromised patients. For example, cytomegalovirus, a virus that can infect up to 90% of humanity, normally only causes mild disease, especially in children, and at its worst in most people, causes a mononucleosis-like illness that runs its course in a few weeks.[138] However, in immunocompromised patients, cytomegalovirus can cause much more severe disease. In bone marrow transplant patients, cytomegalovirus can cause a fatal infection due to cytomegalovirus pneumonia. In patients with AIDS, cytomegalovirus can cause blindness and/or colitis.[138]

The complexities of how a patient's immune status can affect the clinical manifestations of a viral infection are further illustrated by dengue. Dengue, another viral infection that infects a large proportion of humanity, can cause a self-limited flu-like illness the first time a person is infected, but a potentially fatal hemorrhagic fever (bleeding all over the body) the second time.[140] In a small study in China, ten patients with HIV (average CD4 lymphocyte count 254, median count 239; AIDS = <200) and dengue coinfection were compared to 30 patients with dengue alone; hemorrhagic fever was seen significantly less frequently in the coinfected group.[141] The fundamental immunologic defect in AIDS patients is poorly functioning or low numbers of CD4 lymphocytes; perhaps low numbers of CD4 lymphocytes protect against hemorrhagic dengue and its associated cytokine storm. Similarly, could the reason for Case #7's mild course be the low CD4 lymphocyte count? Further work will be necessary to understand the importance of the CD4 lymphocyte in COVID-19 infection.

Another immunocompromised host group that shows the range of the problem is renal transplants. In reports from New York City and Paris, renal transplants were found to have COVID-19 associated mortality of 24–28%, >10 times normal mortality rates.[142,143] Further study will have to be done to understand the effects of COVID-19 on mortality rates in different immuncompromised hosts.

Key Point: Abnormal host immunity will change the natural history of COVID-19 infection, making it less severe in some cases or more severe in others.

---

h. Case #8 — Central nervous system manifestations

A geriatric male with PMH significant for chronic obstructive pulmonary disease, coronary artery disease, heart failure, stroke, atrial fibrillation, hypertension, hyperlipidemia, gout, and amyloidosis, was admitted secondary to generalized weakness, acute kidney injury, and pancytopenia (low red blood cells, white blood cells, and platelets). His presenting manifestations were thought to be most likely due to amyloidosis, and he responded to fluids only. His hospital course was significant for a health-care associated pneumonia on Day 6 of hospitalization, which responded to antibiotics, a gastrointestinal bleed on Day 10, which required one unit of blood and briefly holding his apixaban for his chronic atrial fibrillation, and an incarcerated inguinal hernia on Day 13, which surgery repaired. As part of his preoperative evaluation, he had a SARS-CoV-2 antigen done that was positive and confirmed the next day by PCR. Questioning of his family determined that a few days prior to his positive COVID antigen, he had been visited by his granddaughter, who subsequently became symp-tomatic with a mild COVID-19 infection. On Day 15 of his hospitalization, he had a seizure, and an EEG showed a left temporal lobe seizure focus. A lumbar puncture was done on the same day, which was within normal limits except for an elevated total protein of 127. It was notably negative for herpes simplex virus by PCR, which was a concern because of the seizure. A brain MRI was done, which showed no focal abnormalities in the left temporal lobe or elsewhere. He was diagnosed with COVID-19 encephalopathy (abnormal brain function without identifiable abnormality) and treated only with dexamethasone with steady improvement. Once his post-seizure symptoms had resolved, his son noted that for the first time in many years, he had stopped stuttering.

One of the least common but highly significant COVID-19-associated group of findings is central nervous system (CNS) abnormalities.[144,145] Five major categories have been identified: (1) encephalopathies (Case #1 and #8), (2) inflammatory CNS syndromes (encephalitis, encephalomyelitis — inflammation in the brain or spinal cord), (3) stroke, (4) Guillain-Barre (paralysis that rises from lower extremities toward upper extremities), and (5) miscellaneous.[144] Encephalopathy patients present with confusion and/or delirium/psychosis and negative CNS imaging. Inflammatory CNS syndromes include encephalitis, meningitis, and spinal cord inflammation, with about half of these having associated hemorrhage. This group has been treated with steroids with or without immunoglobulin, with only about 10% making a full recovery. The patients with strokes are clearly hypercoagulable (increased risk of blood clotting), with half of them also having pulmonary emboli. The Guillain-Barre group had partial recovery using traditional treatments. Based on the estimated frequency of strokes shown in Table 4.4 and the relative frequency of the above Groups 2–4 from a single UK hospital study,[144] Groups 2–4 likely occurred with an estimated frequency of 0.5–1% in the pre-vaccine portion of the pandemic. Group 1 may occur at a much higher frequency, as confusion has been noted in up to 28% of hospitalized COVID patients (Table 4.4).

> Key point: Uncommonly, COVID-19 is associated with confusion, encephalitis, strokes, or bleeding in the central nervous system. The cause of such presentations remains to be determined.

i. Case #9 — "Long Haulers" or "Long COVID"

A middle-aged male with PMH significant for exercise-induced asthma (rare use of rescue inhaler), allergic rhinitis, food allergies including shellfish, three melanomas removed without recurrence, developed severe fatigue, weakness, and fever 103°F, and tested SARS-CoV-2 PCR positive in June 2020. Two other family members in his house were also SARS-CoV-2 PCR positive. Over the next two weeks he had a loss of taste and smell, myalgias, diarrhea, cough and mild hypoxia (86% O_2 saturation on room air), pneumonia in both lungs, rash on his toes, and itchiness around old scars. The diarrhea was the most severe manifestation, resulting in his hospital admission for four days due to dehydration and a low serum Na. He was treated with fluids, doxycycline, and azithromycin, but no steroids or specific COVID-19-targeted medications. On discharge, severe fatigue, malaise, myalgias, and shortness of breath remained and caused him to miss eight weeks of work, never having missed work before this. During the two months off from work, he also noted mild relative hypoxia (O_2 saturations in the low 90s), brain fog (difficulty thinking clearly), and a tendency toward easy anger, all of which he had never experienced previously. During the next seven months, his fatigue, myalgias, shortness of breath, and loss of taste and smell slowly improved, but since hospital discharge, he had an increased need for his rescue inhaler and had not returned to baseline exercise tolerance as of nine months after his infection. Recent laboratory testing noted vitamin B12 and vitamin D deficiency and low testosterone and thyroid hormone levels, none of which he had before COVID-19 infection. He also developed hypertension for the first time in his life, three months *after his initial illness, which persisted, requiring him to begin medication. The fatigue is particularly notable, because he played tennis seven days a week before his COVID-19 infection, and the hypertension is notable, because he has always been told he had the blood pressure of a much younger person.*

It is increasingly apparent that symptomatic COVID-19 may result in persistent symptoms, often referred to as long haulers or long COVID. In a large review that looked at 45 studies examining persistent symptoms after COVID-19 infections (follow-up period most commonly 60–90 days), the most common persistent symptoms were shortness of breath (~34%), fatigue (~30%), sleep disturbance (~29%), memory loss (~28%), generalized pain (~25%), and a loss of smell (~23%).[146] A few studies have had at least six months of follow-up. A study from China with follow-up of patients with COVID-19 for six months after hospitalization found that 74% of them had persistent symptoms out to six months. Persistent symptoms included fatigue, muscle weakness, sleep difficulties, anxiety or depression.[147] Whereas in a group of largely outpatient-managed COVID-19 patients followed up for six months, 33% had persistent symptoms, suggesting that more severe COVID-19 results in a higher likelihood of persistent symptoms.[148] There has not yet been a comparably sized group of COVID-19 ICU survivors followed up for six months to test this hypothesis.

Using the US Department of Veterans Affairs healthcare database, it was possible to show that beyond the first 30 days of COVID-19 illness, there was a higher risk of death and health resource utilization than a matched control group, and this persisted out to six months.[149] The Veterans data also showed an increased risk (hazard ratio [HR]: how often an event happens in one group compared to another group, greater than 1 = increased risk) of certain specific clinical manifestations, especially if the patient was hospitalized, to include acute coronary disease (5.59 HR; 11.08 HR, if hospitalized in an ICU), thromboembolic disease (10.84 hospitalized HR, 26.33 ICU HR), stroke (14.1 hospitalized HR, 21.19 ICU HR), and acute kidney disease (2.31 hospitalized HR, 4.5 ICU HR).[149] Comparing the same COVID-19 group with a control group that had seasonal influenza, they found that the COVID-19 group was more likely to be rehospitalized for a variety of reasons than the influenza group (1.3–4 HR).

The explanation for these prolonged symptoms and adverse health outcomes, including other disease processes, is not yet apparent. Possibilities include chronic infection with persistent expression of viral proteins stimulating an ongoing immune response, reinfection (Case #4) or chronic inflammation, such as appears to be the mechanism for MIS-C (Case #5).

> Key Points: After symptomatic COVID-19, patients may experience persistent, sometimes debilitating symptoms, such as fatigue, muscle weakness, sleep difficulties, anxiety or depression, for as long as 9 months (Case 9) and perhaps longer. Whether this is a function of chronic SARS-CoV-2 infection, persistent immune activation analogous to MIS-C, or some as yet unidentified mechanism remains to be shown.

Evidence that there is a persistent immune response after SARS-CoV-2 infection in some individuals is suggested by a recent mRNA vaccine study comparing 109 individuals without pre-existing antibodies to SARS-CoV-2 with 41 individuals with antibodies.[150] The first group required 9–12 days after their first vaccine dose to develop IgG antibodies. The second group required only 5–8 days to develop IgG antibodies, and the antibody levels were 10–20 times higher than those that started off antibody negative (see the next section on pathogenesis). Furthermore, the group with pre-existing antibodies was more likely to have systemic symptoms after vaccination than the antibody-negative group ($P < 0.001$), especially fatigue, headache, chills, myalgias or fever. These findings are consistent with a brisk anamnestic immune response (immunologic memory), a normal response to reexposure to the same antigen. However, as the discussion about MIS-C after Case #5 above suggests, some individuals will have an extreme, prolonged immune response with associated symptoms, suggesting that there is a spectrum of extended immune responses that is associated with prolonged symptoms. Potential drivers of such sustained immune responses will be discussed in the pathogenesis section.

> Key point: Long haulers are a subgroup of COVID-19 patients who have persistent symptoms out to six months or longer. The mechanism for these persistent symptoms may relate to chronic SARS-CoV-2 infection, a persistent immune response causing chronic inflammation or both (see section on pathogenesis that follows).

2. Pathogenesis of COVID-19

Every disease has a unique pathogenesis, i.e. the mechanisms by which it causes disease. An understanding of such mechanisms at the molecular level is required to decide how to treat the disease, develop new drugs and vaccines, and even to explain the disease to patients and families. This section of the chapter will go over current understandings of the ACE2 receptor, lung disease, heart disease, the immune response, the associated coagulopathy, and SARS-CoV-2 mutation in the pathogenesis of COVID-19.

a. ACE2 receptor

i. *Role of binding to ACE2 receptor (angiotensin-converting enzyme 2 receptor)*

For COVID-19 infection to occur, the surface spike protein of SARS-CoV-2 must bind to the ACE2 receptor expressed on nasal goblet cells and ciliated epithelial cells present on the respiratory tract mucosa.[151–154] While SARS-CoV-2 is bound to the ACE2 receptor, it is thought that TMPRSS2, a serine protease (cell surface enzyme), also present on these cell surfaces, will cleave the spike protein on the virus surface, allowing for cell membrane fusion and endocytosis (cell internalization) of the virus.[151–154] The ACE2 receptor has multiple roles and is expressed in multiple tissues throughout the body, including the respiratory tract, heart and circulatory system, gastrointestinal tract, kidneys, central nervous system, reproductive system, and adipose tissue, with the highest density of surface receptors being found in the gastrointestinal tract, and the male reproductive system.[153,155]

Perhaps its most important role the ACE2 receptor has pertinent to COVID-19 infection is its anti-inflammatory effect; it limits the progressive damage associated with heart failure, myocardial infarction, hypertension, diabetes, and obesity, but of particular importance to COVID-19, it protects against acute lung injury, especially due to infection, all likely through the inhibition of inflammation mediated by the renin-angiotensin system (an enzymatic system that regulates blood volume and blood pressure).[153,154,156] Additionally relevant to COVID-19, the ACE2 receptor density varies in a number of human disease states. ACE2 receptor density in the respiratory tract increases with age, smoking, COPD, ventilator support for respiratory failure, use of ACEI (angiotensin-converting enzyme inhibitor)/ARB (angioten-sin 2 receptor blockers) inhibitors for hypertension, coronary artery disease, heart failure, diabetes, and obesity.[157–162] This suggests the possibility that the more of these chronic disease states a patient has, the more likely they will be able to bind SARS-CoV-19 and, therefore, more likely to be infected. Since the ACE2 receptor is internalized (moves inside the cell membrane) associated with SARS-CoV-2 infection, and the ACE2 receptor's role appears to be an inflammation blocking mechanism for the disease states mentioned above, individuals with increased numbers of ACE2 receptors may have a more severe infection and inflammatory reaction in their lungs than individuals without the increased density of ACE2 receptors (Figure 4.56).[163]

Data providing direct support of this hypothesis were recently pro-vided by a large multi-country collaboration that showed that increased plasma ACE2 levels correlated with worse COVID-19 outcomes in hospi-

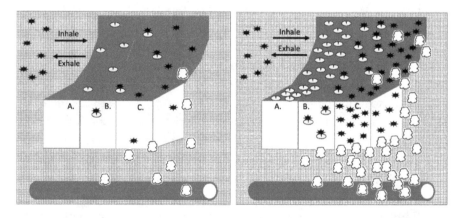

Figure 4.56. Hypothesis: Increased ACE-2 receptor density on bronchial mucosa (curving pink surface) leads to worse inflammation with COVID-19 infection. Left. Patient with min-imal ACE2 receptors (yellow oval with wedge missing; young person without risk factors, see text for details), Right. Patient with increased density of ACE2 receptors (greater than 80 years old, COPD, diabetes, hypertension; see text for details). A. Bronchial mucosa seg-ment of each illustration shows the number of ACE2 receptors prior to infection. B. Bronchial mucosa segment shows ACE2 receptors with SARS-CoV-2 (black circle with spikes) attached to an ACE2 receptor with some internalized below the bronchial mucosal cell surface. C. Bronchial mucosa segment shows replicated intracellular and extracellular SARS-CoV-2. White blood cells are shown as amorphous white shapes that increase in number as the infection progresses; much greater numbers of white blood cells occur around the bronchial mucosa associated with patients having higher numbers of ACE2 receptors. The lower pink cylinder is a blood vessel running below the surface of the bronchial mucosa and the source of the white blood cells. Source: R. Sherertz.

talized patients and elevated plasma ACE2 levels were directly related to underlying hypertension, heart disease, and kidney disease.[164] While this makes logical sense, a recent report did not find increased expression of ACE2 receptors on the surface of alveolar epithelial cells (line air sacs in lungs where gas exchange occurs) in older patients or those with the co-morbidities mentioned above.[165] Further work needs to be done to better understand whether greater ACE2 expression predisposes to a greater risk of COVID-19-related inflammation and death.

One unique manifestation of COVID-19 infection has been the sudden loss of smell and/or taste. Scientists have wondered whether the ACE2 receptor plays a role in the pathogenesis of this clinical finding. A study by Brann and colleagues found that olfactory sensory neurons did not express ACE2 receptors, but immediately adjacent tissues in the nasal epithelium do, suggesting that the effect on smell is mediated by infection/inflammation in adjacent tissues.[166] In contrast, human taste cells have recently been shown to express ACE2 receptors providing direct viral access with the potential for cell damage.[167]

One concern relevant to this discussion is what should be done with COVID-19 patients who are already on an ACEi or ARB drug if they get COVID-19 infection.[168] One study randomized patients already on ACEi or ARB drugs at the time of COVID-19 infection to either a suspension of 30 days (334 patients) versus continuing the medications (325 patients) and found no difference in the clinical outcomes of the COVID-19 infections.[169] The NIH has recommended that at this time, there is no reason to change ACEi or ARB treatment-related acute COVID-19 infection.[170]

b. Lung disease

Nearly all fatal cases (88.5%) of COVID-19 are the result of respiratory failure due to progressive viral pneumonia, with most patients having additional evidence of bacterial pneumonia (57.7%).[171,172] Microscopy of the lungs in fatal cases demonstrated mild to moderate tracheobronchitis and diffuse alveolar damage.[171] The alveolar air sacs, where air exchange occurs, are almost completed denuded of their lining cells, type 1 and 2 pneumocytes, and full of hyaline (protein lining alveolar air sacs) membranes and fibrin deposits.[171,172] Surrounding the alveolar air sacs is a brisk inflammatory response with associated edema. SARS-CoV-2 can be demonstrated by immunohistochemical staining in the upper airways and lungs in 50% and 92% of the patients, respectively.[171] SARS-CoV-2 is not identified in the heart, liver, kidney, spleen or intestine.[171] A total of 75% of the patients have bacterial or viral co-infections.[171]

Ackermann and colleagues compared lung findings from seven patients with fatal COVID-19 infection with seven patients with fatal 2009 pandemic Influenza infection.[172] They found that ACE2 receptor density was similar in COVID-19 and Influenza lungs, and both had greater receptor density than in control lungs. Somewhat surprisingly, they noted COVID-19 lungs had 50% less weight than influenza lungs (the latter had increased weight due to edema fluid). The inflammatory response in COVID lungs had greater numbers of CD4 lymphocytes and lesser numbers of polymorphonuclear (PMN) leukocytes (white blood cells principally responsible for killing bacteria) than influenza lungs (P < 0.05). The latter may relate to the known PMN defect demonstrated by Abramson and colleagues that occurs with influenza infection, which may be the reason for secondary bacterial infections being the predominant cause of death in the 1918 influenza pandemic (Chapter 8).[173] COVID lungs were also found to have nine times greater capillary thrombi (clots) and greater angiogenesis (new blood vessel formation) than influenza lungs.[173] A possible explanation for the latter two findings was suggested by the transmission electron microscope finding of SARS-CoV-2 virus within endothelial cells lining the capillary blood vessels, which might contribute to clot formation and new blood vessels by damaging the capillaries and causing endothelialitis.

A multicountry autopsy study found two different immunopathologic patterns in autopsy lungs in fatal COVID-19 cases.[174] Patients that died early in their ICU stay had high lung SARS-CoV-2 viral loads, high local expression of interferon-stimulated genes and cytokines, and limited pulmonary damage. Those that died later in their ICU stay had lower viral loads, heavy infiltration of CD8 lymphocytes (lymphocytes that mediate adaptive or memory immunity), and severe lung damage. Further investigation will be necessary to confirm the findings of these two small autopsy studies.

c. Heart disease

Multiple studies have now suggested that COVID-19 has both direct and indirect effects on the heart. Several lines of evidence suggest direct

COVID-19 cardiac injury. Up to 28% of the patients admitted to the hospital have troponin elevations (indicates possible cardiac damage, Table 4.6), but this finding says nothing about the potential mechanism of injury. A prospective cardiac MRI study done in Germany evaluated 100 consecutive symptomatic COVID-19 patients on an average of 71 days after diagnosis — 67% had not been admitted to the hospital and 33% had been admitted — in comparison to 50 healthy volunteers and 57 risk factor-matched patients.[175] The COVID-19 patients, in comparison to the two control groups, had lower left ventricular ejection fractions, higher left ventricular volumes, elevated native T1-weighted and T2-weighted values (T1 highlights fat, T2 highlights fat and water), and significantly higher troponin values. The combination of elevated native T1 (73%) and T2 (60%) measures is consistent with inflammation. In three patients with reduced left ventricular ejection fractions (<50%), endomyocardial biopsies were performed, and lymphocytic infiltration of cardiac muscle was seen.

A similar MRI study of 26 competitive college athletes with COVID-19 infection (average age: 19.5 years; 57.7% male, 42.3% female) that did not require hospitalization found that four males (15%) had evidence of active myocardial inflammation.[176] Two of the four males with MRI evidence of inflammation also had pericardial effusions (fluid in sac surrounding heart). A total of 46% of the athletes had evidence of possible inflammation — 10/15 males and 2/11 females (67% vs. 22%, P = 0.02, Fisher's exact test). A study of 789 professional athletes who tested positive for COVID-19 found that 30 of them had either abnormal troponins, electrocardiograms or echo studies, and 5 of the 30 had evidence of cardiac inflammation by cardiac MRI: 3 with myocarditis and 2 with pericarditis.[177] Overall, this suggests the risk of cardiac disease is low, but a much longer follow-up will be necessary to know for sure.

An autopsy study of 39 consecutive COVID-19 patients has provided further evidence of cardiac inflammation.[178] They found that 24 of 39 patients had detectable SARS-CoV-2 virus in the heart muscle, and 16 of 39 patients (41%) had high cardiac SARS-CoV-2 viral loads. They further noted that the expression of 6 inflammatory genes in the heart was greater in the 16 patients with elevated SARS-CoV-2 viral loads (P < 0.05), but this was not associated with increased infiltration of mononuclear cells (lymphocytes, etc.).

Another study looked at the ability of SARS-CoV-2 to infect cardiac cells.[179] They found that the virus can infect cardiomyocytes (heart muscle cells) but not cardiac endothelial cells (cells lining heart blood vessels) or cardiac fibroblasts (cells making up heart scaffolding). As with other tissue types, cardiomyocyte infection was dependent upon ACE2 binding. A comparison of *in vitro* (cells in a test tube) cardiomyocytes with autopsy-derived myocardial cells found similar myofibrillar (muscle fiber) fragmentation, suggesting the *in vitro* model may demonstrate similar effects to *in vivo* infection.

There are also studies that suggest COVID-19 can indirectly affect the heart. A cardiac echo study looked at 100 consecutive COVID-19 patients admitted to the hospital.[180] They found the following abnormalities: right ventricular dilatation/dysfunction (39%), left ventricular diastolic dysfunction (16%), left ventricular systolic dysfunction (10%), valve abnormalities (3%); 32% had normal echos. The lungs were additionally evaluated with ultrasound, where it was claimed that 80% of the lungs had findings consistent with edema due to viral infection, not cardiac-related pulmonary edema. In the 20 patients that deteriorated further, a repeat echo study was done, which demonstrated deterioration of all right ventricular hemodynamic parameters, which did not occur with patients with left ventricular dysfunction, providing possible evidence that pulmonary infection was the biggest driver of right ventricular dysfunction.

A further study looked at 209 consecutive patients (40–80 years old) with COVID-19 who had a chest CT scan at the time of admission and did not have known symptomatic coronary disease.[181] Coronary artery calcium (CAC), a marker of evolving coronary artery disease, was found in half of the patients. Comparing the two groups, those with CAC were much more likely to have mechanical noninvasive or invasive ventilation, extracorporeal membrane oxygenation or death, than patients without CAC (50% vs. 17.5%, $P < 0.0001$). However, in a second study, among 279 patients admitted with COVID-19 infection, CAC was not an independent risk factor for mortality, but peri-coronary adipose tissue attenuation (a measure of peri-coronary inflammation) was an independent risk factor for mortality.[182] For comparison, a group of 591 trauma patients (age greater than 45 years) admitted to the hospital were evaluated as to the predictive risk of CAC versus abdominal artery calcium for in-hospital mortality, and CAC did not increase the risk of dying in this study.[183] While it seems logical that preexisting inflammation with its potential for increased ACE2 receptor cell surface markers, would be the more likely risk factor, further work will be necessary to sort this out.

In either case, this adds further evidence that pre-existing coronary disease (silent or otherwise) is a synergistic risk factor for mortality for COVID-19.

d. Immune response

i. *Are asymptomatic COVID-19 infections due to persistent immunity from prior nonSARS-CoV-2 coronavirus infections?*

COVID-19 is one of many infectious diseases that is associated with a wide spectrum of clinical manifestations, ranging from totally asymptomatic infection to sepsis or septic shock with a "cytokine storm".[184–187] A fundamental question is what role does the immune system play in determining the severity of the inflammatory response. In particular, does prior infection with a nonSARS-CoV-2 coronavirus provide protection against a subsequent SARS-CoV-2 infection? With some viral infectious diseases, such as rubella, prior infection results in life-long immunity whereby antibodies circulating in the blood are sufficient to neutralize future exposure to the same virus and prevent infection. With other viral infections, especially those that mutate rapidly, such as influenza A and HIV (see mutation discussion below for further details), antibodies from prior infection are not sufficient to block subsequent infection.[188] With COVID-19, individuals with preexisting antibodies from prior nonSARS-CoV-2 coronavirus infections were not able to neutralize SARS-CoV-2 and block infection.[189,190] Alternatively, it has been shown that for some infections, like influenza A, that do not result in effective long term neutralizing antibodies, that memory T lymphocytes play a role in minimizing future infection.[191]

Recent evidence suggests that 20–50% of the general population have pre-existing memory T cells, likely from prior non-SARS-CoV-2 coronavirus infections, that have specificity toward SARS-CoV-2 virus and might mitigate the severity of infection.[192,193] To that possibility, one study looking at patients from early in the pandemic found that, among 13 patients with mild COVID-19 versus 11 patients with severe COVID-19, T cells recognizing peptides conserved among coronaviruses were more abundant in the mild COVID-19 group than in the severe group.[194] Looking directly at the severity of illness, another study showed that a recent (less than 441 days), non-SARS-CoV-2 coronavirus infection, was associated with subsequent lower mortality due to SARS-CoV-2 infection, than if no recent coronavirus infection had occurred (<800 days).[195] It has been further shown that pre-existing, cross-reactive CD4+

T lymphocytes enhance SARS-CoV-2 immune responses to both infection and vaccination, providing additional evidence that cell-mediated immunity is important in minimizing the severity of SARS-CoV-2 infection.[196] Preliminary evidence raises the possibility that some of the differential immune responses, comparing those with asymptomatic SARS-CoV-2 infections and those with symptomatic infections, may be manifest in the mucosal immune response.[197] For example, one study from Ethiopia suggests that co-infection with intestinal parasites reduces the severity of COVID-19 infection, possibly through the induction of regulatory T lymphocytes.[197A,197B] There is also some evidence that genetics is important in the severity of COVID-19, but not yet enough to make definitive statements.[59,60,198,199] See Chapter 10 for further discussion.

ii. *Are the most severe COVID-19 pneumonias a consequence of cytokine storm?*

Sepsis and septic shock are well-defined entities and reflect the relative magnitude of the inflammatory response associated with various infectious diseases and other noninfectious diseases.[184] In contrast, cytokine storm has no accepted definition but has become the darling of the scientific and news media to describe severe COVID-19 infection.[184-186] The hyperinflammatory phenotype of Adult Respiratory Distress Syndrome (ARDS), perhaps the prototype of a cytokine storm, includes elevated proinflammatory cytokines (proteins that stimulate inflammation), especially IL-6, shock and adverse clinical outcomes.[187] The ARDS-associated IL-6 levels are 10–200 times higher than those seen with COVID-19 infections.[187] In spite of the apparent lower levels of cytokines, many different treatment agents aimed at cytokines known to be elevated in a cytokine storm have been tried for COVID-19, with the only success so far being the steroids mentioned earlier in this chapter.[186,187] It may turn out that with further study, we will find that cytokine storm is an overcall in most patients with COVID-19 (see Lung Disease discussion above), and the lung manifestations in severe cases more likely represent severe viral pneumonia or added secondary bacterial pneumonia, rather than a consequence of a "cytokine storm".

e. Coagulopathy

At its worst COVID-19 progresses rapidly to respiratory failure, requiring intubation and mechanical ventilation for further treatment.[184–187] One consequence of a true cytokine storm is coagulopathy, commonly associated with disseminated intravascular coagulation (DIC).[200] It is typically mediated by procoagulants secreted by monocyte/macrophages and is often associated with bleeding.[200] The coagulopathy associated with COVID-19 is impressive in terms of the different thrombotic events it can cause (Case #3), but interestingly, bleeding is rare.[200] One study cited earlier in this chapter demonstrated that the clotting seen in the lungs is associated with SARS-CoV-2 in the endothelial cells lining the pulmonary capillaries.[172] Given the very high rate of capillary thrombosis found in this report, it is possible that the high rate of endovascular thrombosis relates to sick endothelial cells, analogous to that seen with Rocky Mountain Spotted Fever and other infectious agents that infect endothelial cells. If this is verified as the pathogenesis of the coagulopathy, it will likely have treatment implications that could include therapeutic anticoagulation.

f. *SARS-CoV-2 mutation*

Case #4 above is remarkable in one particular aspect — 45 days after the patient's initial COVID-19 illness, he developed a second COVID-PCR-positive illness requiring hospitalization, escalation to ICU level care, with eventual death. Although it had been clearly shown that COVID-19 symptoms can persist at least nine months (Case #9), Case #4's second COVID-PCR-positive infection was likely due to a new strain of SARS-CoV-2. At that time reports utilizing genomic sequencing of the causative SARS-CoV-2 strains for each pair of 2 infections in 1 person had unequivocally shown that patients can be infected a second time with a second strain;[81–84] a reinfection case-tracker documenting individuals with two episodes of COVID-19 has shown that this is not uncommon,[201] and a large study from Denmark suggested the reinfection risk could be as high as 20% of the risk of those who are infection naïve.[202] The Denmark study compared COVID-19 infection rates from March through May 2020 (first surge) with rates from September through December (second surge).[202]

At this point in the COVID-19 pandemic the concept of new variants and their origin was poorly understood. In the same time frame that the Denmark study demonstrated that second SARS-CoV-2 infections occurred frequently, Denmark also became aware that SARS-CoV-2 infections were occuring in minks on mink farms, SARS-CoV-2 mutations were occuring, and that some of the mutated variants were then infecting humans. Although there were no data that the second Danish surge had anything to do with the Danish mink farm-associated variant strain with its increased ACE2 receptor affinity, public health recommendations led to 17 million minks being killed to address this possibility.[203–205] Infection with a new strain, at a minimum, suggests two important things: first, immunity does not last long in some individuals, and/or second, the virus is mutating fast enough that the initial immune response soon does not provide protection because the virus has changed sufficiently to evade it. Both of these considerations have implications related to vaccine effectiveness.

Studies looking at antibody levels initially suggested that COVID-19 immunity may not last long. An early study found that the half-life of serum antibodies against SARS-CoV-2 after mild COVID-19 was only 36 days.[206] Similar data exist for other coronavirus infections, including SARS and MERS.[207] However, subsequently, it has been shown that immunologic memory for all four types of immune memory (antibodies, memory B lymphocytes, memory CD8 lymphocytes, memory CD4 lymphocytes) persist after COVID-19 infection for at least six months in 95% of those infected.[208] If that is the case, does it mean that second infections only occur in the 5% who do not have persistent immunologic memory, or is there another possible explanation?

An alternative explanation is the possibility that SARS-CoV-2 can mutate fast enough that a new variant strain can come back into a community already infected by an older strain and cause another wave of infections. By late 2020, it was clear that there were multiple new strains globally causing new waves of infections, most notably the UK variant (B.1.1.7, also known as alpha), the South Africa variant (B.1.351, a.k.a. beta), and the Brazil variant (P.1, a.k.a. gamma).[209,210] Since the identification of these three variants, studies have demonstrated that these variants appear to be more infectious than the original SARS-CoV-2 strain,[211–213] possibly more virulent (cause more severe infection),[213] less likely inhibited by existing convalescent plasma or monoclonal antibodies created to treat the infection,[214–217] and less likely prevented by some existing vaccines (Johnson & Johnson, Novavax).[218,219] Mathematical modeling has estimated that the UK variant has a 43–90% higher R_0 than pre-existing SARS-CoV-strains.[211] The South Africa variant replaced the previous SARS-CoV-2 strains in a matter of weeks, strongly suggesting greater transmission, but hard transmission rate data are not available yet.[212] The Brazil variant has been estimated to be 1.4–2.2 times more transmissible in Manaus than the previous SARS-CoV-2 strains in the area.[213] The study from Manaus, Brazil also suggested the P.1 variant was 1.1–1.8 times more likely to cause death, suggesting greater virulence.[213] That these findings are considered real, and a threat to vaccine efficacy is best indicated by the fact that vaccine manufacturers are already working on boosters that take the variants into consideration.[217–219] For further discussion of the impact of variants on vaccines, see Chapter 5.

Early in the pandemic, researchers speculated that the first appearance of the SARS-CoV-2 virus in China was the result of recombination genetic events with resultant mutations in the spike protein binding domains due to convergent evolution (organisms evolving independently in different geographic regions and reaching the same endpoint).[220] More recently, the appearance of the UK, South Africa, and Brazil variants, all with spike protein mutations, have also been attributed to convergent, adaptive evolution.[221] All three variants became prominent in the time frame when the global number of cases was on a rapid rise. It is an accepted evolutionary concept that the more times an infectious organism experiences a new host to multiply within, the greater the opportunity for mutation. It is quite clear from bat-focused research that coronaviruses have evolved an extraordinary ability to evolutionarily adapt to a new host, as shown best by the finding that virtually all bat species have different species of coronaviruses.[222]

Since coronaviruses can rapidly mutate and adapt in bats, can the same thing happen in humans such that chronic infection can occur? The persistent symptoms for up to 9 months described in Case #9 above and for at least 6 months in literature reports strongly raise the possibility of persistent viral infection. Using viral culture isolation methodologies, it is quite unusual to isolate viruses greater than 30 days after infection (Case #1 discussion), but all culture methodologies have threshold limitations that could easily miss low-grade viral replication. A recent study using subgenomic mRNAs (required for a virus to express its assembly proteins and only present in actively infected cells) suggested that SARS-CoV-2 was replicating in at least 20% of 60 patients with persistent respiratory tract PCR positivity out to at least 101 days.[223] It is also quite possible that persistence is more likely in some tissues than others. A Chinese study found in a group of 289 SARS-CoV-2 pharyngeal PCR-positive patients, 7%

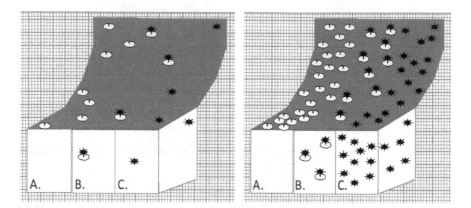

Figure 4.57. Hypothesis: Chronic SARS-CoV-2 infection occurs and is tissue specific. Left panel, respiratory tract epithelial cells: A. ACE2 receptors without attached SARS-CoV-2. B. ACE2 receptors with attached SARS-CoV-2 and early cell internalization. C. Low level viral replication with minimal virus on cell surface. Right panel, intestinal epithelial cells: A. High density ACE2 receptors without attached SARS-CoV-2, B. ACE2 receptors with attached SARS-CoV-2 and early cell internalization, C. High level viral replication with large amount of surface virus apparent. Source: R. Sherertz.

remained PCR-positive at the 8-week mark, but persistent viral replication (based on subgenomic mRNAs) only occurred in the GI tract (18.7%), not in the respiratory tract (0%).[86] Figure 4.57 shows the concept of how different tissues might allow differential SARS-CoV-2 replication. Further research is needed to confirm the possibility of chronic infection, utilizing systematic sampling of different tissues in both symptomatic and asymptomatic patients over a prolonged period of time (greater than one year), such that the mechanism of SARS-CoV-2 persistence can be better understood.

The importance of the human immune system and the possible persistent SARS-CoV-2 human viral infection is probably best suggested by four case reports of persistent viral replication in immunocompromised hosts.[224–227] In a septuagenarian male with immunodeficiency secondary to B cell lymphoma and further compromise of his immune system after vincristine, prednisolone, cyclophosphamide, and anti-CD20B cell depletion therapies, it was shown that there was persistent SARS-CoV-2 viral replication for greater than 100 days and that remdesivir had very little effect on viral evolution, but the administration of convalescent plasma caused a rapid change in the viral genome such that it encoded for a new spike protein.[224] The study further suggested that there were likely spatially distinct viral populations (different variants in different parts of the respiratory tract) and emphasized that these findings may not all represent in-host evolution.[224] In a 45-year-old male with severe antiphospholipid syndrome and immunocompromised status secondary to receiving intermittent treatment with glucocorticoids, cyclophosphamide, rituximab, and eculizumab, it was documented that he had three distinct recurrences over a 5-month period with phylogenetic analysis consistent with persistent infection and accelerated viral evolution.[225] A 71-year-old female, immunocompromised due to chronic lymphocytic leukemia and acquired hypogammaglobulinemia (inability to make normal levels of IgG antibodies), was found to test positive for SARS-CoV-2 by PCR when she was evaluated as part of a rehabilitation facility COVID-19 outbreak.[226] She was tested 14 times by respiratory tract specimen PCR and found to have detectable RNA for 105 days that did not clear until after she had had two infusions of convalescent plasma from recovered COVID-19 donors. Analysis of the 14 isolates found marked within-host genomic evolution of SARS-CoV-2, and all of the different variants were replication competent (able to infect). Finally, a patient with uncontrolled HIV infection developed multiple mutations in the spike protein until his HIV infection was brought under control by three new medications.[227] Collectively, these four case reports strongly suggest the immune system plays an important role in both persistent infection and ongoing viral mutation (evolution).

Given that mutation is important for SARS-CoV-2 to survive, a very important question is how fast does SARS-CoV-2 evolve as a result of its circulation through the human population? For example, the Ebola virus genome (negative sense, single-stranded RNA virus) accumulates mutations at a rate of approximately 10^{-5} (1/100,000) base pair substitutions/site/year, 100,000 times greater than a mouse that has approximately 10^{-10} (1/10,000,000,000) base pair substitutions/site/year.[228] With that frame of reference it is worth comparing SARS-CoV-2 (positive sense, single-stranded RNA virus) with two other important RNA viruses, influenza A (negative sense, single-stranded RNA virus) and HIV (single-stranded RNA retrovirus). The genome size of SARS-CoV-2 is larger in size than Ebola (~30,000 nucleotides versus 19,000 nucleotides) or influenza A — approximately 14,000 nucleotides, and

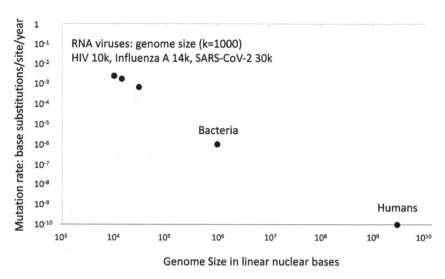

Figure 4.58.   Relationship between mutation rate and species genome size. SARS-CoV-2 vs influenza A vs. HIV vs. bacteria vs. humans.

HIV — approximately 10,000 nucleotides. Estimated mutation rates for these three different RNA viruses are 0.7×10^{-3} base substitutions/site/year for coronavirus, 1.8×10^{-3} for influenza A and 2.5×10^{-3} for HIV, all nearly 100 times faster than Ebola's rate.[229,230] These mutation rates are 1,000 times greater than those seen with most bacteria and 10,000,000 times greater than mutation rates seen with the human genome (Figure 4.58).

Pertinent to SARS-CoV-2 vaccination efforts, which virtually all target the spike protein, the SARS-CoV-2 rate of accumulation of mutations in the spike protein portion of the genome is 1.69×10^{-3}.[230] The rapid rate of the evolution of influenza A viruses results in the need for a new vaccine every year. The rapid occurrence of mutations in HIV necessitates using 3 drugs to suppress the infection, as using only 1 or even 2 drugs can lead to the rapid development of resistance. All of these findings strongly suggest that SARS-CoV-2 vaccines will not have long-lasting protection and may need to be altered and given again, possibly yearly, like influenza. Similarly, antiviral therapy against SARS-CoV-2 may require mulitiple drugs to prevent resistance from developing. And finally, we should expect that the mutations could further change the clinical manifestations seen in patients, as discussed in the above section on new strains.

Key Points: Pathogenesis

1. SARS-CoV-2 attaches to the ACE2 protein on the surface of respiratory tract epithelial cells and other tissues in the body. Some studies suggest there are more ACE2 receptors on tissue surfaces for patients with inflammatory diseases (diabetes, obesity, COPD, etc.), and this may be the explanation for the more severe COVID-19 infections in these patients.

2. The inflammation in the lungs of patients with COVID-19 is primarily lymphocytic, which may be the reason steroids are so beneficial, as they inhibit lymphocytes.

3. COVID-19 causes thrombosis of pulmonary capillaries, which may be the reason why anticoagulation may reduce mortality.

4. COVID-19 causes heart inflammation, but the long-term significance of this is unknown.

5. SARS-CoV-2 mutates nearly as fast as influenza A and HIV, and this may be a problem for long-term vaccine efficacy or the effectiveness of specific antivirals.

References

1. Oran DP, Topol EJ. (2020) Getting a handle on asymptomatic SARS-CoV-2 infection. Scripps Research. https://www.scripps.edu/science-and-medicine/translational-institute/about/news/sarc-cov-2-infection/

2. Mizumoto K, Kagaya K, Zarebski A, Chowell G. (2020) Estimating the asymptomatic proportion of coronavirus 2019 (COVID-19) cases on board the Diamond Princess cruise ship, Yokohama, Japan. *Eurosurveillance* **25**:2000180.

3. Wiersinga WJ, Rhodes A, Cheng AC, *et al.* (2020) Pathophysiology, transmission, diagnosis, and treatment of Coronavirus disease 2010 (COVID-19). *JAMA* **324**(8):782–793. DOI:10.1001/jama.2020.12839

4. Guan W-J, Ni Z-Y, Hu Y, *et al.* (2020) Clinical characteristics of Coronavirus disease 2019 in China. *New England Journal of Medicine* **382**:1708–1720.

5. Suleyman G, Fadel RA, Malette KM, *et al.* (2020) Clinical characteristics and morbidity associated with Coronavirus disease 2019 in a series of patients in metropolitan Detroit. *JAMA* **3**:e2012270. DOI:10.1001/jamanetworkopen.2020.12270

6. Yang BY, Barnard LM, Emert JM, *et al.* (2020) Clinical characteristics of patients with Coronavirus disease 2019 (COVID-19) receiving emergency medical services in King County, Washington. *JAMA* **3**:e2014549. DOI:10.1001/jamanetworkopen.2020.14549

7. Yang W, Cao Q, Qin L, *et al.* (2020) Clinical characteristics and imaging manifestations of the 2019 novel coronavirus disease (COVID-19): A multicenter study in Wenzhou city, Zheijiang, China. *Journal of Infection* **80**:388–393.

8. Goyal P, Choi JJ, Pinheiro LC, *et al.* (2020) Clinical characteristics of COVID-19 in New York City. *New England Journal of Medicine* **382**:2372–2374.

9. Lechien JR, Chiesa-Estomba CM, Hans S, *et al.* (2020) Loss of smell and taste in 2013 European patients with mild to moderate COVID-19. *Annals of Internal Medicine* **173**(8):672–675. https://doi.org/10.7326/M20-2428

10. Lee S, Kim T, Lee E, *et al.* (2020) Clinical course and molecular viral shedding among asymptomatic and symptomatic patients with SARS-CoV-2 infection in a community treatment center in the Republic of Korea. *JAMA Internal Medicine* **180**(11):1447–1452. DOI:10.1001/jamainternmed.2020.3862

11. Bischoff WE, Swett K, Leng I, Peters TR. (2013) Exposure to Influenza virus aerosols during routine patient care. *Journal of Infectious Diseases* **207**:1037–1046.

12. De Jong MD, Simmons CP, Thanh TT, *et al.* (2006) Fatal outcome of human Influenza A (H5N1) is associated with high viral load and hyper cytokinemia. *Nature Medicine* **12**:1203–1207.

13. Ip DKM, Lau LLH, Leung NHL, *et al.* (2017) Viral shedding and transmission potential of asymptomatic and paucisymptomatic Influenza virus infections in the community. *Clinical Infectious Diseases* **64**:736–742.

14. Liu Y, Yan L-M, Wan L, *et al.* (2020) Viral dynamics in mild and severe cases of COVID-19. *Lancet* **20**(6):656–657. https://doi.org/10.1016/S1473-3099(20)30232-2

15. Zhou F, Yu T, Du R, *et al.* (2020) Clinical course and risk factors for mortality of adult inpatients with COVID-19 in Wuhan, China: A retrospective cohort study. *Lancet* **395**:1054–1062.

16. Nguyen LH, Drew DA, Graham MS, *et al.* (2020) Risk of COVID-19 among front-line health-care workers and the general community: A prospective cohort study. *Lancet* **5**(9)E475–E483. https://doi.org/10.1016/S2468-2667(20)30164-X

17. Shields A, Faustini SE, Perez-Toledo M, *et al.* (2020) SARS-Cov-2 seroprevalence and asymptomatic viral carriage in healthcare workers: A cross-sectional study. *BMJ Thorax* **75**(12):1089–1094. DOI:10.1136/thoraxjnl-2020-215414

18. Chou R, Dana T, Buckley DI, Selph S. (2020) Epidemiology of and risk factors for Coronavirus infection in health care workers. *Annals of Internal Medicine* **173**(2):120–136. https://doi.org/10.7326/M20-1632

19. Morawska L, Milton DK. (2020) It is time to address airborne transmission of COVID-19. *Clinical Infectious Diseases* **71**(9):2311–2313. DOI:10.1093/cid/ciaa939

20. Zhang R, Li Y, Zhang AL, Wang Y, Molina MJ. (2020) Identifying airborne transmission as the dominant route for the spread of COVID-19. *Proceedings of the National Academy of Sciences* **117**:14857–14863.

21. Tellier R, Li Y, Cowling BJ, Tang JW. (2019) Recognition of aerosol transmission of infectious agents. *BMC Infectious Diseases* **19**:101–109.

22. Nikitin N, Petrova E, Trifonova E, Karpova O. (2014) Influena virus aerosols in the air and their infectiousness. *Advances in Virology*. http://dx.doi.org/10.1155/2014/859090

23. Yassi A, Bryce E, Moore D. (2004) Protecting the faces of health care workers: Knowledge gaps and research priorities for effective protection against occupationally-acquired respiratory infectious diseases. Occupational Health and Safety Agency for Healthcare in BC. https://www.paho.org/hq/dmdocuments/2009/Protecting%20the%20faces%20of%20health%20care%20workers.pdf

24. Fennelly KP. (2020) Particle sizes of infectious aerosols: Implications for infection control. *Lancet* 8(9):914–924. https://doi.org/10.1016/S2213-2600(20)30323-4

25. Rengasmy S, Miller A, Eimer BC, Shaffer RE. (2009) Filtration performance of FDA-cleared surgical masks. *Journal — International Society for Respiratory Pro* **26**:54–70.

26. Bischoff WE, Reid T, Russell GB, Peters TR. (2011) Transocular entry of seasonal Influenza-attenuated virus aerosols and the efficacy of N95 respirators, surgical masks, and eye protection. *Journal of Infectious Diseases* **204**: 193–199.

27. Chu DK, Akl EA, Duda S, *et al.* (2020) Physical distancing, face masks, and eye protection to prevent person-to-person transmission of SARS-CoV-2 and COVID-19: A systematic review and meta-analysis. *Lancet* **395**:1973–1987.

28. Fischer EP, Fischer MC, Grass D, *et al.* (2020) Low-cost measurement of face mask efficacy for filtering expelled droplets during speech. *Science Advances* **6**(36):eabd3083. DOI:10.1126/sciadv.abd3083

29. Zhao M, Liao L, Xiao W, *et al.* (2020) Household materials selection for homemade cloth face coverings and their filtration efficiency enhancement with triboelectric charging. *Nano Letters* **20**(7):5544–5552. DOI:10.1021/acs.nanolett.0c02211

30. Dharmadhikari AS, Mphahlele M, Stoltz A, *et al.* (2012) Surgical face masks worn by patients with multidrug-resistant tuberculosis. Impact on infectivity of air on a hospital ward. *American Journal of Respiratory and Critical Care Medicine* **185**:1104–1109.

31. Jefferson T, Del Mar C, Dooley L, *et al.* (2009) Physical interventions to interrupt or reduce the spread of respiratory viruses: Systematic review. *BMJ* **339**. https://doi.org/10.1136/bmj.b3675

32. Larson EL, Liverman CT. (2011) *Preventing Transmission of Pandemic Influenza and Other Viral Respiratory Diseases: Personal Protective Equipment for Healthcare Workers: Update 2010*. National Academy of Sciences. http://www.nap.edu/catalog.php?record_id=13027

33. Van Doremalen N, Bushmaker T, Morris DH, *et al.* (2020) Aerosol and surface stability of SARS-CoV-2 as compared with SARS-CoV-1. *New England Journal of Medicine*. DOI:10.1056/NEJMc2004973.

34. Chin AWH, Chu JTS, Perera MRA, *et al.* (2020) Stability of SARS-CoV-2 in different environmental conditions. *Lancet Microbe*. DOI:10.1016/S2666-5247(20)30003-3

35. CDC. (2019) CDC COVID-19. Clean & disinfect. Centers for Disease Control and Prevention. https://www.cdc.gov/coronavirus/2019-ncov/community/organizations/cleaning-disinfection.html

36. CDC. (2019) CDC COVID-19. Hand hygiene recommendations. Centers for Disease Control and Prevention. https://www.cdc.gov/coronavirus/2019-ncov/global-covid-19/hand-hygiene.html

37. Pan F, Zheng C, Ye T, *et al.* (2020) Different computed tomography patterns of coronavirus disease 2019 (COVID-19) between survivors and non-survivors. *Scientific Reports* **10**:11336.

38. Zhang J, Meng G, Li W, *et al.* (2020) Relationship of chest CT score with clinical characteristics of 108 patients hospitalized with COVID-19 in Wuhan, China. *Respiratory Research* **20**:180–190.

39. Alonzo-Fernandez A, Toledo-Pons N, Cosio BG, *et al.* (2020) Prevalence of pulmonary embolism in patients with COVID-19 pneumonia and high D-dimer values: A prospective study. *PLOS One* **15**:e0238216.

40. Roncon L, Zuin M, Barco S, *et al.* (2020) Incidence of acute pulmonary embolism in COVID-19 patients: Systematic review and meta-analysis. *European Journal of Internal Medicine* **82**:29–37. https//doi.org/10.1016/j.ejim.2020.09.006

41. Wikipedia. (nd) COVID-19 testing. https://en.wikipedia.org/wiki/COVID-19_testing

42. Hagen A. (2020) COVID-19 Testing FAQs. American Society for Microbiology, August 19. https://asm.org/Articles/2020/April/COVID-19-Testing-FAQs

43. Wright L. (2021) The plague year. *The New Yorker*, January 4 and 11. https://www.newyorker.com/magazine/2021/01/04/the-plague-year

44. FDA (nd) FDA Emergency Use Authorizations: COVID-19 in vitro diagnostic products. Food and Drug Administration. https://www.fda.gov/emergency-preparedness-and-response/mcm-legal-regulatory-and-policy-framework/emergency-use-authorization

45. FDA (nd) COVID-19 FDA EUA authorized serology test performance. Food and Drug Administration. https://www.fda.gov/medical-devices/coronavirus-disease-2019-covid-19-emergency-use-authorizations-medical-devices/eua-authorized-serology-test-performance. Updated: August 1, 2021.

46. Yang Y, Yang M, Shen C, *et al.* (2020) Evaluating the accuracy of different respiratory specimens in the laboratory diagnosis and monitoring the viral shedding of 2019-nCoV infections. *medRxiv.* https://doi.org/10.1101/2020.02.11.20021493

47. Wang W, Xu Y, Gao R, *et al.* (2020) Detection of SARS-CoV-2 in different types of clinical specimens. *JAMA* **323**:1843–1844.

48. CDC. (2020) Interim guidance for rapid antigen testing for SARS-CoV-2. Centers for Disease Control and Prevention, August 16. https://www.cdc.gov/coronavirus/2019-ncov/lab/resources/antigen-tests-guidelines.html

49. FDA. (2020) EUA authorized serology test performance. Food and Drug Administration, August 26. https://www.fda.gov/medical-devices/coronavirus-disease-2019-covid-19-emergency-use-authorizations-medical-devices/eua-authorized-serology-test-performance

50. Woolf SH, Chapman DA, Lee JH. (2021) COVID-19 as the leading cause of death in the United States. *JAMA* **325**(2):123–124. doi:10.1001/jama.2020.24865

51. Levin AT, Hanage WP, Owusu-Boaitey N, *et al.* (2020) Assessing the age specificity of infection fatality rates for COVID-19: Systematic review, meta-analysis, and public policy implications. *European Journal of Epidemiology* **35**:1123–1138. https://doi.org/10.1007/s10654-020-00698-1

52. Degarege A, Naveed Z, Kabayundo J, Brett-Major D. (2020) Risk factors for severe illness and death in COVID-19: A systematic review and meta-analysis. *medRxIV.* https://doi.org/10.1101/2020.12.03.20243659

53. Goodman KE, Magder LS, Baghdadi JD, *et al.* (2021) Impact of sex and metabolic comorbidities on COVID-19 mortality risk across age groups: 66,646 inpatients across 613 US hospitals. *Clinical Infectious Diseases* **73**(11):e4113–e4123. DOI:10.1093/cid/ciaa1787

54. Huang Y, Lu Y, Huang YM, *et al.* (2020) Obesity in patients with COVID-19: A systematic review and meta-analysis. *Metabolism* **113**:154378. DOI:10.1016/j.metabol.2020.154378

55. Szea S, Pan D, Clareece R, *et al.* (2020) Ethnicity and clinical outcomes in COVID-19: A systematic review and meta-analysis. *EClinicalMedicine* **29**:100630. https://doi.org/10.1016/j.eclinm.2020.100630

56. Seligman B, Ferranna M, Bloom DE. (2021) Social determinants of mortality from COVID-19: A simulation study using NHANES. *PLOS Medicine* **18**(1):e1003490. https://doi.org/10.1371/journal.pmed.1003490

57. Arrazola J, Masiello MM, Joshi S, *et al.* (2020) COVID-19 mortality among American Indian and Alaska Native Persons — 14 states, January–June 2020. *Morbidity and Mortality Weekly Report* **69**:1853–1856. http://dx.doi.org/10.15585/mmwr.mm6949a3external icon

58. CDC (2020) COVID-19 hospitalization and death by race/ethnicity. Centers for Disease Control and Prevention, August 18. https://www.cdc.gov/coronavirus/2019-ncov/covid-data/investigations-discovery/hospitalization-death-by-race-ethnicity.html

59. The Severe Covid-19 GWAS Group. (2020) Genomewide association study of severe Covid-19 with respiratory failure. October 15. *New England Journal of Medicine* **383**:1522–1534. DOI:10.1056/NEJMoa2020283

60. Pairo-Castineira E, Clohisey S, Klaric L, *et al.* (2020) Genetic mechanisms of critical illness in Covid-19. *Nature* **591**(7848):92–98. https://doi.org/10.1038/s41586-020-03065-y

61. Ni W, Yang X, Liu J, *et al.* (2020) Acute myocardial injury at hospital admission is associated with all-cause mortality in COVID-19. *Journal of the American College of Cardiology* **76**:124–125.

62. Solomon MD, McNulty EJ, Rana JS, *et al.* (2020) The COVID-19 pandemic and the incidence of acute myocardial infarction. *New England Journal of Medicine* **383**:7–9.

63. Gluckman TJ, Wilson MA, Chiu S-T, *et al.* (2020) Case rates, treatment approaches, and outcomes in acute myocardial infarction during the Coronavirus disease 2019 pandemic. *JAMA Cardiology* DOI:10.1001/jamacardio.2020.3629

64. Yaghi S, Ishida K, Torres J, *et al.* (2020) SARS-CoV-2 and stroke in a New York healthcare system. *Stroke* **51**:2002–2011.

65. Zhang L, Feng X, Zhang D, *et al.* (2020) Deep venous thrombosis in hospitalized patients with COVID-19 in Wuhan, China. *Circulation* **142**:114–128.

66. Cho ES, McClelland PH, Cheng O, *et al.* (2020) Utility of d-dimer for diagnosis of deep venous thrombosis in coronavirus disease-19 infection. *Journal of Vascular Surgery: Venous and Lymphatic Disorders* **9**(1):47–53. https://doi.org/10.1016/j.jvsv.2020.07.009

67. Nahum J, Morichau-Beauchant T, Daviaud F, et al. (2020) Venous thrombosis among critically ill patients with Coronavirus Disease 2019 (COVID-19). *JAMA Network Open* **3**:e2010478. DOI:10.1001/jamanetworkopen.2020.10478

68. Jevnikar M, Sanchez O, Andronikov, et al. (2020) Prevalence of pulmonary embolism in patients at the time of hospital admission for COVID-19. *Research and Practice in Thrombosis and Haemostasis* **4**(Suppl 1).

69. Poissy J, Goutay J, Caplan M, et al. (2020) Pulmonary embolism in patients with COVID-19. *Circulation* **142**:184–186.

70. Bompard F, Monnier H, Saab I, et al. (2020) Pulmonary embolism in patients with COVID-19 pneumonia. *European Respiratory Journal.* **56**:2001365. DOI:10.1183/13993003.01365-2020

71. Poyiadji N, Cormier P, Patel PY, et al. (2020) Acute pulmonary embolism and COVID-19. *Radiology* **297**(3):E335–E338. https://doi.org/10.1148/radiol.2020201955

72. Hirsch JS, Ng JH, Ross DW, et al. (2020) Acute kidney injury in patients hospitalized with COVID-19. *Kidney International* **98**:209–218.

73. Wu J, Song S, Cao H-C, Li L-J. (2020) Liver diseases in COVID-19: Etiology, treatment and prognosis. *World Journal of Gastroenterology* **26**:2286–2293.

74. Al-Samkari H, Leaf RSK, Dzik WH, et al. (2020) COVID-19 and coagulation: Bleeding and thrombotic manifestations of SARS-CoV-2 infection. *Blood* **136**:489–500.

75. Langford BJ, So M, Raybardhan S, et al. (2020) Bacterial co-infection and secondary infection in patients with COVID-19: A living rapid review and meta-analysis. *Clinical Microbiology and Infection* **26**(12)1622–1629. https://doi.org/10.1016/j.cmi.2020.07.016

76. Mafham MM, Spata E, Goldacre R, et al. (2020) COVID-19 pandemic and admission rates for and management of acute coronary syndromes in England. *Lancet* **396**:381–389.

77. Diegoli H, Magalhaes PSC, Martins SCO, et al. (2020) Decrease in hospital admissions for transient ischemic attack, mild, and moderate stroke during the COVID-19 era. *Stroke* **51**:2315–2321.

78. Lai PH, Lancet EA, Weiden MD, et al. (2020) Characteristics associated with out-of-hospital cardiac arrests and resuscitations during the novel Coronavirus 2019 Pandemic in New York City. *JAMA Cardiology.* DOI:10.1001/jamacardio.2020.2488

79. Baldi E, Sechi GM, Primi R, et al. (2020) Out-of-hospital cardiac arrest during the COVID-19 outbreak in Italy. *New England Journal of Medicine* **383**:496–498.

80. Hall V, Foulkes S, Charlett A, *et al.* (2021) Do antibody positive health-care workers have lower SARS-CoV-2 infection rates than antibody negative healthcare workers?' Large multi-centre prospective cohort study (the SIREN study), England: June to November 2020. *MedRxiv.* Doi. org/10.1101/2021.01.13.21249642

81. To KKW, Hung IF-N, Ip JD, *et al.* (2020) COVID-19 re-infection by a phylogenetically distinct SARS-coronavirus-2 strain confirmed by whole genome sequencing. *Clinical Infectious Diseases.* **73**(9):e2946–e2951. https://doi. org/10.1093/cid/ciaa1275

82. Prado-Vivar B, Becerra-Wong M, Guadalupe JJ, *et al.* (2020) COVID-19 re-infection by a phylogenetically distinct SARS-CoV-2 variant, first confirmed event in South America. SSRN. https://papers.ssrn.com/sol3/papers.cfm?abstract_id=3686174

83. Tillett R, Sevinsky J, Hartley P, *et al.* (2020) Genomic evidence for a case of reinfection with SARS-CoV-2. SSRN. https://doi.org/10.2139/ssrn.3680955 (2020).

84. Gupta V, Bhoyar RC, Jain A, *et al.* (2020) Asymptomatic reinfection in two healthcare workers from India with genetically distinct SARS-CoV-2. *Clinical Infectious Diseases* **73**(9):e2823–e2825. DOI:10.1093/cid/ciaa1451

85. Sabino EC, Buss LF, Carvalho MPS, *et al.* (2021) Resurgence of COVID-19 in Manaus, Brazil, despite high seroprevalence. *Lancet* **397**:452–455. Doi. org/10.1016/S0140-6736(21)00183-5

86. Hu F, Chen F, Ou Z, *et al.* (2020) A compromised specific humoral immune response against the SARS-CoV-2 receptor-binding domain is related to viral persistence and periodic shedding in the gastrointestinal tract. *Cellular & Molecular Immunology* **17**:1119–1125. https://doi.org/10.1038/s41423-020-00550-2

87. NIH. (nd) COVID-19 treatment guidelines. Corticosteroids. National Institutes of Health. Updated: August 27, 2020. https://www.covid19treatmentguide-lines.nih.gov/immune-based-therapy/immunomodulators/corticosteroids/

88. The WHO Rapid Evidence Appraisal for COVID-19 Therapies (REACT) Working Group. (2020) Association between administration of systemic corticosteroids and mortality among critically ill patients with COVID-19. A meta-analysis. *JAMA* **324**(13):1330–1341. https://jamanetwork.com/journals/jama/fullarticle/2770279

89. RECOVERY Collaborative Group; Horby P, Lim WS, Emberson, *et al.* (2021) Dexamethasone in hospitalized patients with COVID-19 — Preliminary report. *New England Journal of Medicine* **384**:693–704. DOI:10.1056/NEJMoa2021436

90. WHO Rapid Evidence Appraisal for COVID-19 Therapies (REACT) Working Group. (2020) Association between administration of systemic corticosteroids and mortality among critically ill patients with COVID-19. A meta-analysis. *JAMA* **324**(13):1330–1341. DOI:10.1001/jama.2020.17023

91. Ranjbar K, Moghadami M, Mirahmadizadeh A, *et al.* (2021) Methylprednisolone or dexamethasone, which one is superior corticosteroid in the treatment of hospitalized COVID-19 patients: A triple-blinded randomized controlled trial. *BMC Infectious Diseases* **21**:337. https://doi.org/10.1186/s12879-021-06045-3

92. NIH. (nd) Coronavirus disease 2019 (COVID-19) treatment guidelines. National Institutes of Health. https://www.covid19treatmentguidelines.nih.gov/. Updated: May 3, 2021.

93. IDSA. (nd) Guidelines on the treatment and management of patients with COVID-19. Infectious Diseases Society of America. https://www.idsociety.org/practice-guideline/covid-19-guideline-treatment-and-management/. Updated: May 3, 2021.

94. Thorland K, Dron L, Park J, *et al.* (nd) Global coronavirus COVID-19 clinical trial tracker. https://www.covid-trials.org/

95. NIH. (nd) Potential antiviral drugs under evaluation for the treatment of COVID-19. Remdesivir. National Institutes of Health. https://www.covid19treatmentguidelines.nih.gov/antiviral-therapy/. Updated: August 27, 2020.

96. NIH. (nd) COVID Treatment guidelines. Anti-SARS-CoV-2 monoclonal antibodies. National Institutes of Health. https://www.covid19treatmentguidelines.nih.gov/anti-sars-cov-2-antibody-products/anti-sars-cov-2-monoclonal-antibodies/

96A. Trump and friends got coronavirus care many others couldn't. New York Times December 23, 2020. nytimes.com/2020/12/09/us/politics/trump-coronavirus-treatments.html.

97. Gordon AC, Mouncey PR, REMAP-CAP Investigators, *et al.* (2021) Interleukin-6 receptor antagonists in critically ill patients with covid-19. *New England Journal of Medicine* **384**(16):1491–1502. DOI:10.1056/NEJMoa2100433

98. Paranjpe I, Fuster V, Lala A, *et al.* (2020) Association of treatment dose anticoagulation with in-hospital survival among hospitalized patients with COVID-19. *Journal of the American College of Cardiology* **76**(1):122–124. https://doi.org/10.1016/j.jacc.2020.05.001

99. Tritschler T, Mathieu M-E, Skeith L, *et al.* (2020) Anticoagulant interventions in hospitalized patients with COVID-19: A scoping review of randomized controlled trials and call for international collaboration. *Journal of*

Thrombosis and Haemostasis **18**(11):2958–2967. https://doi.org/10.1111/jth.15094

100.   Lemos ACB, do Espírito Santo DA, Salvetti MC, *et al.* (2020) Therapeutic versus prophylactic anticoagulation for severe COVID-19: A randomized phase II clinical trial (HESACOVID). *Thrombosis Research* **196**:359–366. DOI:10.1016/j.thromres.2020.09.026

101.   NIH. (2020) NIH ACTIV trial of blood thinners pauses enrollment or critically ill COVID-19 patients. News Release, National Institutes of Health, December 22. https://www.nih.gov/news-events/news-releases/nih-activ-trial-blood-thinners-pauses-enrollment-critically-ill-covid-19-patients

102.   Patell R, Bogue T, Koshy A, *et al.* (2020) Postdischarge thrombosis and hemorrhage in patients with COVID-19. *Blood* **136**:1342–1346.

103.   Roberts LN, Whyte MB, Georgiou L, *et al.* (2020) Postdischarge venous thromboembolism following hospital admission for COVID-19. *Blood* **136**:1347–1350.

104.   NIH. (nd) Blood-derived products under evaluation for the treatment of COVID-19. National Institutes of Health. https://www.covid19treatment-guidelines.nih.gov/immune-based-therapy/blood-derived-products/

105.   Gharbharan A, Jordans CCE, Geurtsvankessel C, *et al.* (2020) Convalescent plasma for COVID-19. A randomized clinical trial. July 3. https://doi.org/10.1101/2020.07.01.20139857

106.   Libster R, Marc GP, Wappner D, *et al.* (2021) Early high-titer plasma therapy to prevent severe COVID-19 in older adults. *New England Journal of Medicine* **384**:610–618. DOI:10.1056/NEJMoa2033700

107.   Joyner MJ, Carter RE, Senefeld JW, *et al.* (2021) Convalescent plasma antibody levels and risk of death from COVID-19. *New England Journal of Medicine* **384**:1015–1027. DOI:10.1056/NEJMoa2031893

108.   Coutinho AE, Chapman KE. (2011) The anti-inflammatory and immunosuppressive effects of glucocorticoids, recent developments and mechanistic insights. *Molecular and Cellular Endocrinology* **335**(1):2–13. DOI:10.1016/j.mce.2010.04.005

109.   Rafiullah M, Siddiqui K. (2020) Corticosteroid use in viral pneumonia experience so far and the dexamethasone breakthrough in coronavirus disease-2019. *Future Medicine*, November 27. https://doi.org/10.2217/cer-2020-0146

110.   Ni, YN, Chen, G, Sun, J, *et al.* (2019) The effect of corticosteroids on mortality of patients with influenza pneumonia: A systematic review and meta-analysis. *Critlcal Care* **23**:99. https://doi.org/10.1186/s13054-019-2395-8

111.   Zhou Y, Fu X, Liu X, *et al.* (2020) Use of corticosteroids in influenza-associated acute respiratory distress syndrome and severe pneumonia: A

systemic review and meta-analysis. *Scientific Reports* **10**:3044. https://doi.org/10.1038/s41598-020-59732-7

112. Tsai MJ, Yang KY, Chan MC, *et al.* (2020) Impact of corticosteroid treatment on clinical outcomes of influenza-associated ARDS: a nationwide multicenter study. *Annals of Intensive Care* **10**:26. https://doi.org/10.1186/s13613-020-0642-4

113. NIH. (nd) COVID-19 Treatment guidelines. Corticosteroids. National Institutes of Health. https://www.covid19treatmentguidelines.nih.gov/immune-based-therapy/immunomodulators/corticosteroids/. Updated: August 27, 2020.

114. The WHO Rapid Evidence Appraisal for COVID-19 Therapies (REACT) Working Group. (2020) Association between administration of systemic corticosteroids and mortality among critically ill patients with COVID-19. A meta-analysis. *JAMA* **324**(13):1330–1341. October 6. https://doi.org/10.1001/jama.2020.17023

115. RECOVERY Collaborative Group; Horby P, Lim WS, Emberson, *et al.* (2021) Dexamethasone in hospitalized patients with COVID-19 — Preliminary report. *New England Journal of Medicine* **384**(8):693–704. DOI:10.1056/NEJMoa2021436

116. WHO Rapid Evidence Appraisal for COVID-19 Therapies (REACT) Working Group. (2020) Association between administration of systemic corticosteroids and mortality among critically ill patients with COVID-19. A meta-analysis. *JAMA* **324**(13):1330–1341. DOI:10.1001/jama.2020.17023

117. Gordon AC, Mouncey PR; REMAP-CAP Investigators, *et al.* (2021) Interleukin-6 receptor antagonists in critically ill patients with covid-19. *New England Journal of Medicine* **384**(16):1491–1502. DOI:10.1056/NEJMoa2100433.

118. Beigel JH, Tomashek KM, Dodd LE, *et al.* (2020) Remdesivir for the treatment of COVID-19 — final report. *New England Journal of Medicine* **383**:1813–1826. DOI:10.1056/NEJMoa2007764

119. Tritschler T, Mathieu M-E, Skeith L, *et al.* (2020) Anticoagulant interventions in hospitalized patients with COVID-19: A scoping review of randomized controlled trials and call for international collaboration. *Thrombosis Haemostasis*, September 5. https://doi.org/10.1111/jth.15094

120. Coleman J. (2021) Biden administration investing billions in antiviral pills for COVID-19. *The Hill*, June 17. https://thehill.com/policy/healthcare/558942-government-spending-billions-for-antiviral-pills-for-covid-19

120A. Niburski K, Niburski O. Impact of Trump's promotion of unproven COVID-19 treatments and subsequent internet trends: observational study. *J Med Internet Res* 2020 Nov 20; **22**(11):e20044. doi:102196/20044

121. Oke J, Howdon D, Heneghan C. (2020) Declining COVID-19 case fatality rates across all ages: Analysis of German data. The Centre for Evidence-Based Medicine, Oxford University, September 9. https://www.cebm.net/covid-19/declining-covid-19-case-fatality-rates-across-all-ages-analysis-of-german-data/

122. Asch DA, Sheils NE, Islam MN, et al. (2021) Variation in US hospital mortality rates for patients admitted with COVID-19 during the first 6 months of the pandemic. JAMA Internal Medicine 181(4):471–478. DOI:10.1001/jamainternmed.2020.8193

123. Robert R, Kentish-Barnes N, Boyer A, et al. (2020) Ethical dilemmas due to the COVID-19 pandemic. Annals of Intensive Care 10:84. https://doi.org/10.1186/s13613-020-00702-7

124. American Academy of Pediatrics. (2020) Children and COVID-19: State-level data reporting. October 29. https://services.aap.org/en/pages/2019-novel-coronavirus-covid-19-infections/children-and-covid-19-state-level-data-report/

125. CDC. (nd) CDC data tracker. COVID-19 hospitalization and death by age. Centers for Disease Control and Prevention. https://www.cdc.gov/coronavirus/2019-ncov/covid-data/investigations-discovery/hospitalization-death-by-age.html

125A. Chung E, Chow EJ, Wilcox NC, et al. (2021) Comparison of symptoms and RNA levels in children and adults with SARS-CoV-2 infection in the community setting. JAMA Pediatr 175(10):e212025. doi:10.1001/jamapediatrics.2021.2025

126. Bixler D, Miller A, Mattison CP. (2020) SARS-Cov-2-associated deaths among person aged <21 years — United States, February 12– July 31, 2020. Morbidity and Mortality Weekly Report 69(37):1324–1329. https://www.cdc.gov/mmwr/volumes/69/wr/mm6937e4.htm

127. Woodruff RC, Campbell AP, Taylor CA, et al. (2021) Risk factors for severe COVID-19 in children. Pediatrics. https://doi.org/10.1542/peds.2021-053418

128. Morris SB, Schwartz NG, Patel P, et al. (2020) Case series of Multisystem Inflammatory Syndrome in Adults associated with SARS-CoV-2 infection — United Kingdom and United States, October 9, 2020. Morbidity and Mortality Weekly Report 69(40):1450–1456. https://www.cdc.gov/mmwr/volumes/69/wr/mm6940e1.htm.

129. CDC. (nd) Health department-reported cases of Multisystem Inflammatory Syndrome in Children (MIS-C) in the United States. Centers for

Disease Control and Prevention. Centers for Disease Control and Prevention. https://www.cdc.gov/mis-c/cases/index.html. Accessed: January, 2021.

130. Stephens DS, McElrath MJ. (2020) COVID-19 and the path to immunity. *JAMA* **324**:1279–1281.

131. Rowley AH. (2020) Multisystem Inflammatory Syndrome in Children and Kawasaki disease; two different illnesses with overlapping clinical features. *Journal of Pediatrics* **224**:129–132. Doi.org/10.1016/j.jpeds.2020.06.057.

132. Henderson LA, Canna SW, Friedman KG, Gorelik M, Lapidus SK, Bassiri H, Behrens EM, Ferris A, Kernan KF, Schulert GS, Seo P, Son MBF, Tremoulet AH, Yeung RSM, Mudano AS, Turner AS, Karp DR, Mehta JJ. (2021) American College of Rheumatology Clinical Guidance for Multisystem Inflammatory Syndrome in children associated with SARS-CoV-2 and hyperinflammation in pediatric COVID-19: Version 2. *Arthritis & Rheumatology* **73**(4): e13–e29. DOI:10.1002/art.41616

133. Godfred-Cato S, Bryant B, Leung J. (2020) COVID-19-associated Multisystem Inflammatory Syndrome in Children — United States, March–July 2020. *Morbidity and Mortality Weekly Report* **69**(32):1074–1080. https://www.cdc.gov/mmwr/volumes/69/wr/mm6932e2.htm

134. Chen L, Li Q, Zheng D, *et al.* (2020) Clinical characteristics of pregnant with COVID-19 in Wuhan, China. *New England Journal of Medicine* DOI:10.1056/NEJMc2009226

135. Woodworth KR, Olsen EO, Neelam V, *et al.* (2020) Birth and infant outcomes following laboratory-confirmed SARS-CoV-2 infection in pregnancy — SET-NET, 16 jurisdictions, March 29–October 14, 2020. *Morbidity and Mortality Weekly Report* **69**:1635–1640. http://dx.doi.org/10.15585/mmwr.mm6944e2.

136. Villar J, Ariff S, Gunier RB, *et al.* (2021) Maternal and neonatal morbidity and mortality among pregnant women with and without COVID-19 infection: The INTERCOVID multinational cohort study. *JAMA Pediatrics* **175**(8):817–826. DOI:10.1001/jamapediatrics.2021.1050

137. Pineles BL, Goodman KE, Pineles L, *et al.* (2021) In-hospital mortality in a cohort of hospitalized pregnant and nonpregnant patients with COVID-19. *Annals of Internal Medicine* **174**(8):1186–1188. https://doi.org/10.7326/M21-0974

137A. Hoyert DL. (2022) Maternal mortality rates in the United States, 2020. *NCHS Health E-stats.* DOI: https://dx.doi.org/10.15620/cdc:113967

138. Griffiths P, Baraniak I, Reeves M. (2015) The pathogenesis of human cytomegalovirus. *Journal of Pathology* **235**:288–297.

139. Simmons CP, Farrar JJ, Van Vinh Chau N, Wills B. (2012) Dengue. *New England Journal of Medicine* **366**:1423–1432.

140. Katzelnick LC, Gresh L, Halloran ME, *et al.* (2017) Antibody-dependent enhancement of severe dengue disease in humans. *Science* **358**: 929–932.

141. Pang J, Thein T-L, Lye DC, Leo Y-S. (2015) Differential clinical outcome of dengue infection among patients with and without HIV infection: A matched case-control study. *American Journal of Tropical Medicine and Hygiene* **92**:1156–1162.

142. Elias M, Pievani D, Randoux C, *et al.* (2020) COVID-19 infection in kidney transplant recipients: Disease incidence and clinical outcomes. *Journal of the American Society of Nephrology* **31**(10):2413–2423. DOI:10.1681/ASN.2020050639.

143. Akalin E, Azzi Y, Bartash R, *et al.* (2020) COVID-19 and kidney transplantation. *New England Journal of Medicine* **382**(25):2475–2477. DOI:10.1056/NEJMc2011117

144. Paterson RW, Brown RL, Benjamin L, *et al.* (2020) The emerging spectrum of COVID-19 neurology: Clinical, radiological and laboratory findings. *Brain* **143**:3104–3120. DOI:10.1093/brainawaa240

145. Huo L, Xu K-L, Xu K-L, Wang H. (2021) Clinical features of SARS-CoV-2-associated encephalitis and meningitis amid COVID-19 pandemic. *World Journal of Clinical Cases* **9**:1058–1078. DOI:10.12998/wjcc.v9.i5.1058

146. Nasserie T, Hittle M, Goodman SN. (2021) Assessment of the frequency and variety of persistent symptoms among patients with COVID-19: A systematic review. *JAMA Network Open* **4**(5):e2111417. DOI:10.1001/jamanetworkopen.2021.11417

147. Huang C, Huang L, Wang Y, *et al.* (2021) 6-month consequences of COVID-19 in patients discharged from hospital: A cohort study. *Lancet* **397**(10270):220–232. DOI:10.1016/S0140-6736(20)32656-8

148. Logue JK, Franko NM, McCulloch DJ, *et al.* (2021) Sequelae in adults at 6 months after COVID-19 infection. *JAMA* **4**(2):e210830. DOI:10.1001/jamanetworkopen.2021.0830

149. Al-Aly Z, Xie Y, Bowe B. (2021) High-dimensional characterization of post-acute sequalae of COVID-19. *Nature*. https://doi.org/10.1038/s41586-021-03553-9

150. Krammer F, Srivastava K, Paris team, *et al.* (2021) Robust spike protein antibody responses and increased reactogenicity in seropositive individuals after a single dose of SARS-CoV-2 mRNA vaccine. *medRxiv*. https://doi.org/10.1101/2021.01.29.21250653

151. Wiersinga WJ, Rhodes A, Cheng AC, *et al.* (2020) Pathophysiology, transmission, diagnosis, and treatment of coronavirus disease 2019 (COVID-19). A review. *JAMA* **324**(8):782–793 DOI:10.1001/jama.2020.12839

152. Sungnak W, Huang N, Becavin C, Berg M, HCA Lung Biological Network. (2020) Sars-CoV-2 entry genes are most highly expressed in nasal goblet and ciliated cells within the human airway. *ArXiv.* arXiv:2003.06122v1

153. Gheblawi M, Wang K, Viveiros A, *et al.* (2020) Angiotensin-converting enzyme 2: SARS-CoV-2. receptor and regulator of the renin-angiotensin system. Celebrating the 20th anniversary of the discovery of ACE2. *Circulation Research* **126**:1456–1474.

154. Kreutz R, Algharably EAE-H, Azizi M, *et al.* (2020) Hypertension, the renin-angiotensin system, and the risk of lower respiratory tract infections and lung injury: Implications for COVID-19. *Cardiovascular Research* **116**(10):1688–1699. DOI:10.1093/cvr/cvaa097

155. Trypsteen W, Van Cleemput J, Snippenberg Wv, Gerlo S, Vandekerckhove L. (2020) On the whereabouts of SARS-CoV-2 in the human body: A systematic review. *PLOS Pathogens* **16**(10):e1009037. https://doi.org/10.1371/journal.ppat.1009037

156. Imai Y, Kuba K, Rao S, *et al.* (2005) Angiotensin-converting enzyme 2 protects from severe acute lung failure. *Nature* **436**:112–116.

157. Bunyavanich S, Do A, Vicencio A. (2020) Nasal gene expression of angiotensin-converting enzyme 2 in children and adults. *JAMA* **323**:2427–2429.

158. Cai G. (2020) Bulk and single-cell transcriptomics indentify tobacco-use disparity in lung gene expression of ACE21, receptor of 2019-nCov. *medRxiv.* https://doi.org/10.1101/2020.02.05.20020107

159. Baker SA, Kwok S, Berry GJ, Montine TJ. (2020) Angiotensin-converting enzyme 2 (ACE2) expression increases with age in patients requiring mechanical ventilation. *medRxiv.* https://doi.org/10.1101/2020.07.05.20140467

160. Smith JC, Sausville EL, Girish V, *et al.* (2020) Cigarette smoke exposure and inflammatory signaling increase the expression of the SARS-CoV-2 receptor ACE2 in the respiratory tract. *Developmental Cell* **53**:514–529.

161. Rao S, Lau A, So H-C. (2020) Exploring diseases/traits and blood proteins causally related to expression of ACE2, the putative receptor of SARS-CoV-2: A mendelian randomization analysis highlights tentative relevance of diabetes-related traits. *Diabetes Care* **43**(7):1416–1426. https://doi.org/10.2337/dc20-0643

162. Patel VB, Zhong J-C, Grant MB, Oudit GY. (2016) Role of the ACE2/Angiotensin 1–7 axis of the renin-angiotensin system in heart failure. *Circulation Research* **118**:1313–1326.

163. Ni W, Yang X, Yang D, *et al.* (2020) Role of angiotensin-converting enzyme 2 (ACE20) in COVID-19. *Critical Care* (2020) **24**:422. https://doi.org/10.1186/s13054-020-03120-0

164. Kragstrup TW, Singh HS, Grundberg I, *et al.* (2021) Plasma ACE2 predicts outcome of COVID-19 in hospitalized patients. *PLOS One* **16**(6):e0252799. https://doi.org/10.1371/journal.pone.0252799

165. Bezara MEO, Thurman A, Pezzulo AA, *et al.* (2020) Heterogeneous expression of the SARS-Coronavirus-2 receptor ACE2 in the human respiratory tract. *bioRxiv.* https://doi.org/10.1101/2020.04.22.056127

166. Brann DH, Tsukahara T, Weinreb C, *et al.* (2020) Non-neuronal expression of SARS-CoV-2 entry genes in the olfactory system suggests mechanisms underlying COVID-19-associated anosmia. *Science Advances* **6**: eabc5801.

167. Doyle ME, Appleton A, Liu QR, Yao Q, Mazucanti CH, Egan JM. (2021) Human taste cells express ACE2: A portal for SARS-CoV-2 infection. *bioRxiv.* DOI:10.1101/2021.04.21.440680

168. South AM, Tomlinson L, Edmonston D, Hiremath S, Sparks MA. (2020) Controversies of renin-angiotensin system inhibition during the COVID-19 pandemic. *Nature Reviews Nephrology* **16**(6):305–307. https://doi.org/10.1038/s41581-020-0279-4

169. Lopes R, on behalf of the BRACE CORONA Investigators. (2020) Continuing versus suspending ACE inhibitors and ARBs: Impact of adverse outcomes in hospitalized patients with COVID-19 — the BRACE CORONA Trial. European Society of Cardiology Congress, September 1.

170. NIH. (nd) COVID-19 treatment guidelines. Considerations for certain concomitant medications in patients with COVID-19. National Institutes of Health. https://www.covid19treatmentguidelines.nih.gov/therapies/concomitant-medications/. Updated: April 21, 2021.

171. Martines, RB, Ritter, JM; COVID-19 Pathology Working Group, *et al.* (2020) Pathology and pathogenesis of SARS-CoV-2 associated with fatal Coronavirus disease, United States. *Emerging Infectious Diseases* **26**(9):2005–2015. https://doi.org/10.3201/eid2609.202095

172. Ackermann M, Verleden S, Kuehnel M, *et al.* (2020) Pulmonary vascular endothelialitis, thrombosis, and angiogenesis in COVID-19. *New England Journal of Medicine* **383**:120–128. DOI:10.1056/NEJMoa2015432

173. Abramson JS, Lyles DS, Heller KA, Bass DA. (1982) Influenza A virus-induced polymorphonuclear leukocyte dysfunction. *Infection and Immunity* **37**:794–799.

174. Nienhold R, Ciani Y, Koelzer VH, *et al.* (2020) Two distinct immunopatho-logical profiles in autopsy lungs of COVID-19. *Nature Communications* **11**:5086. https://doi.org/10.1038/s41467-020-18854-2

175. Puntmann VO, Carerj ML, Wieters I, *et al.* (2020) Outcomes of cardiovascu-lar magnetic resonance imaging in patients recently recovered from Coro-navirus Disease 2019 (COVID-19). *JAMA Cardiology* **5**(11):1265–1273. DOI:10.1001/jamacardio.2020.3557

176. Rajpal S, Tong MS, Borchers J, *et al.* (2020) Cardiovascular magnetic resonance findings in competitive athletes recovering from COVID-19 infection. *JAMA Cardiology* **6**(1):116–118. DOI:10.1001/jamacardio.2020.4916

177. Martinez MW, Tucker AM, Bloom OJ, *et al.* (2021) Prevalence of inflamma-tory heart disease among professional athletes with prior covid-19 infec-tion who received systematic return-to-play cardiac screening. *JAMA Car-diology* **6**(7):745–752. DOI:10.1001/jamacardio.2021.0565

178. Lindner D, Fitzek A, Brauninger H, *et al.* (2020) Association of cardiac infec-tion with SARS-CoV-2 in confirmed COVID-19 autopsy cases. *JAMA Cardi-ology* **5**(11):1281–1285. DOI:10.1001/jamacardio.2020.3551

179. Perez-Bermejo JA, Kang S, Rockwood SJ, *et al.* (2020) SARS-CoV-2 infection of iPSC-derived cardiac cells predicts novel cytopathic features in hearts of COVID-19 patients. *bioRxiv.* https://doi.org/10.1101/2020.08.25.265561

180. Szekely Y, Lichter Y, Taieb P, *et al.* (2020) Spectrum of cardiac manifesta-tions in COVID-19. A systematic echocardiographic study. *Circulation* **142**(4):342–353. DOI:10.1161/CIRCULATIONAHA.120.047971

181. Dillinger JG, Benmessaoud FA, Pezel T, *et al.* (2020) Coronary artery calcifi-cation and complications in patients with COVID-19. *JACC: Cardiovascular Imaging* **13**(11):2468–2470. https://doi.org/10.1016/j.jcmg.2020.07.004

182. Gaibazzi N, Martini C, Mattioli M, *et al.* (2020) Lung disease severity, cor-onary artery calcium, coronary inflammation and mortality in Coronavirus Disease 2019. *medRxiv.* https://doi.org/10.1101/2020.05.01

183. De'Ath HD, Oakland K, Brohi K. (2916) CT screened arterial calcification as a risk factor for mortality after trauma. *Scandinavian Journal of Trauma, Resuscitation and Emergency Medicine* **24**:120. DOI:10.1186/s13049-016-0317-1

184. Hotchkiss RS, Moldawer LL, Opal SM, *et al.* (2016) Sepsis and septic shock. *Nature Reviews* **2**:1–21.

185. Mangalmurti N, Hunter CA.(2020) Cytokine storms: Understanding COVID-19. *Immunity* **53**(1):19–25. https://doi.org/10.1016/j.immuni.2020.06.017

186. Henderson LA, Canna SW, Schulert GS, *et al.* (2020) On the alert for cytokine storm: Immunopathology in COVID-19. *Arthritis & Rheumatology* **72**(7):1059–1063. DOI:10.1002/art.41285

187. Sinha P, Matthay MA, Calfee CS. (2020) Is a "cytokine storm" relevant to COVID-19. *JAMA Internal Medicine* **180**:1152–1154.

188. Murin CD, Wilson IA, Ward AB. (2019) Antibody responses to viral infections: A structural perspective across three different enveloped viruses. *Nature Microbiology* **4**(5):734–747. DOI:10.1038/s41564-019-0392-y

189. Poston D, Weisblum Y, Wise H, *et al.* (2021) Absence of severe acute respiratory syndrome coronavirus 2 neutralizing activity in prepandemic sera from individuals with recent seasonal coronavirus infection. *Clinical Infectious Diseases* **73**(5):e1208–e1211. https://doi.org/10.1093/cid/ciaa1803

190. Anderson EM, Goodwin EC, Verma A, *et al.* (2021) Seasonal human coronavirus antibodies are boosted upon SARS-CoV-2 infection but not associated with protection. *Cell* **184**(7):1858–1864.e10. DOI:10.1016/j.cell.2021.02.010

191. McKinstry KK, Strutt TM, Kuang Y, *et al.* (2012) Memory CD4+ T cells protect against influenza through multiple synergizing mechanisms. *Journal of Clinical Investigation* **122**(8):2847–2856. DOI:10.1172/JCI63689

192. Mateus J, Grifoni A, Tarke A, *et al.* (2020) Selective and cross-reactive SARS-CoV-2 T cell epitopes in unexposed humans. *Science.* **370**(6512):89–94. DOI:10.1126/science.abd3871

193. Braun, J., Loyal, L., Frentsch, M. *et al.* (2020) SARS-CoV-2-reactive T cells in healthy donors and patients with COVID-19. *Nature* **587**:270–274. https://doi.org/10.1038/s41586-020-2598-9

194. Mallajosyula V, Ganjavi C, Chakraborty S, *et al.* (2021) CD8+ T cells specific for conserved coronavirus epitopes correlate with milder disease in COVID-19 patients. *Science Immunology* **6**(61):eabg5669. DOI:10.1126/sciimmunol.abg5669

195. Sagar M, Reifler K, Rossi M, *et al.* (2021) Recent endemic coronavirus infection is associated with less-severe COVID-19. *Journal of Clinical Investigation* **131**(1):e143380. DOI:10.1172/JCI143380

196. Loyal L, Braun J, Henze L, *et al.* (2021) Cross-reactive CD4+ T cells enhance SARS-CoV-2 immune responses upon infection and vaccination. *Science* **374**:1–11. DOI:10.1126/science.abh1823

197. Ravichandran S, Grubbs G, Tang J, *et al.* (2021) Systemic and mucosal immune profiling in asymptomatic and symptomatic SARS-CoV-2-in-

fected individuals reveal unlinked immune signatures. *Science Advances* **7**(42):eabi6533. DOI:10.1126/sciadv.abi6533

197A. Wolday D, Gebrecherkos T, Arefaine ZG, *et al*. Effect of co-infection with intestinal parasites on COVID-19 severity: A prospective observational cohort study. EClinicalMedicine. 2021 Sep;39:101054. doi: 10.1016/j. eclinm.2021.101054.

197B. White PJ, McManus CM, Maizels RM. Regulatory T-cells in helminth infection: induction, function and therapeutic potential. Immunology March 10, 2020. https://doi.org/10.1111/imm.13190

198. Langton DJ, Bourke SC, Lie BA, *et al*. (2021) The influence of HLA genotype on the severity of COVID-19 infection. *HLA*. **98**(1):14–22. DOI:10.1111/tan.14284

199. Castelli EC, de Castro MV, Naslavsky MS, *et al*. (2021) MHC variants associated with symptomatic versus asymptomatic SARS-CoV-2 infection in highly exposed individuals. *Frontiers in Immunology* **28**(12):742881. DOI:10.3389/fimmu.2021.742881

200. Merrill JT, Erkan D, Winakur J, James JA. (2020) Emerging evidence of a COVID-19 thrombotic syndrome has treatment implications. *Nature Reviews* **16**:581–589.

201. BNO News. (2020) COVID-19 reinfection tracker. *BNO News*, August 28. https://bnonews.com/index.php/2020/08/covid-19-reinfection-tracker/

202. Hansen CH, Michlmayr D, Gubbels SM, *et al*. (2021) Assessment of protection against reinfection with SARS-CoV-2 among 4 million PCR-tested individuals in Denmark in 2020; a population-level observational study. *Lancet* **397**(10280):1204–1212. https://doi.org/10.1016/S0140-6736(21)00575-4

203. Bayarri-Olmos R, Rosbjerg A, Johnsen LB, *et al*. (2021) The SARS-CoV-2 Y453F mink variant displays a striking increase in ACE-2 affinity but does not challenge antibody neutralization. *bioRxiv*. https://doi.org/10.1101/2021.01.29.428834

204. Koopmans M. (2021) SARS-CoV-2 and the human-animal interface: outbreaks on mink farms. *Lancet* **21**:18–19. https://www.thelancet.com/journals/laninf/article/PIIS1473-3099(20)30912-9/fulltext

205. Dyer O. (2020) COVID-19: Denmark to kill 17 million minks over mutation that could undermine vaccine effort. *BMJ* **371**:m4338. https://doi.org/10.1136/bmj.m4338

206. Ibarrondo FJ, Fulcher JA, Goodman-Meza D, *et al*. (2020) Rapid decay of anti-SARS-CoV-2 antibodies in persons with mild COVID-19. *New England Journal of Medicine* **383**(11):1085–1087. https://www.10.1056/nejmc2025179

207.   Huang AT, Garcia-Carreras B, Hitchings MDT, *et al.* (2020) A systematic review of antibody mediated immunity to coronaviruses: Antibody kinetics, correlates of protection, and association of antibody responses with severity of disease. *medRxiv.* https://doi.org/10.1101/2020.04.14.20065771

208.   Dan JM, Mateus J, Kato Y, *et al.* (2021) Immunologic memory to SARS-CoV-2 assessed for up to 8 months after infection. *Science* **371**(6529):eabf4063. https://doi.org/10.1126/science.abf4063

209.   CDC. (2021) Science brief: Emerging SARS-CoV-2 variants. Centers for Disease Control and Prevention. https://www.cdc.gov/coronavirus/2019-ncov/science/science-briefs/scientific-brief-emerging-variants.html

210.   Tseng A, Seiler J, Issema R, *et al.* (2021) Summary of SARS-CoV-2 novel variants. Start Center, University of Washington, Washington State Department of Health, Alliance for Pandemic Preparedness, February 5.

211.   Davies NG, Abbott S, Barnard RC, *et al.* (2021) Estimated transmissibility and impact of SARS-CoV-2 lineage B.1.1.7 in England. *Science* **372**(6538). DOI:10.1126/science.abg3055

212.   Tegally H, Wilkinson E, Giovanetti M, *et al.* (2020) Emergence and rapid spread of a new severe acute respiratory syndrome-related coronavirus 2 (SARS-CoV-2) lineage with multiple spike mutations in South Africa. *medRxiv.* https://www.medrxiv.org/content/10.1101/2020.12.21.20248640v1

213.   Faria NR, Mellan TA, Whittaker C, *et al.* (2021) Genomics and epidemiology of a novel SARS-CoV-2 lineage in Manaus, Brazil. *medRxiv.* https://www.medrxiv.org/content/10.1101/2021.02.26.21252554v1.full

214.   Wang, P, Nair, MS, Liu, L. *et al.* (2021) Antibody resistance of SARS-CoV-2 variants B.1.351 and B.1.1.7. *Nature* 593:130–135. https://doi.org/10.1038/s41586-021-03398-2

215.   Cele S, Gazy I, Jackson L, *et al.* (2021) Escape of SARS-CoV-2 401 Y.V2 variants from neutralization by convalescent plasma. Nature. 2021 May; **593**(7857): 142–146. doi: 10.1038/s41586-021-03471-w.

216.   Chen RE, Zhang X, Case, JB, *et al.* (2021) Resistance of SARS-CoV-2 variants to neutralization by monoclonal and serum-derived polyclonal antibodies. *Nature Medicine* **27**:717–726. https://doi.org/10.1038/s41591-021-01294-w

217.   Mahase E. (2021) Covid-19: where are we on vaccines and variants? *BMJ* **372**:n597. DOI:10.1136/bmj.n597

218.   Madhi SA, Baillie V, Cutland M, *et al.* (2021) Efficacy of the ChAdOx1 nCoV-19 Covid-19 vaccine against the B.1.351 variant. *New England Journal of Medicine* DOI:10.1056/NEJMoa2102214

219. GlobalData Healthcare. (2021) COVID-19 vaccine effectiveness affected by variants. https://www.pharmaceutical-technology.com/comment/covid-19-vaccine-effectiveness-affected-by-variants/

220. Patino-Galindo JA, Filip I, AlQuraishi M, Rabadan R. (2020) Recombination and convergent evolution led to the emergence of the 2019 Wuhan coronavirus. *bioRxiv.* https://www.biorxiv.org/content/10.1101/2020.02.10.942748v2

221. Martin D, Weaver S, Tegally H, *et al.* (2021) The emergence and ongoing convergent evolution of the N501Y lineages coincided with a major global shift in the SARS -CoV-2 selective landscape. medRxiv July 25, 2021. https://www/doi:10.1101/2021.02.23.21252268

222. Anthony SJ, Johnson CK; PREDICT Consortium, *et al.* (2017) Global patterns in coronavirus diversity. *Virus Evolution* 3(1):vex012. DOI:10.1093/ve/vex012.

223. Rodriguez-Grande C, Adan-Jimenez J, Catalan P, *et al.* (2021) Inference of active viral replication in cases with sustained positive reverse transcription-PCR results for SARS-CoV-2. *Journal of Clinical Microbiology* 59(2):e02277-20. DOI:10.1128/JCM.02277-20

224. Kemp SA, Collier DA, Datir RP, *et al.* (2021) SARS-CoV-2 evolution during treatment of chronic infection. *Nature* 592:277–282. https://doi.org/10.1038/s41586-021-03291-y

225. Choi B, *et al.* (2020) Persistence and evolution of SARS-CoV-2 in an immunocompromised host. *New England Journal of Medicine* 383:2291–2293.

226. Avanzato VA, *et al.* (2020) Case study: Prolonged infectious SARS-CoV-2 shedding from an asymptomatic immunocompromised cancer patient. *Cell* 183:1901–1912.

227. Karim F, Moosa MYS, Gosnell BI, *et al.* (2021) Persistent SARS-CoV2 infection and intra-host evolution in association with advanced HIV infection. *medRxiv.* https://doi.org/10.1101/2021.06.03.21258228

228. Duffy S. Why are RNA virus mutation rates so damn high? *PLOS Biology* e3000003. https://doi.org/10.1371/journal.pbio.3000003

229. Jenkins GM, Rambaut A, Pybus OG, Holmes EC. (2002) Rates of molecular evolution in RNA viruses: A quantitative phylogenetic analysis. *Journal of Molecular Evolution* 54:156–165. DOI:10.1007/s00239-001-0064-3

230. Xiong C, Jiang L, Chen Y, Jiang Q. (2020) Evolution and variation of 2019-novel coronavirus. *bioRxiv.* https://doi.org/10.1101/2020.01.30.926477

5 Vaccine Salvation?

"The world is on the brink of a "catastrophic moral failure"

WHO Director-General Tedros Adhanom Ghebreyesus
Speaking at the WHO Executive General Assembly meeting,
January 18, 2021

Contents

1. Development of COVID-19 Vaccines
   a. Two recent technologies used to make the SARS-CoV-2 spike protein antigen
      i. Viral-vector vaccines
      ii. mRNA vaccines
2. SARS-CoV-2 Variants
   a. Potential impact of SARS-CoV-2 variants alpha (B.1.1.7) and beta (B.1.351) on transmission, case fatality rate (CFR) and vaccine efficacy
   b. Potential need for repeated vaccination with new variant strains
3. COVID-19 Vaccines — Challenges in Delivery and Distribution
   a. WHO develops programs to create equitable vaccine distribution
      i. Solidarity program and access to COVID-19 tools (ACT)-Accelerator programs
      ii. COVAX — COVID-19 vaccine access program and facility
   b. Prioritizing groups for vaccination
      i. High risk including elderly and healthcare workers
      ii. Do people known to have been infected with SARS-CoV-2 need vaccination or can they wait?
   c. Delivery of vaccines to vaccinations sites
      i. How well did various countries do in rolling out vaccines?
4. Vaccine Hesitancy
   a. Overview of issues impacting vaccine hesitancy
   b. COVID-19 and vaccine hesitancy

      i. Examples of vaccine hesitancy across regions and countries
      ii. How vaccine hesitancy in one region can affect another region
   c. Overcoming vaccine hesitancy
5. Conclusion

1. Development of COVID-19 Vaccines

Vaccines are the most powerful tools available for decreasing the number of COVID-19 cases and deaths, thereby enabling the world to recover faster from the pandemic. Smallpox was the first disease to be impacted by the development of a vaccine. In 1796, a bovine strain of the smallpox virus was used to make a vaccine that prevented smallpox disease in people.[1] Since that time, vaccines have been developed and licensed for use against 27 human diseases, including those due to bacteria (i.e., cholera, diphtheria, H. influenzae type b, meningococcal disease, pneumococcal diseases, pertussis, tetanus, tuberculosis, and typhoid fever) and others due to viruses (i.e., dengue fever, Ebola, hepatitis A, B and E, human papillomavirus infection, influenza, Japanese encephalitis, measles, mumps, rabies, rotavirus, rubella, tick-borne encephalitis, varicella/shingles, and yellow fever). However, unlike during the most recent 2009 influenza pandemic, where there was a lot of experience making vaccines with H1N1 strains, there was no previous vaccine that contained a SARS-CoV-2 virus.[2] This was a major problem because it previously took years to decades to develop, test and obtain regulatory approval for a new type of vaccine[3] (Figure 5.59).

The fact that multiple different vaccines against the SARS-CoV-2 coronavirus species were created, tested in Phase 1, 2 and 3 trials, and approved for Emergency Use Authorization (EUA) within a year is a spectacular achievement that many experts thought was not possible.[4] The development of a successful vaccine requires an investment of hundreds of millions of dollars by the company developing the vaccine. However, for the COVID-19 pandemic, a new approach was initiated by the WHO, in conjunction with the Global Alliance for Vaccines and Immunizations (Gavi), other global partners, and various high-income countries.

By the end of 2020, there were ~180 COVID-19 vaccines in development using various platforms, and over 65 of these vaccines were undergoing Phase 1, 2 or 3 testing in people[5] (Figure 5.60). Nineteen vaccines

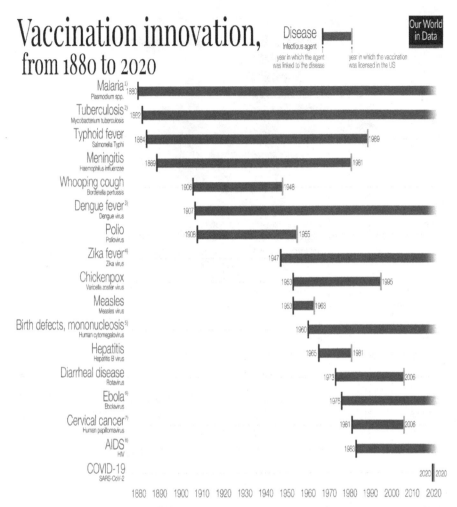

Figure 5.59. Timeline for development of various vaccines.[3]

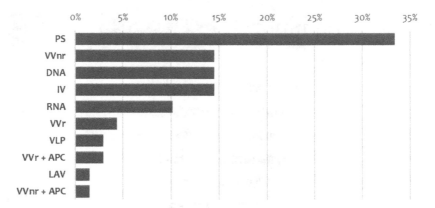

Figure 5.60. The relative percentage of various vaccine platforms for the COVID-19 vaccine that are in clinical trials at the end of 2020.[5] Abbreviations: PS – protein subunit, VVnr – viral vector (non-replicating), DNA – DNA genetic segment, IV – Inactivated Virus, RNA – RNA genetic segment, VV (replicating), VLP – Virus Like Particle, VVr + APC – Virus Vector (replicating) + Antigen Presenting Cell, LAV – Live Attenuated Virus, VVnr + Antigen Presenting – Virus Vector (non-replicating) + Antigen Presenting Cell.

were in ongoing large-scale Phase 3 studies. Four received regulatory and/or government approval and were being used in the general public of one or more countries towards the end of 2020 (Table 5.13). There are other COVID-19 vaccines that could be licensed in 2021, including some that use other platform technologies, including live attenuated viruses and recombinant protein subunits. However, given the large number of vaccines being developed, only the four vaccines that published their Phase 3 results by the beginning of February 2021 and had received EUAs will be discussed in the rest of this chapter. Updated results on other vaccines in clinical trials can be found in regularly updated Vaccine Tracker websites.[5]

The Pfizer-BioNTech, Moderna-NIH and Oxford-AstraZeneca vaccines received EUA by the end of 2020 after submitting their Phase 3 study results to the regulatory agencies in the United States (US) (FDA), United Kingdom (UK) (MHRA) and/or Europe (EMA) (Table 5.14).[6] The vaccine, created by the Gamaleya Research Institute in Russia, was approved in August 2020 by the Russian Ministry of Health on the basis of Phase 1 and 2 studies and started being used soon thereafter.[7] The use of the Russian vaccine was widely criticized for not completing Phase 3 studies before approval, but the vaccine was used in Russia and several other countries[8]; the Phase 3

Table 5.13. Characteristics of COVID-19 vaccines with published Phase 3 trial data being used by the end of 2020.[5]

Vaccine Platform Acronym*	Vaccine Platform Description	Type of Candidate Vaccine	Number of Doses	Dosing Schedule	Route of Administration	Developers
VVnr	Viral vector (Non-replicating)	ChAdOx1-S - (AZD1222)	1–2	Day 0 + 28	IM	AstraZeneca + University of Oxford
RNA	RNA-based vaccine	mRNA -1273	2	Day 0 + 28	IM	Moderna + National Institute of Allergy and Infectious Diseases (NIAID)
RNA	RNA-based vaccine	BNT162 (3 LNP-mRNAs)	2	Day 0 + 21	IM	Pfizer/BioNTech + Fosun Pharma
VVnr	Viral vector (Non-replicating	Gam-COVID-Vac Adeno-based (rAd26-S+rAd5-S)	2	Day 0 + 21	IM	Gamaleya Research Institute; Health Ministry of the Russian Federation

*Abbreviations: VVnr — viral vector (non-replicating), Virus, RNA — RNA genetic segment.

Table 5.14.   Additional COVID-19 vaccines characteristics.[10]*

Vaccine Candidate	Pfizer-Biontech	Moderna-NIH	Astrazeneca-Oxford	Gamaleya
Type	mRNA	mRNA	Non-replicating adenovirus vector	Non-replicating adenovirus vector
Storage and Shelf life	Standard refrigerator for up to 5 days, dry-ice chest for up to 30 days, or ultra-cold freezer (–70°C) up to 6 months.	Room temperature up to 12 hours, standard refrigerator up to 30 days, and a standard freezer up to 6 months.	Can be kept in a standard refrigerator for at least 6 months.	Can be kept in a standard refrigerator, duration unclear
Approximate cost per dose (US)	$20	$15–25	$3	$10
How to administer	2 IM shots, 3 weeks apart	2 IM shots, 4 weeks apart	2 IM shots, 4 weeks apart	2 IM shots, 3 weeks apart
Regulatory status	Received EUA from the MHR and FDA.	Received EUA from the FDA.	Received EUA from the MHR.	Russian government and regulatory agency prior to completing Phase 3 study.
Production capacity	50 million vaccine doses for global distribution by end of 2020, and to 1.3 billion doses in 2021.	20 million doses for US by the end of 2020, and 500 million to 1 billion doses globally in 2021.	Predicts up to 3 billion doses of the vaccine in 2021.	500 million doses in 2021.
Doses ordered (US)	100 million	100 million	300 million	None
Doses ordered (COVAX)	No agreement with COVAX as of the end of 2020.	Agreement signed with COVAX, but details not finalized at end of 2020.	300 million	No COVAX agreement

* Table modified from reference 10. Additional data is from references 11 to 15.

data was published in early 2021.[9] Specific characteristics of these vaccines are noted in Table 5.15.[10-15] The two different platform technologies used to make these four vaccines were developed over the past decade. Two inactivated SARS-CoV-2 vaccines being produced in China are also being used in some countries,[5] but their Phase 3 trial safety and efficacy data were not published as of June 2021. Therefore, these Chinese vaccines are not included in Tables 5.14 or 5.15.

The Coalition for Epidemic Preparedness Innovation (CEPI) played an important role in enabling the development of the new technologies used to make these vaccines. CEPI was formed in 2017 with the support of the Wellcome Trust, Bill & Melinda Gates Foundation, Germany, India, Japan, and Norway with the mission to help stimulate and accelerate the development of vaccines against emerging infectious diseases and enable access to these vaccines for people during outbreaks.[16] Before the emergence of COVID-19, CEPI's priority diseases included Lassa fever, MERS, Nipah, Ebola, Rift Valley Fever, and Chikungunya. CEPI also invested in platform technologies that can be used for rapid vaccine and immunoprophylactic development against yet unknown pathogens.[17]

a. Two recent technologies used to make the SARS-CoV-2 spike protein antigen

i. Viral-vector vaccines

The initial COVID-19 vaccines that received EUA after publishing their Phase 3 data were either a viral vector or mRNA platform, and they are diagrammed in Figure 5.61. The Oxford-AstraZeneca and Gamaleya COVID-19 vaccines use non-replicating virus vector technology. The only previously licensed vaccine using this technology is the Ebola virus vaccine developed by Merck Pharmaceutical Company. Clinical evaluation of this vaccine occurred in the 2014 West Africa Ebola outbreak, and it was also used in the 2018 Ebola outbreak in the Democratic Republic of the Congo. This Ebola vaccine has now been licensed by the European Medicines Agency (EMA) and the US Food and Drug Authority (FDA).[18,19] Similar to the Ebola virus vaccine, the two Covid-19 virus vaccines use an adenovirus strain as a carrier (or "vector") containing the DNA segment that encodes the spike protein on the outer surface of SARS-CoV-2.[20] These adenovirus vectors

Table 5.15. Demographics and characteristics of the Phase 3 studies of the Pfizer, Moderna, AstraZeneca, and Gamaleya vaccines.*

Vaccine	Pfizer-BioNTech n = 37,709	Moderna n = 30,351	AstraZeneca-Oxford**** n = 11,636	Gamaleya***** n = 19,866
Vaccine	50%	50%	49.9%	75.3%
Control	50%	50%	50.1%	24.7%
Male	50.6%	52.7%	39.5%	61.2%
Female	49.4%	47.3%	60.5%	38.8%
Median Age (range)	52 yrs (16–85 yrs)	51.4 yrs (18–95 yrs)	~85% 18–55 yrs, ~10% 55–69 yrs, ~5% >70yrs	45.3 (18–60 yrs)
Race	59% white	79% while	~80% white	98% white
Co-morbidity Conditions Allowed	Stable chronic conditions allowed, including obesity, HIV, and hepatitis B and C	Chronic diseases including lung, cardiovascular, diabetes. Liver, obesity and well-controlled HIV	Chronic diseases including lung, cardiovascular, diabetes, and obesity	Chronic disease including diabetes, hypertension, ischemic heart disease, and obesity
Exclusions**	— Pregnancy — Prior COVID-19 infection, immune suppression treatment	— Pregnancy — Prior COVID-19 infection, immune suppression treatment	— Pregnancy — Prior COVID-19 infection, immune suppression treatment	— Pregnancy — Acute and chronic diseases, immune suppression alcoholism
Country Where Studies Done	Argentina Brazil South Africa US	US	United Kingdom Brazil	25 hospitals and poly-clinics in Moscow, Russia

Local Side Effects***	Pain, redness, and swelling at injection site	Pain, redness, swelling at injection site and lymphadenopathy	See below	Mostly Grade 1 pain, redness, and swelling at injection site
Systemic Side Effects***	Fever, fatigue, headache, chills, muscle and/or joint pain	Fever, fatigue, headache, chills, muscle pain, and joint pain, nausea or vomiting	Not published in 2020. UK MHRA review did not raise concerns	Fever, fatigue, headache, asthenia, muscle, and/or joint pain
Efficacy	95%	94%	70%	92%
References	11	12	13	9,14

*This table highlights some of the characteristics and demographics of the above studies. Further details can be found in the references noted for each vaccine.[10]

**In several of these studies, some patients turned out to have been pregnant or infected prior to vaccination.

***Local and systemic side effects noted in the Table are those that occurred significantly more often in the vaccine than placebo groups after dose 1 and/or 2.

****The AstraZeneca Phase 3 paper was published online on December 8, 2020, as an interim analysis of the efficacy of the vaccine.[13] The data in the paper is noted separately for each of the United Kingdom and Brazil trial sites (a trial was also being conducted in South Africa, but the efficacy data was not included in the interim analysis described in reference 13). The above table shows the data as a combination of studies done in the United Kingdom and Brazil and in some cases is an approximation of the exact results.

*****The Gamaleya Phase 3 study was published online on December 8, 2020, as an interim analysis of the efficacy of the vaccine.[15]

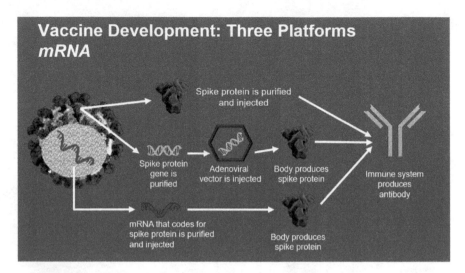

Figure 5.61. Diagram of the three platforms used to make various COVID-19 vaccines.[21] The middle part of the diagram shows a viral vector platform and the lower part of the diagram shows the mRNA platform. The upper part of the diagrams shows the platform for making an inactivated vaccine produced in China, which is not discussed in this chapter because its Phase 3 data has not yet been published.

are non-replicating, meaning that they do not make new virus particles, but rather produce only the spike antigen, which elicits a systemic immune response.[21,22] The CEPI's activities clearly had a catalytic effect on the development of these new platform technologies.

ii. mRNA vaccines

The Moderna and Pfizer-BioNTech vaccines are the first mRNA vaccines to be used outside of a study environment. From the known genetic sequence of the SARS-C0V-2 spike protein, a strand of mRNA is generated that codes for the spike protein. The mRNA strand is protected in a lipid coat and then administered into the muscle, where the muscle cell machinery produces the spike protein that stimulates an immune response[21,22] (Figure 5.62).

Each of the mRNA vaccines received an EUA based on recipients receiving two doses. Other information, including recommended time intervals between dose 1 and 2, storage requirements, anticipated production capacity for each vaccine by the end of 2021, and a number of doses

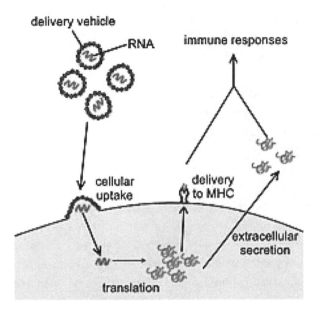

Figure 5.62. Diagram of the operation of an mRNA vaccine. The mRNA is contained in a lipid carrier and enters cells where it is translated into foreign proteins, which trigger an immune response.[21]

contractually available to the US and the COVAX facility are noted in Table 5.14 (see the next section on vaccine delivery and distribution for information on the COVAX facility and program). The ability of these vaccines to decrease asymptomatic infection and the duration of vaccine protection remains to be determined.

Each of these vaccines produces humoral and cell-mediated responses, but at the of 2020 it was still not clear which specific humoral and cell-mediated responses are critical to preventing COVID-19 disease. Therefore, a discussion of the immune response to each vaccine is not included in the discussion of each vaccine. Several excellent reviews of what is known about the immunologic response to SARS-CoV-2 are available.[23,24] The percentage of the population that needs to be infected with the virus or vaccinated to achieve herd immunity is still unknown at the end of 2020. Early on in the pandemic, various public health experts predicted that herd immunity could occur when anywhere between 10% and >70% of people have been vaccinated or infected. The lower end of the prediction has clearly proven incorrect, and most experts now believe the number is likely to be greater than 70%.[25]

The rest of this section focuses on the data from Phase 3 studies for each of these four vaccines.[9-15] The Pfizer-BioNTech Phase 3 studies were done in four countries and included over 37,000 total volunteers in either the vaccine or placebo group[11] (Table 5.15). Participants were 16 years of age and older, and 42% were older than 55 years. The most common local side effect was pain upon injection, which occurred in over 70% of those receiving doses 1 and 2 of the vaccine. Redness and swelling/lymphadenopathy were seen in ~7% of those in the vaccine group. The most common systemic side effects included fever, fatigue, headache, chills, muscle pain, and joint pain. These systemic side effects were seen more frequently after the second dose and in those between 15 and 55 years. These side effects usually were gone within a few days except for the swelling that usually resolved within 10 days. No life-threatening side effects were noted during the study. However, subsequently, anaphylaxis, a severe, potentially life-threatening allergic reaction, was noted at a rate of 11.1 per million doses.[26] The median time from receipt of the vaccine to this event was 13 minutes (range: 2–150 minutes) and it occurred mainly in women. Anaphylaxis is a rare event known to be associated with other vaccines. Healthcare facilities that administer vaccines should be capable of dealing with this if it happens.

The efficacy of the Pfizer vaccine in preventing disease was very good at 94.8% (95% CI- 94.8–97.6%) after 2 doses.[11] Most of those receiving the vaccine who did develop COVID-19 disease had mild to moderate symptoms, and no deaths occurred in any vaccine recipient during the study period, suggesting that the vaccine was particularly good at preventing severe disease. During the interim between doses 1 and 2, the number of COVID-19 cases was less than in the placebo group. The calculated vaccine efficacy a week or more after dose 1 was 52.4% (95% CI- 29.5–68.4%).

Two drawbacks to the Pfizer vaccine relate to its storage requirements and cost (Table 5.14). This vaccine is the only one requiring storage at ultra-cold temperatures ($-70^{\circ}C$), which makes the use of this vaccine in many low and middle-income countries more difficult. In 2021, Pfizer completed the necessary studies to determine that their vaccine could be stored at a refrigeration temperature of $2-8^{\circ}C$. However, the relatively high cost of the vaccine (~US$20 per dose) makes it likely that this vaccine will be used mainly in high-income countries unless a price agreement with the COVAX facility can be reached.

Moderna is a startup US technology company, that in collaboration with the NIH, developed an mRNA vaccine against SAR-CoV-2. The Phase 3 studies of the Moderna vaccine were done at multiple sites in the US and included over 30,000 total volunteers >18 years of age in either the vaccine or placebo group[12] (Table 5.15). Similar to the Pfizer vaccine, the Moderna vaccine uses the mRNA platform, and the safety and efficacy data are similar to those of the Pfizer vaccine. One noteworthy difference is that the second dose of the Moderna vaccine caused a higher rate of systemic side effects, including myalgias and chills, than the Pfizer vaccine.

The Trump administration made a US$1.5 billion commitment to the development of this vaccine as part of "Operation Warp Speed", which helped speed up the development of some of the vaccines, including the Moderna vaccine, which is produced in the US. Over a decade prior to the COVID-19 pandemic, the US government created the Biomedical Advanced Research Development Authority (BARDA), and this agency made significant investments in the development of new platform technologies and also funded the production of the Moderna, Pfizer and Johnson & Johnson (Janssen) vaccines prior to knowing whether the vaccines even worked, making them quickly available after issuance of the EUAs. However, the "America First" policy[27] developed by the Trump administration hindered the use of this vaccine overseas. Moderna has signed an agreement with the COVAX to provide a vaccine, but it is not clear when their vaccine will be available for global use.

The development of the AstraZeneca vaccine was especially important for low-income countries. The vaccine was developed at the University of Oxford in England using a viral-vector platform that had several advantages over mRNA vaccines, in that they are less costly to produce and can be stored in refrigerators for longer time periods (Table 5.14). Oxford had an agreement with AstraZeneca that the vaccine would be sold at or near cost to low-income countries. Indeed, AstraZeneca was the first vaccine company to strike a deal with the COVAX facility that helped ensure these countries would have equitable access to COVID-19 vaccines.

The interim report of the AstraZeneca Phase 3 study[13] published in January 2021[13] noted safety data similar to the Pfizer and Moderna Phase 3 trials. However, one difference among these Phase 3 studies was that the AstraZeneca control group received a quadrivalent meningococcal vaccine while the Pfizer and Moderna placebo group received saline, which makes a direct comparison of differences between vaccine and control groups difficult. Regardless, initially there were not any serious outcomes related to the vaccine.

In contrast to the initial safety data, the efficacy data raised an important issue that needed further analysis. The first dose of the vaccine was mistakenly given at half the normal strength to some participants in the UK Phase 3 trial while the second dose was a standard dose. The efficacy in those who got the lower dose followed by a standard dose at >4 weeks was 90% versus 62% in those who got two standard doses. When the data from all these trials were combined, the overall efficacy was 70%, which was significantly lower than the Pfizer and Moderna mRNA vaccines. This led to many questions, including why did those who received one low and one standard dose have higher efficacy than those who received two standard doses? Initial thoughts centered on the theory that the low dose was acting as a better priming dose than a standard first dose. However, further analysis of the data has led to another conclusion. It turns out that those who got the half dose also had a longer interval of time before getting the second dose. It now appears that delaying the second dose to 12 weeks, rather than 4 weeks, after the first dose, yields better protection (efficacy 82.4%) against the COVID-19 disease.[28]

The first dose of the AstraZeneca and Pfizer vaccines used in the initial phase of the UK's COVID-19 vaccination program (late 2020 and early 2021) was given to all adults before anyone received the second dose.[29] The initial data suggests that the first dose offers ~60% protection against COVID-19 disease and may even be better against severe disease. This may be particularly fortuitous since most people in the UK did not get their second dose for at least 12 weeks, and this might have increased the efficacy of the vaccine program.

The Gamaleya vaccine was developed by the Gamaleya Institute using a virus vector platform with two different adenovirus vectors (i.e., adenovirus 26 for the first dose and adenovirus 5 for the second dose) given

~21 days after the first dose (Table 5.14).[9,14] A potential advantage of using different adenovirus subtypes for each dose is that the adenoviral vectors could potentially induce immune responses against vector components and attenuate antigen-induced responses against the SARS-CoV-2 spike protein being produced by the virus-vector. This risk is potentially decreased in a prime-boost heterologous vaccination using two different viral vectors strains. As noted above, the AstraZeneca vaccine used a single virus-vector strain for both doses, and it is unclear whether the dual vector approach offered any advantage over a single vector for these two vaccines.

The local and systemic safety data from the Gamaleya vaccine study for doses one and two was similar to the three other COVID-19 vaccines noted in Table 5.15. The reported efficacy of the Gamaleya vaccine after two doses was 91.6%,[9] which is similar to both mRNA vaccines and better than the viral-vector AstraZeneca vaccine, which may be due to the need for the AstraZeneca vaccine to have a longer interval between its first and second doses (see above). Initial concern about the reliability of the data[30] has decreased after the peer-reviewed publication in Lancet in February 2021.[9] Development of the Gamaleya vaccine was supported by the Russian government, and Phase 1, 2 and 3 studies were all done in Moscow at laboratories, hospitals or polyclinics with research experience. The cost of the vaccine is expected to be ~US$10, which is more than the AstraZeneca, but less than the two mRNA vaccines (Table 5.14).

Key Point: The development, EUA approval, and initial use of these vaccines within a year of the onset of the pandemic is a remarkable achievement. This was made possible by the use of two new technology platforms (non-replicating viral vectors and mRNA) to produce the SARS-CoV-2 spike proteins, which were crucial to making these safe and effective vaccines.

---

2. SARS-CoV-2 Variants

Most SARS-CoV-2 genetic mutations have no clinical impact, but there are times when a mutation can lead to a variant that increases virus transmission and/or case fatality rate (CFR) while also decreasing the efficacy of vaccines in preventing disease (a variant could have enhanced ability to escape vaccine-induced immune responses).[31] The best way to prevent this is to vaccinate enough of the world's population as quickly as possible to induce herd-immunity. The predominant SARS-CoV-2 virus strain that circulated during the first wave of the pandemic had an estimated R_0 of ~2.2. As previously noted, based on this R_0, most experts believe that at least 60% of the population needs to have immunity from a previous infection or vaccination before herd immunity will occur.[32]

The question of whether a vaccinated person can discontinue their mitigation activities is an important one. While the vaccines discussed in the previous section have proven to have substantial efficacy against disease, especially severe disease, their ability to prevent the nasal carriage of SARS-CoV-2 and thereby prevent transmission/infection of people remains to be determined.[33] The Phase 3 studies done with these vaccines suggest they may decrease transmission; however, many of these studies were done during a time when some or most of the population was in lockdown. Therefore, the US CDC and other public health organizations believe the safest thing for vaccinated people to do is to continue employing mitigation steps, including social distancing and use of masks, until widespread herd immunity has been achieved.[34] Furthermore, herd immunity will not occur at the same time across the globe or within a country. Therefore, decisions on when to discontinue mitigations steps in a particular area should be based on the disease incidence within the community.

a. Potential impact of SARS-CoV-2 variants alpha (B.1.1.7) and beta (B.1.351) on transmission, Case Fatality Rate (CFR) and vaccine efficacy

Several other issues play into the uncertainty about when we will be able to get back to a pre-pandemic "normal" life. The duration of protection offered by COVID-19 vaccines remains to be determined. Additionally, the ability of the current vaccines to protect against the increasing number of variants is also unclear. Towards the end of 2020, variants in Britain alpha (B.1.1.7) and South Africa beta (B.1.351) were detected. Studies showed the alpha variant was ~50% more transmissible than the orginal SARS-CoV-2 strain and spread rapidly to other countries.[31–33] A study also suggested that this variant might cause an increased CFR.[35] Efficacy studies done during the first few months of 2021 by Pfizer, Moderna and AstraZeneca suggest these vaccines maintained their ability to protect against COVID-19 disease in most countries where they were being used.[36] However, data from South Africa suggests that the AstraZeneca vaccine had a ~22% efficacy against mild to moderate COVID-19 disease (studies are ongoing to determine if the vaccine protects against severe disease).[37,38] The antibodies of those vaccinated with the AstraZeneca vaccine showed substantially decreased binding to the B1.351 variant in laboratory studies than previous strains circulating in South Africa earlier in the pandemic. In contrast, those vaccinated had strong cell-mediated T-cell responses, which could mean that the vaccine will still provide good protection against more severe disease.

The AstraZeneca Phase 3 study efficacy results came at the same time the South African government had ordered 1 million doses of this vaccine and was ready to begin immunizing its population.[37,38] Based on the above results, the government decided not to initiate this vaccination program until more data about its protection against severe disease are available. Preliminary data from two other Phase 3 studies in South Africa — Johnson & Johnson COVID-19 viral vector vaccine and a Novovax recombinant nanoparticle vaccine — that were ongoing at that time reported to have 57% and 49% efficacy against the COVID-19 disease, respectively.[38] However, even if these two other vaccines are more effective against the B1.351 variant, they are likely to be more costly than the AstraZeneca vaccine that was purchased for approximately US$3 per dose.

b. Potential need for repeated vaccination with new variant strains

The appearance of variants with increased transmission and/or ability to overcome immune responses have increased the likelihood that even after the COVID-19 pandemic has subsided, there will still be substantial endemic disease due to SARS-CoV-2. During the early phase of the COVID-19 outbreak, it was hoped that the disease would go away if the SARS-CoV-2 virus was contained in the Asian countries where the outbreak first occurred. This is certainly what happened in 2003 when a new strain of coronavirus, SARS-CoV-1, caused an outbreak of SARS with over 8,000 cases within 7 months, but soon thereafter no new cases occurred. However, this is unlikely to occur with SARS-CoV-2 since the disease has caused a global pandemic with >80 million cases by the end of 2020 and virus variants with increased transmissibility and ability to avoid the immune response elicited by previous SARS-COV-2 strains.[39] See the Epilogue (Chapter 10) for further discussion regarding the likelihood of COVID becoming an endemic disease.

The reduced efficacy of certain vaccines to one or more SARS-CoV-2 variants has led vaccine companies to begin the process of modifying their vaccines to more closely match the variants. By mid-2021, Pfizer, Moderna and AstraZeneca started to create new versions of the vaccines to match the alpha and beta variants. The FDA has indicated that it will likely not require large Phase 3 studies for approval of new vaccines against variant strains as long as the companies are using the same platform they used for the already approved vaccine.[40] Smaller safety and immunogenicity studies will still be needed. This will allow the quicker approval of COVID-19 vaccines that more closely match the SARS-CoV-2 strains that are circulating. This incorporation of recent SARS-CoV-2 strains into the vaccine is similar to what the WHO does twice a year when it holds meetings to decide if the influenza A and B strains need to be changed for use in the Southern or Northern hemispheres.[41]

Key Point: While the original strain of SARS-CoV-2 virus mutates at a rate somewhat slower than influenza viruses, it was anticipated that SARS-CoV-2 variants could develop an increased ability to transmit between people, result in higher CFRs, and avoid immune responses that protected against previous versions of the virus. A number of variant strains have emerged with higher transmission and potentially mortality rates. Initial effectiveness data suggests that most of the available COVID-19 vaccines are effective against these variant viruses, particularly against the development of severe disease.

3. COVID-19 Vaccine — Challenges in Delivery and Distribution

a. WHO develops programs to create equitable vaccine distribution

Previous pandemics, including the 2009 influenza pandemic, provided the world with poignant reminders of the severe inequities that occurred between high-income countries and the rest of the world regarding the availability of needed supplies, drugs and vaccines. The WHO was very concerned about these inequities, including the additional impact that increasing nationalism in some high-income countries would have on the ability of middle and low-income countries to acquire needed supplies, treatments and vaccines during the pandemic.[42,43]

i. *Solidarity program and access to COVID-19 tools (ACT)-Accelerator programs*

The WHO began working in early 2020 on the blueprint for a coordinated global response to increase supplies and develop diagnostic tests, treatments and vaccines to deal with the COVID-19 pandemic. They did this by developing two new interconnected programs to help create a coordinated response needed to help all member countries during the pandemic: The Solidarity Call to Action and the Access to COVID-19 Tools (ACT)-Accelerator.

The Solidarity concept provided a mechanism to coordinate the activities needed to deal with the pandemic.[44] The WHO, in collaboration with other global partners, launched the ACT-Accelerator at the end of April 2020. The ACT-Accelerator was created to bring together governments, scientists, businesses, civil society, philanthropists, and global health organizations to speed up the development of tools needed to end the pandemic. The ACT-Accelerator has four pillars (i.e., Diagnostics, Therapeutics, Vaccines and Health Systems) aimed at the development and equitable distribution of tests, therapeutics and vaccines throughout the world, and various global partners oversee these pillars[45] (Table 5.16). This effort focuses on reducing mortality and severe disease, restoring full societal and economic activity globally in the near term, and facilitating high-level control of COVID-19 disease in the medium term.

The Solidarity and ACT programs are meant to overcome nationalism so that all countries can obtain supplies and effective interventions. The specific goals and objectives of these two programs are described in Chapter 2. Additional programs created to specifically support the development of tests, drugs and vaccines are described in the corresponding chapters in this book.

Table 5.16.   Pillars of the ACT-Accelerator.*

Pillar	Purpose	Responsible Global Partners
Diagnostics	By mid-2021: — Bringing to market 2–3 high quality rapid tests — Training 10,000 HCWs in 50 countries — Testing 500 million people in LMIC	FIND Global Fund
Therapeutics	By end of 2021: — Develop, manufacture and distribute 245 million treatments — Helping people recover from COVID-19 disease	Wellcome Unitaid
Vaccines	By the end of 2021: — Speeding up the search for an effective vaccine for all countries — Support the building of manufacturing capabilities — Buying supplies — Distribute 2 billion doses	CEPI Gavi WHO
Health Systems	As the connector to the above pillars, ensure that these tools can reach those who need them.	Global Fund World Bank

*Modified from reference 45.

ii. *COVAX — COVID-19 vaccine access program and facility*

Vaccines are one of the four pillars of the ACT-Accelerator plan[44,45] (Table 5.16). The plan called for the Global Alliance for Vaccines and Immunization (Gavi), which is the organization with the primary responsibility for purchasing vaccines for low-income countries, to work in partnership with United Nations Children's Fund (UNICEF) and CEPI to administer the COVID-19 Vaccine Access (COVAX) Program and Facility. COVAX was created to provide a global mechanism to coordinate and develop the resources needed to meet the demand for COVID-19 vaccines. The purpose of this effort was to accelerate the availability and equitable access to safe and efficacious vaccines to all countries that became members of the COVAX program.[46] This was done in conjunction with the establishment of the Gavi COVAX Advanced Market Commitment (AMC), a newly developed financing mechanism to help ensure that all countries that signed onto the plan had equitable access to COVID-19 vaccines.

Gavi was particularly well suited to oversee this process since its mission is to save children's lives and protect people's health by increasing equitable use of vaccines in lower-income countries.[46,47] Gavi was created in 2000 and currently supplies WHO-recommended vaccines to almost half the world's children by purchasing large amounts of vaccines at substantially reduced prices. This is done in partnership with UNICEF, who is responsible for delivering vaccines to those living in low-income countries. CEPI is the third organization responsible for the vaccine pillar, and they bring expertise in the development of new vaccines against microbes that have the potential to cause large infectious disease outbreaks.[48]

The COVAX Program and Facility was designed to enable the ACT-Accelerator Vaccine Pillar's stated goal for procurement and purchasing of sufficient volumes of the vaccine to end the acute phase of the pandemic. COVAX was financed with contributions from high-income countries and 28 donor organizations that signed onto the program.[46,47] This funding enabled the sharing of monetary risks with vaccine companies attempting to develop and manufacture COVID-19 vaccines. Using this mechanism enabled vaccines to be manufactured in large quantities before regulatory approval and then rapidly deployed as soon as regulators issued an EUA for a specific vaccine. By the end of 2021, the goal was to have 2 billion doses of various COVID-19 vaccines distributed to both high-income countries capable of paying the cost of COVID-19 vaccines and the 92 COVAX AMC-eligible countries. While most of the money for the COVAX program comes from high-income countries and donors, the AMC-eligible countries also financially contribute to the program on a sliding scale. The COVAX facility functions as a pass-through mechanism for equitably matching limited vaccine supply in 2021 with expressed demand.

A total of 184 countries (of which 76 were high-income) and 6 territories had signed agreements to be part of COVAX and therefore are eligible to access vaccine doses in 2021.[49,50] By the end of 2020, COVAX had agreements with a number of vaccine companies to access nearly 2 billion doses of several promising vaccine candidates. This aligned with the COVAX goal to distribute 2 billion doses to countries by the end of 2021. Of these 2 billion vaccine doses, at least 1.3 billion would be made available to 92 economies eligible for the Gavi COVAX AMC reduced pricing.

Meeting this target would allow approximately 20% of the population in all COVAX countries (high, middle, and low-income) to be vaccinated by the end of 2021. The COVAX initiative raised US$2.4 billion in 2020, exceeding its funding target of US$2 billion. For 2021, it was estimated that COVAX needed an additional US$6.8 billion which would allow US$800 million for research and development, US$4.6 billion for the COVAX AMC, and US$1.4 billion for delivering vaccines to everyone designated to be vaccinated.

Despite all the efforts to make sure that there was equitable vaccine distribution across the globe, problems with getting timely access to the COVID-19 vaccines occurred in many countries dependent on the COVAX agreement. The high-income countries make up ~14% of the world's population, but as of December 2020, had contracted for ~50% of the vaccine doses.[51] England provides one example of a high-income COVAX-committed country taking a nationalistic approach. England was experiencing a high level of disease towards the end of 2020 and on December 8 initiated a mass vaccination program for their adult population using the AstraZeneca vaccine instead of equitably sharing the vaccine as promised in the COVAX equity agreement it signed in September 2020.[52] Another example of a nationalistic approach occurred in the US, where the Trump administration refused to sign onto the COVAX agreement and stated that it would only donate the vaccine once it had fully immunized all its citizens.[53] Indeed, the US contracted for 800 million doses, which was more than two doses for its entire population. This nationalistic approach is one of the major reasons why the COVAX-AMC-eligible African countries did not start receiving their vaccines until the second half of February 2021.[54]

There is evidence suggesting that this type of nationalistic approach is detrimental to all countries. While the cost of the COVAX program and facility is high, the overall health and economic benefit will accrue to all countries participating in the COVAX program. Recent modeling by Northeastern University examined how many lives an equitable distribution of COVID-19 vaccines could save. The study found that if high-income countries buy up the first 2 billion doses of the vaccine instead of making sure they are distributed in proportion to the global population, approximately twice as many people could die from COVID-19.[55] The economic ramifications of this approach are also consequential. A RAND Europe analysis found that if some countries insist on having first access to vaccines and initially immunize only their own populations, there would be a negative economic impact for themselves as well as the wider global population of up to US$1.2 trillion a year in GDP.[56] Additionally, for every US$1 spent by high-income countries procuring vaccines for lower-income countries, they would get back an economic benefit of ~US$4.80. This is due in large part to the shift of most countries to a global economy.

As 2020 came to a close, approximately 10 million doses of various COVID-19 vaccines had been used in 15 high-income countries[57] (Figure 5.63). These numbers do not include doses being given as part of clinical trials. The Pfizer/BioNTech (Germany), Moderna/NIH (US), and AstraZeneca/ Oxford (England) vaccines are the main vaccines contributing to this total, but Sinovac (China) and Gamaleya (Russia) vaccines were also being used in their respective countries as well as some other places. Each of these vaccines requires two doses, and therefore, essentially, no one was yet fully immunized. No African country had started to vaccinate its population by the end of January 2021.

Low-income countries dependent on the COVAX facility for their vaccines did not receive their COVID-19 vaccine doses at the end of 2020 (Figure 5.63). The first shipments of the COVAX vaccine were sent to Ghana on February 23, 2021, and soon thereafter to the Ivory Coast.[58] During the first week of March 2021, UNICEF shipped vaccine doses to 20 other countries. These shipments also included vaccines needed for routine childhood vaccination programs of each country to help impact the decrease in routine immunizations that occurred in almost every country in 2020 due to COVID-19. UNICEF is planning to deliver ~2 billion COVID-19 vaccine doses in 2021, which, as noted, will provide the COVID-19 vaccine to ~20% of the population in these countries.[47]

The development of safe and effective COVID-19 vaccines was only the first critical step to getting people immunized. When supplies are limited, the process of prioritizing who gets the COVID-19 vaccine and the logistical planning of delivering vaccines to immunization sites should be ready to implement as soon as vaccines have received an EUA. Most high and upper-middle-income countries plan this process on their own, but many low and low-middle-income countries rely on UNICEF to help with vaccine delivery. Some of the major issues that countries encountered are discussed in this section.

UNICEF has a long and successful history of delivering vaccines to children in ~100 low and middle-income countries, and for this reason, UNICEF was asked by the WHO to be one of the three global organizations assigned to oversee the COVAX initiative.[46] Since the pandemic began, UNICEF had been working to prepare for the release of COVID-19 vaccines for distribution. UNICEF had been stockpiling the other necessary components needed to vaccinate people (e.g., single-dose syringes, safety boxes for syringe disposal, etc.). UNICEF had also installed hundreds of solar-powered refrigerators in countries that have little access to electrical power. Additionally, UNICEF also worked with airlines, freight operators, shipping lines, and other logistics partners to help enable the rapid and safe delivery of vaccines.

UNICEF's pandemic mission was not solely focused on vaccines. It had already delivered supplies such as masks, gowns, oxygen concentrators, and other items to help countries respond to the pandemic. UNICEF is also responsible for the delivery of 245 million therapeutics and 500 million diagnostic test kits by the end of 2021.

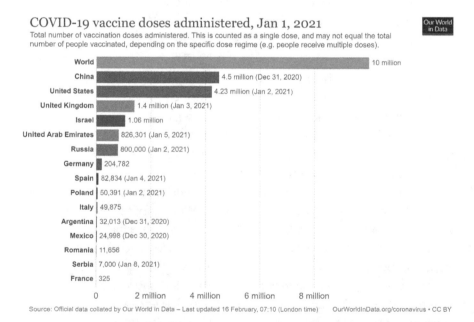

COVID-19 vaccine doses administered, Jan 1, 2021

Total number of vaccination doses administered. This is counted as a single dose, and may not equal the total number of people vaccinated, depending on the specific dose regime (e.g. people receive multiple doses).

Our World in Data

World	10 million
China	4.5 million (Dec 31, 2020)
United States	4.23 million (Jan 2, 2021)
United Kingdom	1.4 million (Jan 3, 2021)
Israel	1.06 million
United Arab Emirates	826,301 (Jan 5, 2021)
Russia	800,000 (Jan 2, 2021)
Germany	204,782
Spain	82,834 (Jan 4, 2021)
Poland	50,391 (Jan 2, 2021)
Italy	49,875
Argentina	32,013 (Dec 31, 2020)
Mexico	24,998 (Dec 30, 2020)
Romania	11,656
Serbia	7,000 (Jan 8, 2021)
France	325

0   2 million   4 million   6 million   8 million

Source: Official data collated by Our World in Data – Last updated 16 February, 07:10 (London time)   OurWorldInData.org/coronavirus • CC BY

Figure 5.63. Countries that began vaccinating its population with a COVID-19 vaccine prior to January 1, 2021.[57]

Key Point: One year after the start of the COVID-19 pandemic, there were already multiple COVID-19 vaccines that received EUAs from one or more regulatory authorities. Simultaneously, the WHO and its global partners created a program that would allow the equitable distribution of vaccines to all countries across the globe. By the end of 2020, almost all the high, middle and low-income countries had signed onto the COVAX plan, however achieving the goal of equitable delivery of 2 billion doses of these vaccines globally by the end of 2021 remains in doubt.

b. Prioritizing groups for vaccination

The process for determining how much of the available COVID-19 vaccines are delivered to a country participating in the COVAX program is determined by a Fair Allocation mechanism. This mechanism was set up by the WHO and Gavi with consultation from the participating COVAX member countries. The two groups that determine the allocation amount are the Joint Allocation Taskforce (JAT) composed of WHO and Gavi staff and the Independent Allocation Vaccine Group (IAVG), which is made up of 12 independent committee experts that validate the JAT staff recommendations.[59]

Each country across the globe is responsible for developing policies for how their vaccine supply will be prioritized. Initially, most countries prioritized COVID-19 vaccines for those at the highest risk of developing serious disease, along with front-line health and social workers.[60] The prioritization policies for the timing of who gets vaccine doses vary across the globe based on the availability of the vaccine and the impact of the pandemic on various groups (Figure 5.64). Prioritizing vaccines based on the risk of being infected with SARS-COV-2 and the severity of disease for those who are infected can be complex. There are many facets to each individual's risk, including the interface between the risk of age (i.e., the greater the age, the greater the risk), underlying high-risk conditions (e.g., obesity, diabetes, cardiovascular disease, cancer, HIV), racial disparities (e.g., higher risk of infection and/or severe disease in Black and Hispanic populations), essential occupations (e.g., healthcare workers, food handlers) and other characteristics.

The WHO published two documents in September 2020 to provide guidance to all countries on these issues, and both have been endorsed by the WHO's Strategic Advisory Group of Experts on Immunization (SAGE). The Values Framework offers guidance on the allocation of COVID-19 vaccines among countries and the prioritization of groups for vaccination within countries while supply is limited.[61] The Framework is intended to be helpful to policymakers and expert advisors at the global, national and regional levels as they make allocation and prioritization decisions about COVID-19 vaccines. The Framework articulates the overall goal of the COVID19 vaccine deployment, provides six core principles to guide distribution and 12 objectives that further elucidate the six principles[61] (Table 5.17). The Values Framework listed over 20 population subgroups that, if vaccines need to be prioritized due to limited supply, would advance one or more of its principles and objectives that are noted in the Framework.

The Values Framework did not rank the subgroups in any order. To assist in developing recommendations for the use of COVID-19 vaccines, SAGE proposed a Prioritization Roadmap of COVID-19 vaccines that considers priority groups based on epidemiologic settings and vaccine supply scenarios,[62] as well as recommendations for priority cases for COVID-19 vaccines in the context of limited supply. These scenarios suggest priority groups based on the epidemiology of virus transmission (no cases, sporadic/cluster of cases and community transmission) and varying vaccine supplies for the population (three stages: very limited vaccine supply of 1–10%, limited supply for 11–20%, and moderate supply for 21–50% of the population).

Table 5.17. WHO's values framework for allocation and prioritization of COVID-19 vaccination.[61]

Goal Statement	COVID-19 vaccines must be a global public good. The overarching goal is for COVID-19 vaccines to contribute significantly to the equitable protection and promotion of human well-being among all people of the world.
Principles	**Objectives**
Human Well-being	— Reduce societal and economic disruption by containing transmission, reducing severe disease and death, or a combination of these strategies. — Protect the continuing functioning of essential services, including health services.

Table 5.17. *(Continued)*

Equal Respect	— Treat the interests of all individuals and groups with equal consideration as allocation and priority-setting decisions are being taken and implemented. — Offer a meaningful opportunity for the vaccine to all individuals and groups who qualify by prioritization criteria.
Global Equity	— Ensure that vaccine allocation takes into account the special epidemic risks and needs of all countries, particularly low-and middle-income countries. — Ensure that all countries commit to meeting the needs of people living in countries that cannot secure vaccine for their populations on their own, particularly low- and middle-income countries.
National Equity	— Ensure that vaccine prioritization within countries takes into account the vulnerabilities, risks and needs of groups who, because of underlying societal, geographic or biomedical factors, are at risk of experiencing greater burdens from the COVID-19 pandemic. — Develop the immunization delivery systems and infrastructure required to ensure COVID-19 vaccine access to priority populations and take proactive action to ensure equal access to everyone who qualifies under a priority group, particularly socially disadvantaged populations.
Reciprocity	Reciprocity protects those who bear significant additional risks and burdens of COVID-19 to safeguard the welfare of others, including healthcare and other essential workers.
Legitimacy	Employ best available scientific evidence, expertise, and significant engagement with relevant stakeholders for vaccine prioritization between various groups within each country, using transparent, accountable, and unbiased processes to engender deserved trust in prioritization decisions.

i. *High risk including elderly and healthcare workers*

The Roadmap also contains guidance on how to apply the recommendations for different contingencies based on vaccine safety, efficacy and uptake; number of vaccine types, epidemic conditions and immune status of the population; and social, economic and legal considerations. An example of guidance provided by the Roadmap is that in a country with substantial community transmission with a very limited supply of vaccine (<10%), the vaccine should first be given to healthcare workers (HCWs) at high risk of contracting disease and thereafter to the elderly populations with age cut-offs based on vaccine supply. This Roadmap is applicable to low-middle and high-income countries as guidance, but countries are free to alter it as they deem appropriate. The US used this same approach during the initial rollout of vaccine in December 2020,[63] while the Ivory Coast modified it to also include their armed forces and teachers.[64] Substantial variation in the policies of countries determining who should get priority for COVID-19 vaccines is shown in Figure 5.64.

Which groups should be prioritized often raises a myriad of ethical issues as the available vaccine increases. Once all those who are >65 years have been offered the vaccine, many countries add on other risk groups to be prioritized, but choosing which groups can be problematic. For example, should it be those with chronic diseases that put them at high risk for severe COVID-19 disease, caretakers of people who cannot provide for themselves, or other important occupations that were initially not included? Each of these groups may not only compete for vaccine doses against other groups but also within their own group. For example, for those with chronic underlying disease, should someone with cystic fibrosis be given higher priority than someone with pulmonary fibrosis or chronic liver disease? In some instances, there is sufficient data to determine who is at greatest risk from COVID-19 (e.g., an obese person with diabetes and cardiovascular disease is known

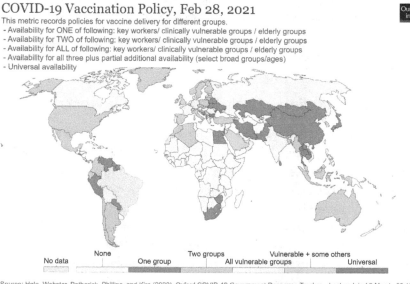

COVID-19 Vaccination Policy, Feb 28, 2021

This metric records policies for vaccine delivery for different groups.
- Availability for ONE of following: key workers/ clinically vulnerable groups / elderly groups
- Availability for TWO of following: key workers/ clinically vulnerable groups / elderly groups
- Availability for ALL of following: key workers/ clinically vulnerable groups / elderly groups
- Availability for all three plus partial additional availability (select broad groups/ages)
- Universal availability

Our World in Data

| | None | | Two groups | | Vulnerable + some others | |
| No data | | One group | | All vulnerable groups | | Universal |

Source: Hale, Webster, Petherick, Phillips, and Kira (2020). Oxford COVID-19 Government Response Tracker – Last updated 9 March, 03:15 (London time)
OurWorldInData.org/coronavirus • CC BY

Figure 5.64. Vaccination prioritization policies of various countries.[60]

to be at very high risk). However, for most chronic diseases, the relative risk amongst different chronic diseases has not yet been determined.[65] In many instances, determining which chronic disease gets the vaccine first is dependent on the effectiveness of particular advocacy groups.

ii. *Do people known to have been infected with SARS-CoV-2 need vaccination or can they wait?*

Various ideas were proposed on how the number of people vaccinated within the confines of inadequate numbers of doses could be increased. The question of whether those who had already had COVID-19 disease really needed two doses of vaccine was considered. Most countries initially took the approach that everyone, including those known to have gotten the disease, should still get two doses since there was insufficient data to recommend doing otherwise. However, England took an alternative approach: they immunized everyone with the first dose before anyone was given the second dose but still immunized those who had previously had the disease. This was done to first provide some protection to everyone but was not really a dose sparing strategy. In February 2021, a non-peer-reviewed study was published, suggesting that those who had previously gotten the disease had a robust antibody response to the first dose of vaccine.[66] Some countries considered giving only one dose of a COVID-19 vaccine to those who are known to have been infected, but no country has yet made this decision.

c. **Delivery of vaccines to vaccinations sites**

The delivery of the COVID-19 vaccine to sites where people can be immunized is another critical step in the process of implementing the COVID-19 vaccination programs. Countries that are not part of UNICEF's supply chain must plan and implement all the logistic steps, including ensuring the vaccine arrives and is stored at the appropriate temperature. Once the vaccine arrives at the vaccination site, there needs to be a registration and appointment process as well as sufficient number of trained vaccinators to give the vaccine. To ensure that the vaccination process does not become a super-spreader event, long queues need to be avoided.

Planning the logistic steps needed to immunize a large number of people has proven to be difficult for many countries. In many low and middle-income countries, UNICEF has substantial experience that will help deal with delivery problems. However, there are longstanding problems that will be difficult to overcome even with the increased resources available due to the pandemic. The pandemic has resulted in further problems with routine immunization, but even in 2019, prior to the onset of the COVID-19 pandemic, only ~85% of all eligible children worldwide received their third dose of diphtheria, tetanus toxoids and pertussis-containing vaccine (DTP), polio, and the first dose of measles-containing vaccines.[67] Even more startling, there were ~14 million eligible children who did not receive even their first dose of DTP vaccine (i.e., zero-dose children). Many under-immunized children live in hard-to-reach, fragile and/or conflict settings. While children will not be prioritized to get COVID-19 vaccines in 2021, many of the reasons why these children are not vaccinated will also apply to their adult family members. The specific logistic issues surrounding vaccine delivery as well as the acceptance of vaccines, including COVID-19, by various communities, will need to be solved (see the next section on vaccine hesitancy).

Many high-income countries also had major logistic problems with the timely delivery of vaccines. Some of these problems are shared across the globe, including insufficient needles, syringes and other supplies needed for vaccination. Other problems such as adequate cold storage capacity are less of a problem in high-income countries. However, some of the most important issues relate to the competence of the government to create a comprehensive cohesive plan.

i. *How well did various countries do in rolling out vaccines?*

Israel was the most successful country in vaccinating its population in a timely manner, with ~90% of its Jewish population having received at least one dose of vaccine by the end of February 2021.[68] The vaccination rates of the various countries that are highlighted in Chapter 3 are shown in comparison to Israel, which vaccinated a much greater percentage of its population as of the end of February 2021[68] (Figure 5.65). Israel's success was based on a number of factors, including having contracted with Pfizer for accelerated access to their vaccine in exchange for paying a higher price for the vaccine than paid by other high-income countries. Israel's government

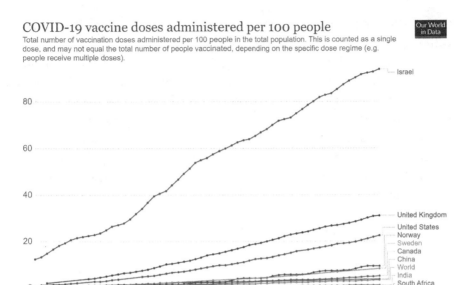

COVID-19 vaccine doses administered per 100 people

Total number of vaccination doses administered per 100 people in the total population. This is counted as a single dose, and may not equal the total number of people vaccinated, depending on the specific dose regime (e.g. people receive multiple doses).

Source: Official data collated by Our World in Data   CC BY

Figure 5.65. COVID-19 vaccines administrated per 100 people by the end of February 2020 in the countries highlighted in Chapter 3, except for Jordan and Iran (who had not yet received any vaccines at that time).[68]

also agreed to give Pfizer anonymized data on those who were vaccinated, which allowed the company to collect more detailed data on the safety and effectiveness of the vaccine in people with various underlying health conditions. Israel was able to provide these data because it has universal healthcare with digitized data on each person.[69] This increased supply of vaccines in conjunction with their healthcare system, which has very good logistic capability, allowing for the rapid vaccination of their population. Israel's government felt the extra price paid for the vaccine was worthwhile since they believed it would allow them to decrease the number and duration of lockdowns in their country and thereby help the economy.

However, two ethical issues arose with this approach.[69] Allowing Pfizer access to healthcare data on each citizen enabled Pfizer to gather information about how its vaccine functioned in various age groups and individuals with a variety of medical conditions, which is helpful to not only Pfizer but those groups making vaccine recommendations. However, the agreement also raises privacy issues in that the Pfizer data on ~140,000

COVID-19-positive patients was turned over to Israel's security division without the consent of COVID-19-infected individuals.

The other ethical issue raised by Israel's vaccination program was that the vaccine went only to its own citizens. Palestinians living in Israel's occupied territories were not included in the initial program. The government insisted that this was the responsibility of the Palestinian Authority: however others argued that the Fourth Geneva Convention indicates that the duty falls on the occupying country. Substantial global pressure finally persuaded Israel to start vaccinating these Palestinians in early March 2021.[70]

Most of the countries in the European Union had major problems with the timely receipt and delivery of vaccines.[71,72] The European Commission was responsible for negotiating advance purchase agreements with the vaccine companies for all 27 member countries. This was done to help ensure a more equitable distribution of the vaccine once a vaccine is approved by the EMA. While the Commission was able to buy COVID-19 vaccines at a somewhat cheaper price than some other high-income countries (~10–20% less), the rollout of the vaccine was slower. European Union President Ursula von der Leyen was fiercely criticized for the slow rollout of COVID-19 vaccines.[72] She admitted that the Commission was late in granting authorization for the vaccine and too optimistic about the ability to mass-produce and deliver COVID-19 vaccines. This issue was heightened by the rapid rollout of the Pfizer and AstraZeneca vaccines in the UK in early December 2020 (the UK was no longer a member of the European Union at that point). By the middle of February 2021, 23% of the population in the UK had received one dose of the vaccine compared to <1% of those living in the European Union. The UK had signed an earlier contract with AstraZeneca that had assured high priority for their vaccine, while the European Union reached an agreement with the company months later and the contract did not guarantee high priority for the delivery of the doses. The Pfizer vaccine was made in plants within the European Union, and in January 2021, the European Commission threatened to withhold delivery of Pfizer's COVID-19 vaccine to the UK. However, the Commission quickly backed off from this threat after intense criticism from Ireland's government and others.

Not everyone feels the criticism is justified. Some experts believed the UK rushed the process. They felt it was better to thoroughly examine the data before pushing out the vaccine, noting that a problem with the vaccine would cause the public to lose confidence in it. Others felt the European Commission was doing a reasonably good job in very difficult circumstances and adapting as needed. It also needs to be pointed out that the approach the UK took violated the COVAX agreement it had previously signed onto.[52]

The US and a few other high-income countries that did not sign the COVAX agreement had a greater supply of vaccines for use than countries that signed with the COVAX program. Despite this, the US was less successful than Israel in vaccinating its population. The US Operation Warp speed focused on getting high numbers of doses manufactured but lacked a nationwide cohesive plan to get the vaccines delivered to immunization centers that had trained personnel prepared to rapidly identify and vaccinate large numbers of people prioritized to get the vaccine. There were multiple bottlenecks blocking the ability of states to immunize those prioritized to receive the vaccines.[73,74] Once the vaccines were manufactured, the federal government determined how many vaccine doses each state received, and there was not a sufficient number of doses to meet the initial high demand. Furthermore, many states were unsure when the vaccine would arrive, how many doses they would receive, and when they would get more doses. This led vaccine centers to hold onto a second dose for every dose they gave, to assure those who had gotten their first dose would get the second dose a month later.

Each state had a website where people could determine if they were eligible for the vaccine, and if so, schedule an appointment. However, the software used for these websites differed in various states, and in some states, the website frequently crashed due to large numbers of queries. Most states also had a phone number to call, but people often could not get through. Many states also did not have a centralized dashboard that enabled knowing how many vaccine doses were given each day and to whom, thus making it hard to anticipate when to order more vaccines from the federal government. In various places across the US, people had to stand in long lines for hours to get the vaccine, increasing the risk of the SARS-CoV-2 virus being transmitted between people.[74]

Under the Biden administration, these issues are now being resolved, and it is anticipated that by May 2021, there will be enough vaccines available to all states for any adult who wants one.[74,75] During the first quarter of 2021, as vaccine production increased, the state and local Public Health systems were able to administer the vaccines in a timely manner after they arrived. Furthermore, state and local Public Health workers and others are reaching out to communities to make it easier on those who have difficulties getting to vaccine centers and/or are hesitant about getting the vaccine.

The Israel, Europe, US and COVAX vaccine delivery programs each provide an example of the many logistical problems and ethical issues raised by trying to produce vaccines and immunize large populations of people in a short period of time. The approach taken by Israel was clearly the most successful in rapidly immunizing its population, but it cost the most and raised important ethical issues. The European approach resulted in somewhat lower prices for the vaccine but also resulted in intense criticism from some experts and the public for delays in rolling out the vaccine program. The US COVID-19 vaccination program had the potential to be delivered as quickly as in Israel, but the rollout was very fragmented and, therefore, slower. The COVAX program solves some of the equity problems previously seen in the 2009 influenza pandemic in low and middle-income countries, but the slow rollout leaves these countries and the entire globe at risk for the development of new variants and other problems. Much remains to be learned about the best approach to implementing a vaccine program during this and future pandemics.

Key Point: The initial vaccines that received EUAs had better efficacy than expected, but until they are injected into the arms of people, this does not matter. During the first six months after the vaccine approval, the demand for vaccines far exceeded the supply in almost every country across the globe. There are many reasons this happened and many lessons to be learned.

---

4. Vaccine Hesitancy

a. Overview of issues impacting vaccine hesitancy

Vaccine hesitancy is a general term with a large number of causes. Over the past several decades, the WHO has become very concerned that vaccine hesitancy is increasing across the globe and in 2019 listed vaccine hesitancy as one of the top ten threats to global health.[76] Previously SAGE formed a Vaccine Hesitancy working group in 2012 to help determine the various causes of vaccine hesitancy and suggest potential solutions. The findings were presented at the SAGE biannual meeting on October 23, 2014, and published in 2015.[77] The working group noted that the term "vaccine hesitancy" included a wide spectrum of beliefs: full acceptance, delaying vaccination, refusal of some vaccines, and refusal of all vaccines despite the availability of vaccines and vaccination services. They noted that vaccine hesitancy is complex and context-specific, varying across time, place and vaccines. It is influenced by factors such as: complacency (increases if the individual perceives the risk of the disease to be low), convenience (how easy it is to get the vaccine), confidence (trust in the effectiveness and safety of vaccines), the system that delivers them (including the reliability and competence of the health services and health professionals), and the motivations of policymakers who decide on the need for the vaccine. These reasons for vaccine hesitancy can be present in low, middle and high-income countries. Those who are opposed to the use of vaccines for use against all diseases often use one or more of these issues to spread doubt about the safety and/or effectiveness of vaccines, including COVID-19 vaccines.

The SAGE Vaccine Hesitancy working group developed a vaccine Hesitancy Matrix Table that notes many of the issues that affect why an individual or group may be hesitant[77] (Table 5.18). They noted that while higher socioeconomic status and education lead to better health, these two determinants do not influence hesitancy in only one direction. Indeed, there are individuals and groups within the higher education category who span the spectrum from accepting all vaccines to rejecting all vaccines.

b. COVID-19 and vaccine hesitancy

Concerns about the impact that vaccine hesitancy would have on the uptake of COVID-19 vaccines were raised at the beginning of the pandemic, and surveys began to look at this issue months before the first EUA COVID-19 vaccines became available. For example, a survey of 13,426 people in 19 countries across Asia, the Americas, Europe and Africa was done in June 2020 to examine potential acceptance rates and factors influencing the acceptance of a COVID-19 vaccine.[78] Overall, approximately 72% of the

Table 5.18.   Vaccine Hesitancy Determinants.[77]

Contextual Influences Influences arising due to historic, socio-cultural, environmental, health system/institutional, economic or political factors	a. Communication and media environment b. Influential leaders, immunization program gatekeepers, and anti- or pro-vaccination lobbies c. Historical influences d. Religion/culture/gender/socioeconomic e. Politics/policies f. Geographic barriers g. Perception of the pharmaceutical industry
Individual and Group Influences Influences arising from personal perception of the vaccine or influences of the social/peer environment	a. Personal, family and/or community members' experience with vaccination, including pain b. Beliefs, attitudes about health and prevention c. Knowledge/awareness d. Health system and providers — trust and personal experience e. Risk/benefit (perceived, heuristic) f. Immunization as a social norm vs. not needed/harmful
Vaccine/vaccination — specific issues directly related to vaccine or vaccination	a. Risk/benefit (epidemiological and scientific evidence) b. Introduction of a new vaccine or new formulation or a new recommendation for an existing vaccine c. Mode of administration d. Design of vaccination program/Mode of delivery (e.g., routine program or mass vaccination campaign) e. Reliability and/or source of supply of vaccine and/or vaccination equipment f. Vaccination schedule g. Costs h. The strength of the recommendation and/or knowledge base and/or attitude of healthcare professionals

participants reported that they would be "very" or "somewhat likely to accept" a COVID-19 vaccine.

A more recent survey done from October 21 to December 16, 2020, in 32 countries from all regions revealed a wide range in the prevalence of vaccine hesitancy across the globe.[79] (Table 5.19). Overall the Asian countries had the highest percentage of people willing to receive COVID-19 vaccines, while Europe had the highest prevalence of vaccine hesitancy. This survey differs from the survey done in the middle of 2020 since several COVID-19 vaccines were known to be under consideration for EUA approval. While there are some commonalities between regions and countries, what makes vaccine hesitancy so difficult to deal with is that many of the reasons are individual- and/or community-specific.

Table 5.19. Survey of the willingness of those living in various countries in different regions to be vaccinated with a COVID-19 vaccine.[79]*

Country	Region	% Willing to be Vaccinated	% Unwilling to be Vaccinated
China	Asia	91%	9%
India	Asia	91%	9%
Brazil	Americas	83%	17%
UK	Europe	81%	19%
Canada	Americas	77%	23%
Hong Kong	Asia	74%	26%
USA	Americas	66%	34%
Nigeria	Africa	64%	36%
Lebanon	EMRO	44%	56%
France	Europe	44%	56%

*The Table is modified to show 10 of the 32 countries that were surveyed for vaccine hesitancy. The countries shown for each region were reasonably representative in showing the prevalence of vaccine hesitancy in their region.

i. Examples of vaccine hesitancy across regions and countries

Prior to the pandemic, there were already important lessons learned on the impact community concerns might have on vaccine uptake. During the 2018 Ebola outbreak in the Democratic Republic of the Congo, many people living in the affected areas were refusing the Ebola vaccine for various reasons, including mistrust of the government and false rumors being spread by militant groups and others about the vaccine. The militants did not want outside organizations such as the WHO and Doctors without Borders providing care within their area. Solving this problem was greatly aided by the engagement of community leaders and anthropologists who understood the issues.[80] Additional approaches to reducing hesitancy are discussed at the end of this chapter.

The Americas region typically has a higher vaccination rate than other regions. The Pan American Health Organization (PAHO) has a revolving fund mechanism where most countries in the region pay into a fund that allows the purchase of large quantities of vaccines at reduced prices compared to high-income countries. However, PAHO has a substantial number of zero-dose or under-immunized children living in hard-to-reach areas.[81] Additionally, during the past decade, PAHO has seen increased levels of vaccine-preventable diseases due to political disruption (e.g., Venezuela) and, in the case of the COVID-19 vaccine, attempts by some politicians to discourage vaccination (e.g., Brazil's President Bolsonaro).[82]

The US provides another example of where one of the most important reasons for vaccine hesitancy has a unique aspect. A monthly survey done from April 1, 2020, through December 8, 2020, initially showed that ~75% of the people were likely to be vaccinated, but by December 2020, this was down to <60%.[83] One major factor that is highly correlated with whether a person intends to take the vaccine is their political party affiliation. A national poll done in March 2021 showed over 33% of those who identify with the Republican Party indicated they would not be vaccinated compared to 10% of the Democrats.[84] Although President Trump promoted Operation Warp Speed which helped rapidly develop COVID-19 vaccines, his public downplaying of the seriousness of the pandemic and his disparaging of public health measures contributed to many of his followers indicating that they would not be vaccinated. In December 2020, Trump rescinded plans for White House staff to be vaccinated, and he waited until March 2021 to announce that he had gotten the vaccine, and only then did he encourage others to get the vaccine.[85] The correlation between whether a person accepts or rejects the vaccine is not a direct effect of either party's political platform. Rather, it more likely relates to how those who identify themselves as Republicans or Democrats weigh the importance of individual rights versus public good and their view of the role of government in making recommendations for individuals.

Since President Biden took over the US Presidency on January 20, 2021, polls show that an increasing percentage (~70%) of the US population is willing to be vaccinated.[86] Another big problem that the Biden administration is trying to overcome is that while the burden of COVID-19 disease is significantly higher in minority and other socioeconomically disadvantaged populations, these groups have substantially lower vaccination rates due to various issues discussed later in this section.[87]

Europe appears to be the WHO region with the highest rate of vaccine hesitancy.[88] The European Centre for Disease Prevention and Control (ECDC), in collaboration with the Rapid European COVID-19 Emergency

Response research (RECOVER) Social Sciences team, published a policy brief based on their latest study of the public's views of COVID-19 vaccination in seven European countries — France, Germany, Belgium, Italy, Spain, Sweden, and Ukraine.[89] The data shows that <50% of the respondents in each country believed that COVID-19 vaccines were safe. Furthermore, even if the vaccines were found to be safe and effective and provided at no cost, only 44–66% of the respondents would agree to be vaccinated.

Those accepting vaccination emphasized the benefits of protecting the health of themselves, their families, and society. They also highlighted the importance of vaccination to put an end to the pandemic, to resume a normal life, and to restore the economy. Nevertheless, vaccine safety concerns were important in all countries, with many respondents from France, Spain and Sweden convinced that safety considerations were being bypassed in vaccine development. While trust in medical personnel was consistently high across all countries, mistrust of global and national authorities and pharmaceutical companies, who are thought to pursue financial and political interests above those of public health, was a widely held view.

The Asian region has three countries (i.e., Vietnam, India and China) where >90% of the populations indicate they would accept COVID-19 vaccines[79] (Table 5.19). This certainly suggests that this region has the least vaccine hesitancy. However, vaccine hesitancy has not yet been widely studied or characterized in Asia.[90] Some Asian countries, including Bangladesh, Bhutan, India, Myanmar, Nepal, Pakistan, and Sri Lanka, have high numbers of zero-dose and under-vaccinated children. While part of this problem relates to reaching hard-to-access areas, vaccine hesitancy clearly exists in various countries relating to religious beliefs, conspiracy stories, and poor communication about the benefits of vaccines and safety concerns.

ii. *How vaccine hesitancy in one region can affect another region*

Vaccine hesitancy issues that arise in one region can have a substantial impact in other regions. Many African countries had little or no vaccines during the first quarter of 2021. Most of these countries were awaiting shipment of the AstraZeneca vaccine, which was the main vaccine initially purchased by the COVAX facility, since the price was substantially lower than the other vaccines, and less-stringent cold-chain requirements made them easier to ship. This inequity in vaccine supply was in large part due to a number of the high-income countries not honoring their equity commitment.

Some of the AstraZeneca vaccines in Europe became available to Africa when the population of various European countries became concerned that the AstraZeneca vaccine might be less effective than the Pfizer vaccine and might cause blood clots. Many of these countries put a hold on the AstraZeneca vaccine and asked the EMA to reconsider its approval of the vaccine. Less than a week later, the EMA met to review recent data and concluded that the available data supported the continued use of the vaccine. Despite a third wave causing an increasing number of COVID-19 cases in various European countries, the concerns about the AstraZeneca vaccine had substantially decreased the demand for this vaccine in Europe.[91] The WHO Regional Director for Africa used this situation to acquire a sizeable supply of the AstraZeneca vaccine for Angola, Ethiopia and Ghana, who had little vaccine supply but a substantial pent-up demand.[92]

At the same time, South Africa decided to sell its supply of the AstraZeneca vaccine since it was found that it did not protect against mild-moderate disease caused by the B.1.135 SARS-CoV-2 variant strain that was predominant in that country (studies of the efficacy of the AstraZeneca vaccine against severe disease caused by B.1.135 had not been completed at that point). Five other African countries where the B.1.135 strain was not predominant received the vaccine and South Africa began purchasing the Johnson-Johnson vaccine that had ~50% efficacy against this strain.[93] Thus, while Europe (for reasons related to vaccine hesitancy), and South Africa (for reasons of decreased vaccine efficacy against the predominant SARS-CoV-2 strain in their country) used less of the AstraZeneca vaccine, other African countries were happy to receive the vaccine.

The irony is that soon after the EMA once again indicated that the AstraZeneca vaccine was safe and effective on March 18, 2021,[91] and most European countries again started to use it, the European Union banned the export of all vaccines made in Europe.[94] This ban was mainly aimed at AstraZeneca, which had decreased the number of doses that Europe had been receiving, but it also affected the other COVID-19 vaccines with manufacturing sites in Europe.

c. Overcoming vaccine hesitancy

Over the past decade, our understanding of both the scope and reasons for vaccine hesitancy has improved. Studies note that there are many reasons for vaccine hesitancy and that careful listening and good communication are two keys to overcoming public concerns and distrust.[95] Governments and other organizations (e.g., regulators, public health authorities, etc.) involved in making vaccine recommendations need to be transparent and clear on why they made the recommendations. Also, those involved in implementing the vaccine program (e.g., physicians, nurses, community workers, etc.) need to understand what the concerns are at the community and individual levels and help address these concerns.

The European Centre for Disease Control and Prevention, in collaboration with the RECOVER social science team, has noted four approaches for promoting the COVID-19 or other vaccines used in an emergency to the European Union public and overcoming misleading information that is inadvertently or purposefully spread.[88] The approaches include messages focusing on the many benefits of mass vaccination in an emergency, targeted messages that deal with specific concerns that have been raised, providing support to health care workers to promote vaccination, and working with journalists from a range of media to facilitate accurate and comprehensive coverage of vaccination issues.

Negative media coverage of the pandemic, including about vaccines, can be detrimental and lead to hesitancy.[96] Figure 5.66 shows the percentage of negative media pandemic coverage in the US versus internationally. The media coverage in the US was more negative than most other places over the first half of 2020. Negativity was estimated using supervised machine learning on article phrases coupled with a training data set. Articles were manually downloaded from LexisNexis for the period January 1, 2020, to July 31, 2020. The US media coverage continued to be negative even when the number of COVID-19 cases was decreasing. In contrast, in other countries, the negative media coverage decreased as cases decreased. The negative coverage in the US did not significantly change over the study period and was similar in both liberal and conservative media outlets. The reasons why US coverage is more negative remain to be determined.

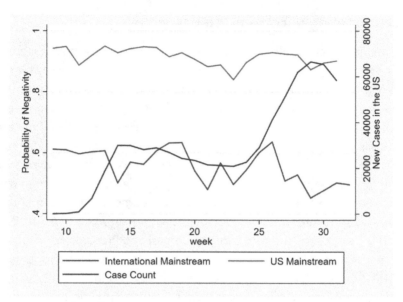

Figure 5.66.   Percentage of negative media coverage in the US versus international media coverage. "Negativity" was estimated using supervised machine learning on article phrases coupled with a training data set. Articles were manually downloaded from LexisNexis from January 1, 2020, to July 31, 2020. The red line shows the weekly average of daily newly confirmed COVID-19 cases. From NBER Working Paper Series, WHY IS ALL COVID-19 NEWS BAD NEWS?[96]

Regardless, studies clearly show that negative media coverage, whether on mainstream or social media sites, can increase vaccine hesitancy.[97–99]

Another issue critical to controlling the pandemic in the US and other countries is that minority populations are often less likely to get vaccinated. Through March 1, 2021, the percentage of the White, Black and Hispanic populations in the US that had received at least one dose of a COVID-19 vaccine was 25%, 15%, and 13%, respectively.[100] There are a multitude of reasons for this, including concerns about being deported if they are not US citizens, previous mistreatment by the government, lack of transport to vaccination sites, lack of access to the Internet, lack of information in Spanish, and a loss of pay if they miss work.[100,101] Dealing with these and other issues requires knowledge of the specific issues that individuals and communities are facing, along with clear answers from people they trust, whether they are healthcare, community workers or other people they trust. This all takes time and effort but is vital to overcoming vaccine hesitancy.

Key Point: There are many reasons for vaccine hesitancy, and behavioral science-based studies are helping to provide answers on various steps that can be taken to overcome this problem. Countries and organizations throughout the world are paying more attention to vaccine hesitancy, not only for emergency situations but also routine times, to help increase the uptake of recommended vaccines.

5. Conclusion

The availability of multiple COVID-19 vaccines by the end of 2020 is nothing short of remarkable, and in the future, some of these new vaccine platforms will help us deal with new disease outbreaks. However, we have yet to learn how to equitably deal with worldwide pandemics. At the end of June 2021, high-income countries had 70% of the global COVID-19 vaccine supply despite having only 16% of the world's population (Figure 5.67). While the world is well aware of the inequity of vaccine distribution that occurred in the

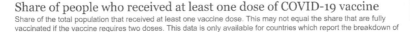

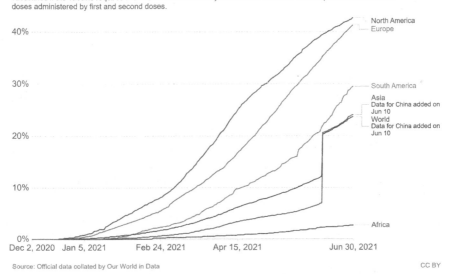

Figure 5.67. Share of people vaccinated with at least one dose of COVID-19 vaccines, as of June 30, 2021.[57]

2009 influenza pandemic, the equitable distribution of COVID-19 vaccines was not achieved despite the development of the COVAX program that was meant to overcome this issue.[102] It will serve us well in the future to figure out a workable solution to overcome this equity problem along with some of the other ethical considerations regarding the development and use of pandemic vaccines. Some of these other ethical issues are highlighted in Chapter 6 and potential solutions to the inequitable global distribution of vaccines are discussed in Chapter 9.

References

1. Jenner E. (1801) *An Inquiry into the Causes and Effects of the Variolae Vaccinae: A Disease Discovered in Some of the Western Counties of England, Particularly Gloucestershire, and Known by the Name of the Cow Pox.* Ashley & Brewer, London.

2. Wikipedia. (nd) Vaccine-preventable diseases. https://en.wikipedia.org/wiki/Vaccine-preventable_diseases. Accessed: December 31, 2021.

3. Richie H, Ortiz-Opsina E, Bellekian D, *et al.* (nd) Vaccine Innovations from 1880 to 2020. OurWorldinData.org. https://ourworldindata.org/vaccination#vaccine-innovation. Accessed: February 10, 2020.

4. Ball P. (2020) The lightning-fast quest for COVID vaccines — and what it means for other diseases. *Nature*, December 18. https://www.nature.com/articles/d41586-020-03626-1

5. WHO. (nd) Draft landscape and tracker of COVID-19 candidate vaccines. World Health Organization. https://www.who.int/publications/m/item/draft-landscape-of-covid-19-candidate-vaccines. Accessed: February 16, 2021.

6. Miller J. (2020) Explainer: How does AstraZeneca's vaccine compare with Pfizer-BioNTech? *Reuters*, December 30. https://www.reuters.com/article/uk-health-coronavirus-vaccines-astrazene/explainer-how-does-astrazenecas-vaccine-compare-with-pfizer-biontech-idUKKBN2941PE?edition-redirect=uk

7. Sutton S. (2020) When fast science spells bad science. *The Medicine Maker*, September 2. https://themedicinemaker.com/manufacture/when-fast-science-spells-bad-science

8. Nikolskaya P, Ivanova P. (2020) Exclusive-Russia ships only first part of COVID-19 vaccine to Argentina — sources. *Reuters*, December 28. https://www.reuters.com/article/us-health-coronavirus-russia-vaccine-arg/

exclusive-russia-ships-only-first-part-of-covid-19-vaccine-to-argentina-sources-idUSKBN2920XP

9. Logunov DY, Dolzhikova IV, VShcheblyakov D, *et al.* (2021) Safety and efficacy of an rAd26 and rAd5 vector-based heterologous prime-boost COVID-19 vaccine: An interim analysis of a randomized controlled phase 3 trial in Russia. *Lancet* **397**:20–22. DOI:10.1016/S0140-6736(21)00234-8.

10. Jibilian I. (2020) Here's how the top 3 coronavirus vaccines compare when it comes to efficacy, cost, and more. *Insider*, December 7. https://www.businessinsider.com/how-covid-vaccines-compare-cost-astrazeneca-oxford-pfizer-biontech-moderna-2020-11

11. Polack FP, Thomas SJ, Kitchin N. *et al.* (2020) Safety and efficacy of the BNT162b2 mRNA covid-19 vaccine. *New England Journal of Medicine* **383**:2603–2615. DOI:10.1056/NEJMoa2034577

12. Baden LR, El Sahly HM, Essink B, *et al.* (2021) Efficacy and safety of mRNA-1273 SARS-CoV-2 vaccine. *New England Journal of Medicine* **384**:403–416. DOI:10.1056/NEJMoa2035389. https://www.nejm.org/doi/full/10.1056/NEJMoa2035389

13. Voysey M, Costa Clemens SA, Madhi SA *et al.* (2021) Safety and efficacy of the ChAdOx1 nCoV-19 vaccine (AZD1222) against SARS-CoV-2: an interim analysis of four randomized controlled trials in Brazil, South Africa, and the UK. *Lancet* **397**:99–111. DOI:https://doi.org/10.1016/S0140-6736(20)32661-1

14. Logunov DY, Dolzhikova IV, Zubkova OV, *et al.* (2020) Safety and immunogenicity of an rAd26 and rAd5 vector-based heterologous prime-boost COVID-19 vaccine in two formulations: Two open, non-randomized phase 1/2 studies from Russia. *Lancet* **396**:887–897.

15. Taylor P. (2020) Russian Sputnik COVID-19 vaccine "will cost less than $10 a dose". *PharmaPhorum*, November 24. https://pharmaphorum.com/news/russian-sputnik-covid-19-vaccine-will-cost-less-than-10-a-dose/

16. CEPI. (2021) A world in which epidemics and pandemics are no longer a threat to humanity. https://cepi.net/about/whyweexist/

17. CEPI. (2021) Priority Diseases https://cepi.net/research_dev/priority-diseases/

18. EMA. (2019) Ebola virus. European Medicines Agency, October 18. https://www.ema.europa.eu/en/human-regulatory/overview/public-health-threats/ebola

19. FDA. (2020) First FDA-approved vaccine for the prevention of Ebola virus disease, marking a critical milestone in public health preparedness and response. News Release, Food and Drug Administration, December 19.

https://www.fda.gov/news-events/press-announcements/first-fda-approved-vaccine-prevention-ebola-virus-disease-marking-critical-milestone-public-health

20. Mendonça, S.A., Lorincz, R., Boucher, P. *et al.* (2021) Adenoviral vector vaccine platforms in the SARS-CoV-2 pandemic. npj Vaccines 6, 97 (2021). https://doi.org/10.1038/s41541-021-00356-x

21. Wikipedia. (nd) COVID-19 vaccines. https://en.wikipedia.org/wiki/COVID-19_vaccine. Accessed: February 19, 2020.

22. Forni G, Mantovani A; COVID-19 Commission of Accademia Nazionale dei Lincei. (2021) COVID-19 vaccines: Where we stand and challenges ahead. *Cell Death & Differentiation* **28:**626–639. https://doi.org/10.1038/s41418-020-00720-9

23. Chowdhury MA, Hossain N, Kashem MA, *et al.* (2020) Immune response in COVID-19: A review. *Journal of Infection and Public Health* **13:**1619–1629. DOI:10.1016/j.jiph.2020.07.001. https://pubmed.ncbi.nlm.nih.gov/32718895/

24. Poland GA, Ovsyannikova IG, Kennedy RB. (2020) SARS-CoV-2 immunity: Review and applications to phase 3 vaccine candidates. *Lancet* **396:**1595–1606. https://www.thelancet.com/action/showPdf?pii=S0140-6736%2820%2932137-1

25. Aschwanden C. (2020) The false promise of herd immunity for COVID-19. *Nature* **587:**26–28. https://doi.org/10.1038/d41586-020-02948-4

26. CDC COVID-19 Response Team; Food and Drug Administration. (2020) Allergic reactions including anaphylaxis after receipt of the first dose of Pfizer-BioNTech COVID-19 vaccine — United States, December 14–23, 2020. *Morbidity and Mortality Weekly Report* **70**(2):46–51. https://www.cdc.gov/mmwr/volumes/70/wr/mm7002e1.htm

27. Higgins T. (2020) Trump to sign "America First" executive order on Covid-19 vaccines, *CNBC News*, December 7. https://www.cnbc.com/2020/12/07/trump-to-sign-covid-19-vaccine-executive-order-prioritizing-americans.html

28. Wise J. (2021) Covid-19: New data on Oxford AstraZeneca vaccine backs 12 week dosing interval. *BMJ* **372:**n326. https://doi.org/10.1136/bmj.n326

29. Department of Health and Social Care. (2020) Priority groups for coronavirus (COVID-19) vaccination: Advice from the Joint Committee on Vaccination and Immunization (JCVI). Department of Health and Social Care, United Kingdom, 30 December. https://www.gov.uk/government/publications/priority-groups-for-coronavirus-covid-19-vaccination-advice-from-the-jcvi-30-december-2020

30. Mueller B. (2021) One AstraZeneca dose substantially reduced the risk of getting sick with Covid-19 for the elderly, a new study shows. NY Times Coronavirus Briefing, March 1. https://www.nytimes.com/live/2021/03/01/world/covid-19-coronavirus#one-astrazeneca-dose-substantially-reduced-the-risk-of-getting-sick-with-covid-19-for-the-elderly-a-new-study-shows

31. Monroe JP, Offit PA. (2021) SARS-C0V-2 vaccines and the growing threat of viral variants. *JAMA* **325**:821–822.

32. Altmann DM, Douek DC, Boyton RJ. (2020) What policy makers need to know about COVID-19 protective immunity. *Lancet* **395**:1527–1529. DOI:10.1016/S0140-6736(20)30985-5

33. Iati M, Fritz A, Hawkins D. (2021) What you need to know about the coronavirus variants. *Washington Post*, November 19. https://www.washingtonpost.com/health/interactive/2021/01/25/covid-variants/. Updated: March 1, 2021.

34. CDC. (2021) CDC issues first set of guidelines on how fully vaccinated people can visit safely with others. Press Release. March 8. https://www.cdc.gov/media/releases/2021/p0308-vaccinated-guidelines.html

35. Challen R, Brooks-Pollock E, Read JM. (2021) Risk of mortality in patients infected with SARS-CoV-2 variant of concern 202012/1: Matched cohort study. *BMJ* **372**:n579. https://doi.org/10.1136/bmj.n579

36. Pilishvili T, Fleming-Dutra KE, Farrar JL, *et al.* (2021) Interim estimates of vaccine effectiveness of Pfizer-BioNTech and Moderna COVID-19 vaccines among health care personnel — 33 U.S. sites, January–March 2021. *Morbidity and Mortality Weekly Report*, **70**:753–758. http://dx.doi.org/10.15585/mmwr.mm7020e2external icon

37. Madhi SA, Baillie V, Cutland CL. (2021) Efficacy of the ChAdOx1 nCoV-19 Covid-19 Vaccine against the B.1.351 Variant. *New England Journal of Medicine* **384**:1885–1898. DOI:10.1056/NEJMoa2102214.

38. Cohen J. (2021) South Africa suspends use of AstraZeneca's COVID-19 vaccine after it fails to clearly stop virus variant. *Science*, February 8. https://www.science.org/content/article/south-africa-suspends-use-astrazenecas-covid-19-vaccine-after-it-fails-clearly-stop

39. Adam D. (2021) SARS-CoV-2 isn't going away, experts predict. *The Scientist*, January 25. https://www.the-scientist.com/news-opinion/sars-cov-2-isnt-going-away-experts-predict-68386

40. FDA. (2021) Coronavirus (COVID-19) update: FDA issues policies to guide medical product developers addressing virus variants. FDA News Release, Food and Drug Administration, February 22. https://www.fda.gov/news-

events/press-announcements/coronavirus-covid-19-update-fda-issues-poli-cies-guide-medical-product-developers-addressing-virus

41. WHO. (nd) WHO recommendations on the composition of influenza virus vaccines. World Health Organization. https://www.who.int/influenza/vaccines/virus/recommendations/en/. Accessed: March 29, 2021.

42. Bieber F. (2020) Global nationalism in times of the COVID-19 pandemic. Nationalities Papers, First View, Cambridge University Press, pp. 1–13. DOI:10.1017/nps.2020.35

43. Pierson D. (2020) WHO is struggling against COVID-19 and a divided world testing its authority. *Los Angeles Times*, April 1. https://www.latimes.com/world-nation/story/2020-04-01/coronavirus-who

44. WHO. (2020) The access to COVID-19 Tools (ACT) accelerator. World Health Organization, April. https://www.who.int/initiatives/act-accelerator

45. WHO. (2020) ACT-accelerator pillars. World Health Organization, April. https://www.who.int/initiatives/act-accelerator/about

46. Gavi. (nd) COVAX. Global Alliance for Vaccines and Immunizations. https://www.gavi.org/covax-facility. Accessed: February 11, 2020.

47. Gavi. (nd) Alliance strategy. Global Alliance for Vaccines and Immunizations. https://www.gavi.org/our-alliance/strategy. Accessed: February 11, 2020.

48. CEPI. (nd) COVAX: CEPI's response to COVID-19. Coalition for Epidemic Preparedness Innovation. https://cepi.net/

49. WHO. (2020) COVAX announces additional deals to access promising COVID-19 vaccine candidates; plans global rollout starting Q1 2021. World Health Organization News, December 18. https://www.who.int/news/item/18-12-2020-covax-announces-additional-deals-to-access-promising-covid-19-vaccine-candidates-plans-global-rollout-starting-q1-2021

50. Kelland K. (2020) Exclusive: Vaccine group says 76 rich countries now committed to "COVAX" access plan. *Reuters*, September 15. https://www.reuters.com/article/health-coronavirus-vaccines-covax-exclus/exclusive-vaccine-group-says-76-rich-countries-now-committed-to-covax-access-plan-idUSKBN25T39T

51. Kuehn BM. (2021) High-income countries have secured the bulk of COVID-19 vaccines. *JAMA*. **325**(7):612. DOI:10.1001/jama.2021.0189

52. Worley W. (2020) UK joins COVAX scheme on deadline day. Devex, September 18. https://www.devex.com/news/uk-joins-covax-scheme-on-deadline-day-98132#:~:text=LONDON%20E2%80%94%20The%20United%20Kingdom%20on,signing%20up%20to%20the%20scheme

53. Rauhala E, Abutaleb Y. (2020) U.S. says it won't join WHO-linked effort to develop, distribute coronavirus vaccine. *Washington Post*, September 1. https://www.washingtonpost.com/world/coronavirus-vaccine-trump/2020/09/01/b44b42be-e965-11ea-bf44-0d31c85838a5_story.html

54. ReliefWeb. (2021) COVAX expects to start sending millions of COVID-19 vaccines to Africa in February. *Reliefweb*, February 4. https://reliefweb.int/report/world/covax-expects-start-sending-millions-covid-19-vaccines-africa-february

55. Eschner K. (2020) A coronavirus vaccine will save more lives if we share it widely. *Popular Science*, September 17. https://www.popsci.com/story/health/coronavirus-vaccine-bill-gates-report/

56. Hafner M, Yerushalmi E, Fays C, *et al.* (2020) COVID-19 and the cost of vaccine nationalism. Rand Europe, October 28. https://www.rand.org/randeurope/research/projects/cost-of-covid19-vaccine-nationalism.html

57. Richie H, Ortiz-Opsina E, Bellekian D, *et al.* (nd) COVID-19 vaccine doses administered. OurWorldinData.org. https://ourworldindata.org/covid-vaccinations

58. WHO. (2021) COVID-19 vaccine doses shipped by the COVAX Facility head to Ghana, marking beginning of global rollout. World Health Organization Newsletter, February 24. https://www.who.int/news/item/24-02-2021-covid-19-vaccine-doses-shipped-by-the-covax-facility-head-to-ghana-marking-beginning-of-global-rollout#:~:text=Today%2C%20Ghana%20became%20the%20first,and%20supply%20operation%20in%20history

59. WHO. (2021) COVAX published first round of allocation. World Health Organization, March 2. https://www.who.int/news/item/02-03-2021-covax-publishes-first-round-of-allocations

60. Richie H, Ortiz-Opsina E, Bellekian D, *et al.* (nd) Vaccination policies. OurWorldinData.org. https://ourworldindata.org/covid-vaccinations#vaccination-policies

61. WHO. (2020) WHO SAGE values framework for the allocation and prioritization of COVID-19 vaccination. World Health Organization, September 14. https://apps.who.int/iris/bitstream/handle/10665/334299/WHO-2019-nCoV-SAGE_Framework-Allocation_and_prioritization-2020.1-eng.pdf?ua=1

62. WHO. (2020) WHO SAGE roadmap for prioritizing uses of COVID-19 vaccines in the context of limited supply. World Health Organization, November 13. https://www.who.int/docs/default-source/immunization/sage/

covid/sage-prioritization-roadmap-covid19-vaccines.pdf?Status=Temp&
sfvrsn=bf227443_2

63. CDC. (2020) The advisory committee on immunization practices' ethical
    principles for allocating initial supplies of COVID-19 vaccine — United
    States, 2020. *Morbidity and Mortality Weekly Report*, November 23. https://
    www.cdc.gov/mmwr/volumes/69/wr/mm6947e3.htm

64. N'Gotta T. (2021) Ivory Coast begins its vaccination campaign with COVAX
    doses. *AP News*, March 1. https://apnews.com/article/health-coronavi-
    rus-pandemic-abidjan-africa-west-africa-ee77cd5f8aa5e1051e9eaddab-
    0b6c542

65. CDC. (2021) People with certain medical conditions. Centers for Disease
    Control and Prevention, February 22. https://www.cdc.gov/coronavi-
    rus/2019-ncov/need-extra-precautions/people-with-medical-conditions.
    html

66. Krammer F, Srivastava K; the PARIS team, Simon V. (2021) Robust spike
    antibody responses and increased reactogenicity in seropositive individu-
    als after a single dose of SARS-CoV-2 mRNA vaccine. *medRxiv*. https://doi.
    org/10.1101/2021.01.29.21250653

67. Chard AN, Gacic-Dobo M, Diallo MS. (2020) routine vaccination cover-
    age — worldwide. *Morbidity and Mortality Weekly Report* **69**:1706–1710.
    https://www.cdc.gov/mmwr/volumes/69/wr/mm6945a7.htm

68. Richie H, Ortiz-Ospina E, Bellekian D, *et al.* (nd) Country by country data on
    COVID-19 vaccination. OurWorldinData.org. https://ourworldindata.org/
    covid-vaccinations#

69. Aditya Goenka, A. (2020) Israel's vaccine rollout has been fast, so why is it
    controversial and what can other countries learn? *The Conversation*, Jan-
    uary 27. https://theconversation.com/israels-vaccine-rollout-has-been-fast-
    so-why-is-it-controversial-and-what-can-other-countries-learn-153687

70. Aljazeera. (2021) Israel starts vaccinating Palestinian workers after delays.
    March 8. https://www.aljazeera.com/news/2021/3/8/israel-starts-vaccinat-
    ing-palestinian-workers-after-delays

71. Hyde R. (2021) Von der Leyen admits to covid-19 vaccine failures. *Lancet*
    397(10275):655–656. doi.org/10.1016/S0140-6736(21)00428-1

72. The New York Times. (2021) Europe's vaccination slip-ups. NY Times Coro-
    navirus Briefing, February 10. https://www.nytimes.com/2021/02/10/us/
    coronavirus-today.html

73. Mohta NS, Weinstraub R. (2021) Covid-19 vaccine distribution: One of the most complex tasks in American public health history. *New England Journal of Medicine*, February 10. https://catalyst.nejm.org/doi/full/10.1056/CAT.21.0050

74. The New York Times (2021) The pace of US vaccination begins to rebound after recent winter storms. NY Times Coronavirus Briefing, February 25. https://www.nytimes.com/live/2021/02/25/world/covid-19-coronavirus#the-pace-of-us-vaccination-begins-to-rebound-after-recent-winter-storms

75. Osterholm M. (2021) Can President Biden's team speed vaccine delivery? Human Vaccine Project, January 22. https://www.humanvaccinesproject.org/covid-post/issue-25-can-president-bidens-team-speed-vaccine-delivery/

76. WHO. (2019) The ten threats to global health in 2019. World Health Organization. https://www.who.int/news-room/spotlight/ten-threats-to-global-health-in-2019

77. MacDonald NE; SAGE Working Group on Vaccine Hesitancy. (2015) Vaccine hesitancy: Definition, scope and determinants. *Vaccine* **33**(34):4161–4164. DOI:10.1016/j.vaccine.2015.04.036

78. Lazarus JV, Ratzan SC, Palayew A, *et al.* (2021) A global survey of potential acceptance of a COVID-19 vaccine. *Nature Medicine* **27**:225–228. https://doi.org/10.1038/s41591-020-1124-9

79. de Figueiredo, Alexandre, and Heidi J. Larson. (2021) Exploratory study of the global intent to accept COVID-19 vaccinations. *Communications medicine* **1**(1):1–10.

80. Carter S, Mobul L, Samaha A, Ahuka SM. (2020) Community engagement and vaccinations during the Ebola outbreak in Democratic Republic of Congo. *World Bank Blogs*, October 22. https://blogs.worldbank.org/health/community-engagement-and-vaccinations-during-ebola-outbreak-democratic-republic-congo

81. Muhoza P, Danovaro-Holliday MC, Diallo MS, *et al.* (2021) Routine vaccination coverage — worldwide, 2020. *Morbidity and Mortality Weekly Report* **70**:1495–1500. http://dx.doi.org/10.15585/mmwr.mm7043a1external icon

82. Savarese M. (2020) Brazil's Bolsonaro rejects COVID-19 shot, calls masks taboo. Associated Press, November 27. https://abcnews.go.com/International/wireStory/brazils-bolsonaro-rejects-covid-19-shot-calls-masks-74428885

83. Szilagyi PG, Thomas K, Shah MD, *et al.* (2021) National trends in the US public's likelihood of getting a COVID-19 vaccine — April 1 to December 8, 2020. **325**(4):396–398. DOI:10.1001/jama.2020.26419

84. The New York Times. (2020) Refusing Vaccines. NY Times Coronavirus Briefing, March 16. https://www.nytimes.com/2021/03/16/us/coronavirus-today.html

85. Karni A, Haberman M. (2020) Trump rescinds plan for White House Staff to be quickly vaccinated. *NY Times*, December 13. https://www.nytimes.com/2020/12/13/us/politics/white-house-coronavirus-vaccine-trump.html

86. Fink G, Tyson A. (2021) Growing share of Americans say they plan to get a COVID-19 vaccine — or already have. Pew Research Center, March 5, 2021. https://www.pewresearch.org/science/2021/03/05/growing-share-of-americans-say-they-plan-to-get-a-covid-19-vaccine-or-already-have/

87. Hughes MM, Wang A, Grossman MK, *et al.* (2021) County-level COVID-19 vaccination coverage and social vulnerability — United States, December 14, 2020 to March 1, 2021. *Morbidity and Mortality Weekly Report* DOI: http://dx.doi.org/10.15585/mmwr.mm7012e1external icon

88. RECOVER. (2021) COVID-19 vaccine hesitancy is striking, shows RECOVER Social Science study. European Centre for Disease Prevention and Control, Rapid European COVID-19 Emergency Response research, February 1. https://www.recover-europe.eu/covid-19-vaccine-hesitancy-is-striking-shows-recover-social-science-study/

89. Giles-Vernick T, Vray M, Heyerdahl L *et al.* (2021) Public views of COVID-19 vaccination in seven European countries: Options for response. Rapid European COVID-19 Emergency Response research (RECOVER), February 1. https://www.recover-europe.eu/covid-19-vaccine-hesitancy-is-striking-shows-recover-social-science-study/

90. JHSPH. (2020) Vaccine hesitancy in Southeast Asia. International Vaccine Access Center, John Hopkins Bloomberg School of Public Health. https://www.jhsph.edu/ivac/wp-content/uploads/2020/12/SAVI-Vaccine-Hesitancy-in-South-Asia-White-Paper.pdf

91. Kupferschmidt K, Vogel G. (2021) European countries resume use of Astra-Zeneca's COVID-19 vaccine, hoping pause has not dented confidence. *Science*, March 18. https://www.sciencemag.org/news/2021/03/european-countries-resume-use-astrazenecas-covid-19-vaccine-hoping-pause-has-not-dented

92. Opali O. (2021) African countries stick with AstraZeneca in shots rollout. *China Daily*, March 23. https://www.chinadailyhk.com/article/161227

93. Reuters. (2021) South Africa sells AstraZeneca COVID-19 vaccines to other African countries. *Reuters*, March 21. https://www.reuters.com/article/us-health-coronavirus-safrica-vaccine/south-africa-sells-astrazeneca-covid-19-vaccines-to-other-african-countries-idUSKBN2BD0K4

94. Stevis-Gridneff M. (2021) E.U. will curb covid vaccine exports for 6 weeks, *NY Times*, March 23. https://www.nytimes.com/2021/03/23/world/europe/eu-curbs-vaccine-exports.html

95. Walllis C. (2021) The best evidence for how to overcome COVID vaccine fears. *Scientific American*, January 7. https://www.scientificamerican.com/article/the-best-evidence-for-how-to-overcome-covid-vaccine-fears1/

96. Sacerdote B, Sehgal R, Cook M. (2021) Why Is all Covid-19 news bad news? Working Paper 28110, National Bureau Of Economic Research. https://www.nber.org/system/files/working_papers/w28110/w28110.pdf

97. Catalan-Matamoros D, Peñafiel-Saiz C. (2020) Exploring the relationship between newspaper coverage of vaccines and childhood vaccination rates in Spain. *Human Vaccines & Immunotherapeutics*. **165**:1055–1061. DOI:10.1080/21645515.2019.1708163

98. Wilson SL, Wiysonge C. (2020) Social media and vaccine hesitancy. *BMJ Global Health* **5**:e004206.

99. Smith TC. (2017) Vaccine rejection and hesitancy: A review and call to action. *Open Forum Infectious Diseases* **4**(3):ofx146. DOI:10.1093/ofid/ofx146

100. Ndugga N, Pham O, Hill L. (2021) Latest data on COVID-19 vaccinations race/ethnicity. *KFF*, March 31. https://www.kff.org/coronavirus-covid-19/issue-brief/latest-data-on-covid-19-vaccinations-race-ethnicity/

101. CDC. (2021) County-level COVID-19 vaccination coverage and social vulnerability — United States, Dec control and prevention. December 14, 2020–March 1, 2021. *Morbidity and Mortality Weekly Report* **70**(12):431–436. https://www.cdc.gov/mmwr/volumes/70/wr/mm7012e1.htm

102. Lancet. (2021) Access to COVID-19 vaccines: Looking beyond COVAX. *Lancet* **397**(10278):941. DOI:10.1016/S0140-6736(21)00617-6

6 Collateral Damage

"There are things that can be far more detrimental to health than this virus. These things are loneliness at the end of one's life, the loss of years of healthy life due to a poorly treated chronic or acute illness or a tumor that is diagnosed months too late. The discussion about coronavirus interventions still does not take sufficient account of the collateral damage. There are no daily updated dashboards for unemployment, cancer and heart attacks. ... In autumn and winter the following rule must apply: the old and dying must not be left alone and cut off from the rest of the world. And those who are seriously ill must be able to see a doctor. This is what people must take to heart."

Bernadette Redl, *Der Standard*
August 31, 2020

Contents

1. Introduction
2. Impact on Birth Rate
3. Impact on Other Diseases
    a. Drug shortages
    b. Declining outpatient visits and elective surgeries
    c. Increasing TB, malaria, HIV, and sexually transmitted infections
    d. Decrease in vaccination rate for routine preventable diseases
    e. Decreased in incidence of influenza and RSV infections
    f. Psychological impact: Community and healthcare workers
    g. Excess deaths due to COVID-19 versus other causes
4. Misinformation, Countering Misinformation
5. Ethical Issues
    a. Drug trials
    b. Equipment shortages
    c. Racial disparities

     d. Prisoners

     e. Immigrants

     f. Vaccines

        i. Exclusion of pregnant women

        ii. Vaccine passports

        iii. Jumping the line for vaccines

        iv. Should vaccines be mandated?

        v. Countries using vaccines to advance their foreign policy agenda

     g. School closure — Impact on children, families and teachers

6. Conclusion

1. Introduction

The previous chapters in this book focused on issues that can be directly attributed to SARS-CoV-2 and the COVID-19 pandemic. However, the pandemic also resulted in a multitude of collateral (indirect) consequences.[1] The known or potential impact of some of these collateral effects during the first two years of the pandemic, will be briefly highlighted in this chapter. In Chapter 10, The Epilogue, further information on some of the collateral damage during the first six months of 2022 will be noted.

2. Impact on Birth Rate

It has been speculated that there would be a decline in the global birth rate as a consequence of the Coronavirus Pandemic.[2,3] Early in the pandemic, the Brookings Institute predicted that the United States (US) would have 300,000 fewer births.[3] Actual data from the US gathered by the US CDC demonstrated a 4% reduction in the birth rate during 2020, 142,309 births lower than the previous year.[4] Data from the beginning and end of 2020 in Italy, France, Spain and Germany found a similar decline.[5,6] Data from Asia during 2020 suggested this will likely be a global phenomenon.[7] Some think that such fertility cycles relate to economic uncertainty.[8] It has also been noted in a systematic review looking at the effect of the COVID-19 pandemic on maternal and perinatal outcomes that there has been a global increase in maternal deaths, stillbirths, ruptured ectopic pregnancies, and maternal depression.[9] Additionally, while one study in the Netherlands suggested that COVID-19 reduced the incidence of preterm birth, three other studies from the US showed an increase in preterm births associated with COVID-19 infection.[10-13] Whether these negative effects on maternal fetal outcomes are due to stress, economic uncertainty, a direct effect of SARS-CoV-2 on the mother or child, or even an unappreciated effect of a SARS-CoV-2 variant, will require further research.

3. Impact on Other Diseases

a. Drug shortages

In addition to overwhelming hospitals in many parts of the world, the pandemic also had significant effects on other areas of the healthcare system. For example, the COVID-19 pandemic caused significant shortages in the US and other parts of the world for a number of drugs used for either COVID-19 or non-COVID-19 indications.[14-16] Critical drug shortages developing as a consequence of treating COVID patients have occurred with propofol, albuterol, midazolam, hydroxychloroquine, cisatracurium, fentanyl, azithromycin, and vancomycin. Other drugs that were affected as an offshoot of the pandemic included insulin, amoxicillin, heparin, vincristine, phenytoin, and acetaminophen. Some of these shortages were due to the consumption of drugs by COVID-19 patients; others were due to indirect effects that the stress of COVID-19 placed on the drug supply chain, especially in China and India. The pandemic also affected materials availability, production capacity, transport, and other parameters that were already maximally stressed prior to the pandemic. Within the past decade, 160 new drug shortages were documented in the US alone, so clearly, additional work is necessary to buttress the global drug supply chain against future global disasters.

b. Declining outpatient visits and elective surgeries

In many countries in the world, including the US, various countries in Europe and elsewhere, the COVID-19 pandemic led to a dramatic reduction in outpatient clinic visits (40–70%), pediatric vaccination visits (more than 50%), and non-COVID Emergency Department visits (40–60%).[17-23] When adults were queried about this trend, 40% of those surveyed said they avoided medical care because they were afraid of COVID-19.[24] Elective surgeries also declined after the pandemic began in most countries.[25]

c. Increasing TB, malaria, HIV, and sexually transmitted infections

In developing countries, modeling studies suggested that deaths due to HIV, tuberculosis and malaria would likely increase due to interruptions in usual interventions (medication, timely diagnosis, net campaigns, respectively).[26,27] Similarly, for sexually transmitted infections, modeling suggested that the number of cases of STIs would also increase.[28] These modeling studies may be difficult to confirm due to the global reduction in clinic visits, but data should eventually be available to address these predictions.

d. Decrease in vaccination rate for routine preventable diseases

Routine vaccination decreased dramatically in high, middle and low-income countries in 2020 due to COVID-19.[29] Based on a poll done during the first quarter of 2020, the WHO estimated that 80 million children under the age of 1 would be at risk for vaccine-preventable diseases, including diphtheria, measles and polio due to the pandemic disrupting routine vaccination efforts.

A second poll done during June 2020 further examined the impact of the pandemic on routine immunizations.[30] These polls were developed by the WHO, UNICEF and Gavi, in collaboration with the Sabin Vaccine Institute's Boost Community, the Johns Hopkins International Vaccine Access Center (IVAC), and the Global Immunization Division/US CDC. The second poll had 260 respondents from 82 countries (roughly half of them working at the national level, the other half at the sub-national level). The poll showed that disruptions to routine immunization services continued to be widespread. National level respondents from 61 of these countries reported that 52 of these 61 countries had a lower vaccination rate in May 2020 than in early 2020 when the first poll was done. The most common reasons for disruption to immunization services were: short supply of personal protection equipment for health workers (49%), travel restrictions (40%), and low availability of health workers (43%).

The above studies also showed that demand by families for immunization services also decreased. Survey responders from 73% of the countries indicated that the decrease in demand was highest for respondents from countries in the WHO African (89%), Americas (75%) and Eastern Mediterranean (73%) regions. Among respondents, 48% noted that families were concerned about the risk of exposure to COVID-19 if they went for vaccination, and 33% indicated that the main factors related to limited public transport, lockdown and physical distancing policies. Approximately, 75% of respondents indicated that plans to "catch-up" people who missed vaccine doses were in place.

In September 2020, the University of Washington, in collaboration with the Gates Foundation, reported that global routine immunization had decreased from 84% in 2019 to 70% during the pandemic. The report warned that if this is not corrected, there would be a marked increase in vaccine-preventable deaths in children in the next few years.[31]

e. Decreased in incidence of influenza and RSV infections

Not all the collateral consequences of the COVID-19 pandemic had a negative impact. One of the more unexpected impacts of COVID-19 was the dramatic decrease in seasonal influenza in both the Southern and Northern hemispheres in 2020. As the first wave of COVID-19 spread from Asia during the first half of 2020, a remarkable finding was noted: there was very little influenza disease being detected in the Southern Hemisphere. This occurred even though widespread testing was occurring while countries were trying to determine if the increase in the number of people with respiratory diseases had influenza or COVID-19. For example, in the Southern Hemisphere, from April to July 2020, in Australia, Chile and South Africa, a total of just 51 cases of influenza were detected despite more than 83,000 tests being done.[32]

This finding surprised many public health experts across the globe. The WHO, US CDC and other groups still recommended increasing the effort to have people in the Northern Hemisphere vaccinated with the influenza vaccines due to the concern that a moderate or severe influenza season would overwhelm hospitals already under tremendous stress caring for patients with COVID-19. It turned out that the incidence of influenza in the Northern Hemisphere during the 2020–2021 season was also very low. For example, the incidence of influenza disease in the US was substantially lower than in any previous year during the past decade.[33]

While the decreased incidence of influenza disease was clearly help-ful in decreasing the stress on the healthcare systems, it remains unclear why this happened. A number of explanations have been proposed for this fortuitous circumstance.[34] The lockdowns imposed by many countries, along with social distancing and mask wearing, likely played a role in the decrease in respiratory diseases due to non-COVID-19 microbes. However, numerous countries did not enforce or even recommend these containment or mitigation steps and still had very little influenza disease. The enhanced efforts to increase the use of influenza vaccines were successful in some countries, but the incidence of influenza disease also decreased remarkably in countries that do not have an annual influenza vaccine program. Addi-tionally, the incidence of some other viral respiratory diseases for which there are no currently licensed vaccines also decreased. For example, an abrupt decline in respiratory syncytial virus (RSV), a virus that can cause a respiratory illness requiring hospitalization in a large number of young children, also occurred. While containment and mitigation policies certainly played a role in decreasing the incidence of these other viral infections, other potential mechanisms have also been proposed (e.g., COVID-19 could interfere with the ability of influenza, RSV, and some other viruses to infect people either by affecting local and/or systemic immunity).[34]

Some public health experts worry that influenza will come back with a vengeance in 2021–2022.[35] One concern is that the scarcity of influenza during the first year of the pandemic will make it more difficult to know what strains of influenza virus to put into the vaccine for the coming year. Hope-fully, this will not be the case, but the COVID-19 pandemic has reminded us that hope is not a plan, and we should do everything possible to be better prepared for the next influenza season to be severe.

f. Psychological impact: Community and healthcare workers

The COVID-19 pandemic has been associated with significant increases in anxiety and depression in adults of all ages, especially among healthcare workers.[36–41] Although there is so far no evidence that this has led to a rise in suicide rates in the elderly or any other group, it is likely that further analysis will find increased rates of suicide in as yet unidentified subgroups. Doctors and nurses, in particular, are experiencing extraordinary levels of stress, as was shown in the physician's first-person account in the prelude, especially when they were asked to make life and death decisions, such as who and who not to place on a ventilator. This decision was sometimes made by an individual physician caring for the patient but usually was formalized through the so-called "God Committees" (see the discussion below under equipment shortages).[40] Even without the extreme equipment and drug shortages, the tremendous difficulties associated with taking care of patients whose family members were not allowed to stay with them, and in some cases, personnel shortages that led to extended shifts and working weeks in a row without a break, all took their toll and wore out even the strongest healthcare workers. Some newscasts have encapsulated this well, for example, showing a nurse crying while trying to describe the frustration she felt as one patient after another dies despite all their collective efforts, or a physician in India, who cried as he begged in front of a camera for more oxygen supplies for his patients to keep them alive. This sustained intensity has been associated with signs of healthcare workers "burning out" at alarming rates (>30%).[42–46] Factors increasing the risk of COVID burn out have included being younger of age, being female, redeployment from their usual role to a COVID-19 ward, and having a prior history of depression.[46] It is likely that the stresses felt by healthcare workers related to losing patients and colleagues to COVID-19 and concerns about taking COVID-19 home to their loved ones will only improve when there are more clinical staff, fewer COVID-19 patients at their particular hospital, and less perceived risk, such as being vaccinated against SARS-CoV-2.

g. Excess deaths due to COVID-19 versus other causes

Global data during 2020 has shown excess mortality in many countries, compared with previous years, with the US being a good example (Figure 6.68).[47–49] The top figure notes the number of deaths due to COVID-19 in 2020 and the bottom Figure compares this to what happened during the five year period prior to the onset of the pandemic (2015–2019). At first pass, this data suggests non-COVID-19 mortality might have included undocumented or diagnosed COVID-19 cases as the former tracks very tightly with the latter. However, as discussed in Chapter 4 and this chapter related to non-COVID-19 diseases (e.g., heart attacks, strokes, untreated TB, etc.), it is likely that many patients with non-COVID-19 diseases did not go to the

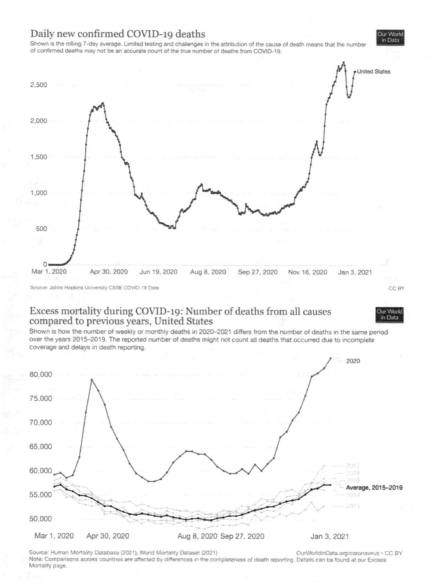

Daily new confirmed COVID-19 deaths

Shown is the rolling 7-day average. Limited testing and challenges in the attribution of the cause of death means that the number of confirmed deaths may not be an accurate count of the true number of deaths from COVID-19.

Source: Johns Hopkins University CSSE COVID-19 Data   CC BY

Excess mortality during COVID-19: Number of deaths from all causes compared to previous years, United States

Shown is how the number of weekly or monthly deaths in 2020–2021 differs from the number of deaths in the same period over the years 2015–2019. The reported number of deaths might not count all deaths that occurred due to incomplete coverage and delays in death reporting.

Source: Human Mortality Database (2021), World Mortality Dataset (2021)   OurWorldInData.org/coronavirus • CC BY
Note: Comparisons across countries are affected by differences in the completeness of death reporting. Details can be found at our Excess Mortality page.

Figure 6.68. COVID-19 deaths compared with all-cause mortality in the US. Top. Rolling 7-day average of COVID-19 deaths, March 1, 2020 – January 3, 2021. Limited testing and challenges in the attribution of the cause of death meant that the number of confirmed deaths was not an accurate count of the true number of deaths from COVID-19. Bottom. The number of weekly or monthly all-cause deaths in March 1, 2020 – January 3, 2021. differs from the number of deaths in the same period over the years of 2015–2019. The reported number of deaths might not include deaths due to incomplete coverage and delays in death reporting.[49]

hospital out of fear of being exposed to SARS-COV-2 or were not cared for in a hospital due to hospital capacities being exceeded by COVID-19 patients.[47] Thus, it is likely that the high number of total deaths are a combination of deaths due directly and indirectly due to COVID-19.[48] The excess death data is updated through June 2022 in the Epilogue (Chapter 10), but the full magnitude of this discrepancy will likely take years to uncover.

4. Misinformation, Countering Misinformation

Another important problem during the pandemic was the difficulty that many people had in finding reliable information about the pandemic. News personalities, politicians and private citizens commonly reached different conclusions from the same data, or worse yet, made up data to fit their agenda.[50-57] Although many individuals, all the way up to the Secretary-General of the WHO, have called out those who were thought to be spreading misinformation, very little has changed, and misinformation continues to be a major problem. The resultant confusion that such misinformation engendered made the public susceptible to being misled or becoming victims of scams. Two examples of politically motivated misinformation were: President Trump claiming that hydroxychloroquine could prevent COVID-19, resulting in a run on buying the drug, and injecting a disinfectant might be a treatment for COVID-19, which led to disinfectant poisonings.[58,59] Such high-level misinformation spread has occurred in many other countries, including Brazil, Russia and China.[60-62] (see Chapter 3 for more details). In some countries, aggressive efforts have been made to combat misinformation, but so far, it has been difficult to determine the impact of such efforts.[63]

Misinformation also made many people susceptible to con artists who attempted to make money off the pandemic.[53,54] Some examples of the growing list of scams perpetrated on the US public included imposters posing as IRS (Internal Revenue Service) agents or faking law enforcement calls. There were also fake government assistance programs, loans, debt relief, coupons, anti-COVID products (including treatments), and home test kits.[53,54]

5. Ethical Issues

a. Drug trials

The first drug-related ethical issue that came up at the beginning of the COVID pandemic was whether existing medications approved for treating other diseases might be repurposed against COVID-19.[64] Examples of repurposed drugs or vaccines that turned out to have *in vitro* activity against SARS-CoV-2 or *in vivo* activity in animal models against similar viruses included lopinavir/ritonavir, remdesivir, favipiravir, chloroquine, hydroxychloroquine, and the BCG vaccine.[64] All of these drugs experienced early surges of usage related to the COVID-19 pandemic with very little oversight as to what this would mean for those with other diseases that required treatment with these drugs. In an attempt to minimize such occurrences early in the pandemic, the WHO set up the Solidarity Trials (i.e., global treatment trials designed to let as many countries as possible participate in determining the efficacy/effectiveness of various drugs to treat COVID-19).[49] Drugs studied under the Solidarity Trials included remdesivir, hydroxychloroquine and lopinavir/ritonavir.[49] Thoughtful planning about how this can be done better in the future needs to occur.[65–67]

Other ethical questions related to drugs that surfaced during the pandemic included the following:[68–70] Was informed consent adequate for experimental drugs? When should a study be closed due to futility? When should a study having inconclusive, but very promising early results be expanded? Should studies have a placebo arm when patients are dying? Should parts of the world with poor infrastructure be excluded from clinical trials? Is it acceptable to do studies in parts of the world, where they can be done easily but have poor oversight? It will likely take years of retrospective analysis to fully appreciate all of the drug treatment ethical issues raised by this pandemic and how this can be done better.

b. Equipment shortages

It became clear early in the pandemic that there were global shortages in the availability of PPE[71–79] and lifesaving equipment used in ICUs and elsewhere (e.g., ventilators, dialysis machines, O_2 canisters).[80–86] The shortage in PPE forced healthcare workers to reuse masks, gowns and other

PPE, increasing their risk of becoming infected (Chapter 4). This led some healthcare workers to improvise and use plastic bags, bandanas, etc., none of which have proven efficacy. The shortage of ventilators led in many cases to healthcare workers attaching two patients to one ventilator (see the Prologue) and increased the risk of equipment malfunction. The shortage of both ventilators and dialysis machines led to extremely difficult decisions about which patients were more likely to survive, and which were not. In some hospitals where they were overwhelmed with patients (e.g., New York and Italy), these decisions happened daily. Constantly making decisions about who lived or died placed severe stress on the physicians making these decisions.[87] Multiple countries around the world experienced shortages in O_2 canisters that resulted in patient deaths, including Mexico, Peru, Brazil, and India.[85,86] Other countries were at risk of such a crisis at various times.[88] It will be very important in the aftermath of this pandemic to rethink how this could be approached better in the future.[89]

c. Racial disparities

Data from multiple areas in the world, including Brazil, Asian countries, Nordic countries, the United Kingdom (UK), and the US, have shown greater COVID-19 mortality in nonwhite than white populations.[90–96] In Brazil, individuals identifying themselves as of African descent had a 1.5 times greater risk of death than "white" Brazilians.[94] Somalians in Norway had COVID-19 infection rates ten times higher than the national average.[95] In the UK, individuals of Bangladeshi, Pakistani, Chinese, or mixed ethnic descent had a 1.8 times greater mortality than whites, and blacks had a 4 times greater mortality than whites.[96]

In the US, data suggest that COVID-19 mortality occurred disproportionally among nonwhite races.[90–93] The disparities were even greater when the data were adjusted for age.[90] In Michigan, a study looking at data through the end of October 2020, showed that blacks experienced age-adjusted mortality rates that were 5.5 times greater than for whites.[97] The same Michigan study showed that age-adjusted case fatality rates (CFRs) were only slightly higher for blacks than whites. The large discrepancy between overall age-adjusted mortality and age-adjusted CFRs could be explained by the much greater infection rates in the black population

(1626/100,000 versus 297/100,000), especially in those greater than 50 years of age.[97] In a New York City study, among those testing positive for SARS-CoV-2, the hospitalization odds were similar among blacks and whites, but the former were less likely to have a severe illness (i.e., an odds ratio of 0.6 as compared to the latter) and to die or be discharged to hospice (i.e., a hazard ratio of 0.7 compared to the latter), even after adjustment for age, sex, insurance status, and comorbidities.[98] While these data clearly demonstrated that nonwhite populations had greater mortality rates in the US, at least for the black population, this was more likely due to a greater frequency of underlying disease, not differences in susceptibility to developing more severe Coronavirus infection. Similar findings have been found in the UK,[99] but no other data have been provided as yet for racial disparities in COVID-19 deaths outside the US and the UK that have been adjusted for co-morbidities, age, etc.

d. Prisoners

The global jail and prison population was estimated to be around 11,000,000 in 2020. Because of the crowded circumstances in many prisons, there was a high risk for SARS-CoV-2 transmission. Unfortunately, relatively few countries publish data on deaths from infections in prison. In the UK during 2020, the mortality rate from COVID-19 within their prison system was reported to be slightly greater than 1%.[100] In US prisons, COVID-19 infection rates were reported to be as high as one in three. Across the US, the rates were more than five times higher than for the general population.[101,102] The cumulative raw mortality rate in US prisons from COVID-19 was approximately 0.6% less than the general population, reflecting a lower average age of prisoners, but when it was adjusted for age, the mortality rate was >3 times higher than for the general population, and as much as 5–11 times greater in some states.[102–104] This strongly suggested the possibility that care provided to COVID-19-infected prisoners in the US was either less effective or delayed in comparison to that provided to the general population. In a pre-COVID-19 study of US prisoners, age-adjusted mortality for white males in prison was nearly identical to white males outside of prison, compared with black males who actually had a lower mortality rate in prison than outside of prison.[105] At present, less data is available for prison populations in other countries, so comparisons with other countries besides the UK and US are not feasible.[106]

e. Immigrants

Another high-risk population in many countries is immigrant groups. Data from the European OECD group have found that among the confirmed cases, immigrants make up a disproportionally higher percentage of the total COVID-19 infections in many countries (Norway, 31% foreign-born; Sweden, 32%; Denmark, 18%; Portugal, 24%; Canada, 44%).[107] The WHO attempted to tabulate data on COVID-19 in refugees and asylum seekers, and by February 2021, had identified 450 deaths out of a global population of 80 million refugees and displaced people, likely a massive underestimate.[108] In the US, a high-risk site for COVID infection was immigrant detention centers.[109] The percentage of SARS-CoV-2-positive individuals among those tested in US detention centers was 17% higher than the general US population, and commonly dwarfed those of surrounding communities.[109–110] Notably, the Immigration and Customs Enforcement (ICE) group enacted policies inconsistent with US CDC guidelines, which resulted in the spread of COVID-19 from these detention centers to surrounding communities. In the US, it was further shown that there was a disproportionate impact of COVID-19 on immigrant communities outside of detention centers, which was similar to that documented with H1N1 in 2009.[111] It was clear from a preliminary analysis of the US pandemic response and its impact on immigrants, that many things could have been done better.[112]

f. Vaccines

A number of important ethical issues arose during the planning and implementation of the COVID-19 vaccine studies. Additional ethical issues surfaced as these vaccines received EUAs and were used in the general population. Some of these are discussed in Chapter 5, while others are noted in this section. The issues are both important and complex, and the purpose of this section is to note what concerns were raised, and hopefully, ethicists will be able to give further guidance before we face these questions again.

i. *Exclusion of pregnant women*

Pregnant women are at a higher risk for complications from a number of infectious diseases, and this turned out to be the case for COVID-19 (see Chapter 4, Case #6 for more COVID-19 details).[113–116] Up until the last decade, there has been a reluctance by vaccine companies to include pregnant women in vaccine trials due to liability concerns, and therefore many vaccines were not labeled by regulators for use in pregnant women. The lack of data on the use of vaccines in pregnant women caused a number of problems for vaccine-recommending bodies. However, over the past several decades, the WHO, the Advisory Committee on Immunization Practices (ACIP) and other groups have become more amenable to the use of certain vaccines, including influenza and pertussis vaccines, in pregnant women based on retrospective data obtained on already licensed vaccines that are not labeled for use in pregnant women.[114,115] Most recently, several vaccine companies have initiated clinical trials for pregnant women using new vaccines created to protect their infants against Group B strep and respiratory syncytial virus.

However, this has not solved the issue of the use of vaccines in pregnant women during disease outbreaks and pandemics. A recent example of this issue arose during a large outbreak of yellow fever in the Democratic Republic of the Congo in 2013. Due to a large number of deaths caused by the yellow fever virus in pregnant women, SAGE considered the use of the yellow fever vaccine in pregnant women, even though live-virus vaccines are usually not considered for use in pregnant women because of the possibility the virus in the vaccine could infect their fetus. SAGE concluded: "Noting that yellow fever is a live virus vaccine, a risk-benefit assessment should be undertaken for all pregnant and lactating women. In areas where yellow fever is endemic, or during outbreaks, the benefits of yellow fever vaccination are likely to far outweigh the risks of potential transmission of vaccine virus to the fetus or infant. Pregnant women and nursing mothers should be counseled on the potential benefits and risks of vaccination so that they may make an informed decision about vaccination. Lactating women should be advised that the benefits of breastfeeding far outweigh alternatives."[115] During this and subsequent yellow fever outbreaks, the vaccine has been offered to pregnant and lactating women.

The Zika virus outbreak that started in Brazil in April 2015 and then spread throughout the Americas further highlighted the issues involving the development of new vaccines for use in pregnant women. While the US and others attempted to develop a vaccine, there was a debate over whether a Zika virus vaccine should be tested in pregnant women, despite the fact that they were the group who had the greatest stake in the development of an effective vaccine that could prevent the disease from occurring in their unborn child. The Pregnant Women & Vaccines against Emerging Epidemic Threats (PREVENT) group was established to consider the ethical questions that surround testing new vaccines in pregnant women and to give guidance on when pregnant women should be offered an opportunity to participate in studies of vaccines under development.[116] The group concluded that the "current way of treating pregnant women in vaccine research and deployment is not acceptable. Business as usual can no longer continue". The group then went on to make 22 recommendations on ways to improve the situation.

This summary of the history of vaccine use in pregnant women brings us to the current situation where COVID-19 vaccine trials are underway. Despite the recommendations of the PREVENT group, pregnant women were not included in the initial Phase 3 studies being done by any of the COVID-19 vaccine-developing companies. Once again, this caused serious problems since healthcare workers, including those who were pregnant, were in the first priority groups in all countries to get the EUA COVID-19 vaccines as they become available. Since there were no studies that examined the use of COVID-19 vaccines in pregnant women, the WHO and other organizations could not issue clear guidance.[116-119] For example, the WHO noted that "while pregnancy puts women at higher risk of severe COVID-19 disease, very little data are available to assess vaccine safety in pregnancy. Nevertheless, based on what we know about this kind of vaccine, we do not have any specific reason to believe there will be specific risks that would outweigh the benefits of vaccination for pregnant women. For this reason, those pregnant women at high risk of exposure to SARS-CoV-2 (e.g. health workers) or who have comorbidities that add to their risk of severe disease, may be vaccinated in consultation with their health care provider."[117] The US CDC and other groups offered similar guidance.[118] If the WHO and CDC cannot give clear guidance it is hard to fathom how individual doctors are going to do better. All of this leaves the burden of making a decision to the pregnant woman.

While no one should ever put pressure on pregnant women to be in vaccine studies, what is still happening at this point is that they are not being offered the chance to decide if they want to be part of the studies. The US CDC has started a registry of pregnant women vaccinated with the COVID-19 vaccine, and as of May 2, 2021, 4,776 pregnant women are participating.[119] However, this does not provide the same strength of evidence on the safety and efficacy of a prospective study. The PREVENT recommendations provide guidance on how to overcome these issues,[116] and the fact that Pfizer has now started a global phase 2/3 study to evaluate the safety, tolerability and immunogenicity of their vaccine in pregnant women ≥18 years of age indicates that further progress can be made.[120]

ii. *Vaccine passports*

Vaccine cards are government-issued documents indicating an individual's vaccine status. In the US, they are small, white cards containing the recipient's name, date of birth, and the type and lot number of the vaccine administered. As of the end of April 2021, they documented whether someone had been fully vaccinated, but this did not affect a person's ability to travel or go to restaurants, sporting events or other public places. In a few countries, they were used for these purposes and, in effect, become travel passports (see Chapter 5 where the rapid vaccination of Israel's population was done in conjunction with the use of vaccine passports, which did impact the ability to travel and be in public places).

There are a number of pros and cons concerning the use of vaccine passports by countries, involving scientific, technical, legal and ethical issues. Vaccine passports have the potential to increase the percentage of a population that chooses to be vaccinated by offering them the freedom to travel to countries that make vaccine passports a prerequisite to enter the country. On the con side, vaccine passports could worsen ongoing equity issues. Many high-income countries are currently considering whether to issue vaccine passports that enable freedom of movement, and this section focuses mainly on the ethical arguments of doing so.

The WHO has issued interim guidance on the use of vaccine passports for those who have been immunized with a COVID-19 vaccine. This guidance was mainly aimed at travel between countries and discusses some of the ethical issues.[121] The WHO noted that currently the great majority of those vaccinated live in high or high-middle-income countries and that vaccine passports have the potential to further worsen the inequity by hindering equitable distribution of the limited supply of vaccine and thereby is unlikely to improve overall global health. Furthermore, if vaccination status becomes a condition for entry to or exit from a country, it could unfairly impede the freedom of movement. Therefore, the WHO position was that proof of COVID-19 vaccination should not be a requirement for international travel, given that there are still critical unknowns regarding the efficacy of vaccination in reducing transmission. In addition, due to the limited availability of vaccines, preferential vaccination of travelers could result in further increasing the inadequate supplies of vaccines for priority populations considered at high risk of severe COVID-19 disease. The WHO also recommended that people who are vaccinated should not be exempt from complying with other travel risk-reduction measures.

Various high-income countries are currently debating the use of vaccine passports. This debate is an important one, and the *Journal of the American Medical Association* sponsored a podcast in which Dr. Jana Shaw (Professor of Pediatrics and Clinical Associate Professor of Public Health and Preventive Medicine at SUNY Upstate Medical University in Syracuse, New York), Lawrence Gostin (Professor at Georgetown University in Washington, D.C. and Director of the O'Neill Institute for National and Global Health Law and Director of the World Health Organization Collaborating Center on National and Global Health Law), and Glenn Cohen (Harvard Law School Deputy Dean, Professor and Director of the Petrie-Flom Center for Health Law Policy Biotechnology and Bioethics) discussed some of the controversies.[122] The discussion centered on the use of vaccine passports in the US, but also would be germane to many other countries. The discussion highlighted various issues, including those that are technical (e.g., moving away from cards to digital health passes since cards are more likely to result in forgeries), scientific (e.g., what is the duration of protection of the various vaccines), legal (e.g., would states or the federal government oversee the vaccine passports in the US, and if the former, would all states agree to have vaccine passports), and ethical concerns.

The ethical discussion focused on two main problems posed by vaccine passports. The first relates to how these passports could affect minority groups living within high-income countries. Depending on what benefits the passports afforded a person (e.g., freedom to travel abroad), this could hurt those who were not vaccinated. This was particularly concerning for minority groups who have substantially lower vaccination rates. Part of the problem related to the decreased availability and delivery of vaccines to minority populations in those areas of the country where they work and live. There was also an increased hesitancy of minority groups to get the vaccine, which in part is due to a higher level of distrust of government-based on past programs.

The second major ethical issue relates to those living in low and middle-income countries around the globe who wanted to come to the US or another high-income country. Many of these poorer countries currently have little-to-no vaccines and may not be able to get them for a prolonged period of time. Until there is a clear commitment from high-income countries to an equitable distribution of COVID-19 vaccines, this issue remains problematic. As noted by the WHO, the commitment to equity is really in the best interest of all countries since it is likely that the negative health and economic impact of the pandemic will continue until most of the global population is vaccinated or infected.[121]

iii. *Jumping the line for vaccines*

There have been many instances in high, middle and low-income countries of wealthy people jumping the line to get the vaccine before they would have if they followed the prioritization rules. For example, in early 2021, hospitals in Washington State and South Florida faced criticism for offering invitation-only vaccine slots to private donors.[123] This example is just one of many, and on the surface, it would seem that jumping the line to get a vaccine is never ethical, but the views of two well-known ethicists give a somewhat more nuanced view and are briefly summarized below.

Katherine Parker, a legal ethicist based at Littler CaseSmart in North Carolina, has substantial expertise in this area.[123] She notes that the unfairness of getting a vaccine before one is eligible based on the established prioritization criteria for the COVID-19 pandemic was created because the demand for vaccine was greater than the amount available. Jumping the line further compounds other inequalities associated with the pandemic (e.g., minorities and others who are poor have greater numbers of cases and deaths due to SARS-CoV-2). Furthermore, building trust in the fairness of the line, alongside trust in the vaccine itself, is critical to the success of the immunization program. Those who skip the line not only displace those waiting behind them, they flout the priority rules that make the rollout fairer than any market or lottery-based alternatives.

Arthur Caplan, a bioethicist at New York University, believes that the pandemic has caused us to go beyond established medical ethics and consider public health ethics that look at treating whole communities as "patients".[124] Ethical principles for distributing vaccines are much more about maximizing lives saved rather than looking at what is best for the individual. If people feel that something is not fair, they are less likely to follow the rules. Vaccine rollouts in the US and many other countries have been inefficient and frustrating. This has resulted in some people feeling that they cannot trust their governments. However, Caplan notes there are instances when something looks unfair, but in reality is not. For example, if a clinic has vaccine doses that will expire by the end of the day, then it is reasonable to make the vaccine available to whoever can come in that day. His answer to improving the problem is to make the prioritization system as fair and transparent as possible and to better communicate the process to the public.

iv. *Should vaccines be mandated?*

The question of whether vaccines can be mandated has been around for a long time and has both legal and ethical aspects.[125] Many countries mandate routine childhood vaccines and use various mechanisms of enforcement, including restricting the ability of a child to attend school and fining parents who do not have their children vaccinated.[126] Vaccination can also be a requirement for employment. For instance, in the US, some hospitals require their healthcare workers to receive annual influenza vaccination as a condition of employment. There are arguments on both sides of the debate about whether forcing healthcare workers to be vaccinated can be ethically justified, but the courts have supported mandatory vaccination with influenza and other vaccines (e.g., MMR).

Recently, a number of US colleges have made it mandatory for students who want to attend college on campus to be immunized with a COVID-19 vaccine. Some hospitals have also required their healthcare workers to do the same.[127] A major difference between mandating routine vaccines and COVID-19 vaccines is that the latter is being used under EUAs and are not yet licensed. There are court cases pending over the issue of mandating the use of COVID-19 vaccines.

v. *Countries using vaccines to advance their foreign policy agenda*

While some countries were refusing to export COVID-19 vaccines made in their country, China, India and Russia were offering to donate or sell vaccines they made to countries where they thought it would help their foreign policy agendas.[128] For example, both China and India promised to donate vaccines they produced to Sri Lanka and Nepal, two neighboring countries important to both China and India. The two Chinese companies, Sinopharm and Sinovac, had each developed an inactivated SARS-CoV-2 vaccine that had been approved for use by the government. However, their Phase 3 studies had not been published, and at the time they donated the vaccine to various countries, the vaccine had not been used widely in China. The Chinese vaccines ran into problems with the late delivery of vaccines to countries. Furthermore, as some countries started using these vaccines, which the Chinese indicated had an efficacy of ~80%, public health officials and physicians were concerned that the vaccine was less effective than what they were led to believe and questioned why the Phase 3 trial safety and efficacy results had not been published.[129,130] For example, in Brazil, the public health authorities reported that the vaccine was only ~50% effective and questioned whether the vaccine should continue to be used in their country.[131]

A different issue occurred with the COVID-19 AstraZeneca vaccine being manufactured in India. The Serum institute in India had reached an agreement with COVAX to produce the viral vector vaccine developed by

AstraZeneca. The Serum Institute has a long history of producing vaccines for domestic and global use, and currently, ~60% of the routine childhood vaccines used worldwide are made by the Serum Institute. Their agreement with the COVAX facility was to produce very large quantities of the vaccine on an annual basis that would then be equitably distributed through the COVAX facility to the countries that were part of the COVAX program (see Chapter 5 for more details about the COVAX program and facility). Initially, the Serum Institute was making progress to meet its obligations to the COVAX facility, but as the second wave of the pandemic in India became more severe towards the end of the first quarter of 2021, Prime Minister Modi required that most of the vaccine doses remain in India to vaccinate its citizens. The government also assumed more control over which countries would receive exported vaccine doses.[132] The actions of the Indian government hampered the ability of the COVAX facility to meet its commitments to other countries.[133]

The Gamaleya Institute in Russia had developed a viral vector COVID-19 vaccine that showed 95% efficacy in a Phase 3 study (see Chapter 5 for more details on this vaccine). The Russian government began offering the vaccine to its own citizens in August 2020. At that point, the Phase 3 study results had not been peer published, and many people in Russia were reluctant to get the vaccine even after the data was published. During the second half of 2020, the Russian government began offering to sell the vaccine to various countries, and over time an increasing number of countries requested the vaccine. In March 2021, Russia had contractual agreements to supply various countries with ~400 million doses of the vaccine. However, Russia experienced major problems producing enough vaccines to meet its commitments.[134]

While offering to supply COVID-19 vaccines to other countries can be a win-win for the countries supplying and receiving the vaccines, a substantial downside occurs when the promises cannot be met. However, it is important to note that while the concept of the COVAX program was altruistic, COVAX also encountered problems meeting its obligation. What is truly needed is a unified global vaccine equity plan that all countries stay committed to. Whether that is even possible and how it might be accomplished is discussed in Chapter 9.

g. School closure — Impact on children, families and teachers

The COVID-19 pandemic caused a major disruption to the education system in all countries, and this greatly impacted not only those going to school but also their families. A UN policy brief reported that the pandemic was responsible for the largest disruption of education systems in history, affecting 94% (~1.7 billion) of learners in more than 200 countries.[135]

A literature review of the impact of COVID-19 on education globally looked at how school closing along with mitigation policies (e.g., social distancing) have impacted traditional education and social learning and caused the need for digital learning.[136] The requirement for digital learning is dependent on the availability of the internet. Virtual learning is hard enough in high-income countries where the ability to connect to the Internet is more widely available, albeit this is another area where socioeconomic groups living in these countries are disadvantaged. The problem is even worse in middle- and low-income countries where Internet accessibility and adequate bandwidth are less available. Broadly identified challenges with virtual learning are accessibility, affordability, flexibility, learning pedagogy, lifelong learning, and educational policy.

Teachers in this low- and middle-income setting have less experience with digital teaching tools, and this further hinders the ability to implement these programs.[136] Furthermore, the availability of digital platforms comes at a relatively high price for most school and family budgets. Transitioning from traditional face-to-face learning to online learning is often an entirely different experience for both the learner and educator, which they must adapt to with little or no other alternatives available. Lack of parental guidance, especially for young learners, is another challenge, especially when both parents work.[137] While there is a substantial amount being learned about how to improve digital learning, effective solutions to these problems will take years to devise and implement.

Various countries have tried different approaches to dealing with the problems caused by school closings. Some countries in Europe kept schools open most of the time during the pandemic, even when the country was otherwise in lockdown.[138] In the US, most schools stayed closed in 2020, but as increasing numbers of studies suggested that children, particularly those in elementary school, transmitted the virus less often than adults. The US CDC developed criteria and protocols for schools to reopen.[139] However, these protocols were relatively expensive to implement, and most schools were only able to open on a partial basis (i.e., children attended school a few days a week). A more radical solution was formulated in Kenya where the government felt they could not equitably introduce digital learning throughout the country and announced that all students would have to repeat the grade once school was reopened.[140]

There is a high level of concern that student learning, as well as their socialization and mental health, will be substantially affected even in places with ready access to the Internet.[140] While the highly motivated student will likely be less affected by reduced contact with teachers, the impact on learning will be greater in students that are less motivated, and those with learning difficulties will need additional support and guidance. However, a study done by the non-profit Northwest Evaluation Association on over 4 million US children in Grades 3 to 8 found that children, overall, had done better than predicted when comparing their scores in the first half of 2019 (pre-pandemic) to the first half of 2020 (when children were either learning virtually or in limited classroom time due to the pandemic). The Association had earlier predicted that students' testing scores would decrease by 50% and 30% in mathematics and reading, respectively, when compared to the previous year. However, the testing results instead showed gains in both subjects, although less than in a typical year. While this was encouraging, the Association noted that 25% of children in the study group did not take the test, and these were mainly minority students and/or those living in poverty.[141] Determining the full impact of the school disruption on learning will likely take several years.

The impact of the pandemic on student education not only affects learning but also can cause emotional stress for the whole family. For students, social skills are further developing as they interact with their peers at school, and the pandemic decreased these interactions and likely slowed their social maturation. The impact of the pandemic on families was examined in Italy via a survey done with parents of children between 2 and 14 years of age that examined the effect of the COVID-19 pandemic experience on parents' and childrens' well-being.[142] Parents who reported more difficulties in dealing with being part of government-imposed lockdowns felt more stress. Dealing with the lockdown was a particularly stressful experience for parents who found it difficult to balance personal life, work and raising children. This, in turn, increased the problems their children experienced. The lack of support some of these children received likely increased their psychological symptoms.

The negative impact of the pandemic has been particularly hard on working mothers, many of whom left the workplace because they lost their jobs at a higher rate than males and/or the closure of daycare centers for their children.[143] The pandemic also increased the pressure on working mothers more than working fathers. One out of four women who became unemployed during the pandemic reported the job loss was due to a lack of childcare, twice the rate of men surveyed. A survey done in the US between February and August 2020, revealed that mothers with children ≤12 years of age had lost 2.2 million jobs compared to 870,000 jobs lost by fathers.[143] Additionally, those who were able to work from home had to also care for or help teach their children in the case of inaccessible childcare or limited in-person instruction at schools.

We are only beginning to understand the full impact of closing schools during the pandemic. Further studies are needed to examine not only the educational and psychological toll that occurred but whether children and teachers are really at higher risk of COVID-19 disease if schools stay open using recommended mitigation policies. This information is critical for the ongoing and future pandemics.

6. Conclusion

This section contains only some of the ethical issues that occurred during the pandemic. The issue of inequitable distribution of vaccines in low and middle-income countries is discussed in detail in Chapter 5 and further updated in Chapter 10. Another intensely debated issue was whether it was ethical to infect human volunteers with the SARS-CoV-2 virus after giving them a vaccine for which the efficacy was not yet known. The rationale for doing so was it would likely speed up the development of the COVID-19 vaccines since Phase 3 studies would require fewer subjects. However, the fact that there was no highly effective drug to treat the virus was a major issue. The WHO set up a committee to develop criteria for considering this question, but the issue remains contentious.[144,145] Additional publications on this and other ethical issues that pertain to the development and testing of COVID-19 vaccines are available.[146,147]

References

1. Kaczorowski L, Del Grande C. (2021) Beyond the tip of the iceberg: direct and indirect effects of COVID-19. *Lancet* **3**:E205–E206. https://doi.org/10.1016/S2589-7500(21)00024-8

2. Ullah MA, Moin AT, Araf Y, *et al.* (2020) Potential effects of the COVID-19 pandemic on future birth rate. *Frontiers in Public Health*, December 12. DOI:10.3389/fpubh.2020.578438

3. Kearney MS, Levine PB. (2020) The coming COVID-19 baby bust: Update. The Brookings Institution, December 17, 2020. https://www.brookings.edu/blog/up-front/2020/12/17/the-coming-covid-19-baby-bust-update/

4. Hamilton BE, Martin JA, Osterman MJK. (2021) Births: Provisional data for 2020. Report No. 012, US Department of Health and Human Services CDC. https://www.cdc.gov/nchs/products/index.htm

5. De Rose AF, Mantica G, Ambrosini F, *et al.* (2021) COVID-19 impact on birth rates: First data from Metropolitan City of Genoa, Northern Italy. *IJIR: Your Sexual Medicine Journal.*

6. Mallet V, Dombey D, Arnold M. (2021) Pandemic blamed for falling birth rates across much of Europe, March 9. https://www.ft.com/content/bc825399-345c-47b8-82e7-6473a1c9a861

7. UNFPA. (2021) The impact of COVID-19 on human fertility in the Asia-Pacific region. Asia-Pacific Regional Office, UNFPA, January, 36 pp. https://asiapacific.unfpa.org

8. Chabe-Ferret B, Gobbi P. (2019) Economic uncertainty and fertility cycles: the case of the post-WWII baby boom. *VoxEU*, january 26, 2019. https://voxeu.org/article/economic-uncertainty-and-fertility-cycles

9. Chmielewska B, Barratt I, Townsend R, *et al.* (2021) Effects of the COVID-19 pandemic on maternal and perinatal outcomes: A systematic review and meta-analysis. *Lancet Global Health* **9**:e759–e772.

10. Been JV, Burgos Ochoa L, Bertens LCM, *et al.* (2020) Impact of COVID-19 mitigation measures on the incidence of preterm birth:

A national quasi-experimental study. *Lancet Public Health*. **5**(11):e604-e611. DOI:10.1016/S2468-2667(20)30223-1

11. Karasek D, Baer RJ, McLemore MR, *et al.* (2021) The association of COVID-19 infection in pregnancy with preterm birth: A retrospective cohort study in California. *Lancet Regional Health*. **2**:100027. https://doi.org/10.1016/j.lana.2021.100027

12. Ellington S, Strid P, Tong VT, *et al.* (2020) Characteristics of women of reproductive age with laboratory-confirmed SARS-CoV-2 infection by pregnancy status — United States, January 22–June 7, 2020. *Morbidity and Mortality Weekly Report* **69**:769–775. http://dx.doi.org/10.15585/mmwr.mm6925a

13. Woodworth KR, Olsen EO, Neelam V, *et al.* (2020) Birth and infant outcomes following laboratory-confirmed SARS-CoV-2 infection in pregnancy — SET-NET, 16 jurisdictions, March 29–October 14, 2020. *Morbidity and Mortality Weekly Report* **69**:1635–1640. http://dx.doi.org/10.15585/mmwr.mm6944e2

14. Scholndelmeyer SW, Seifert J, Margraf DJ, *et al.* (2020) Part 6: Ensuring a resilient US prescription drug supply. *The CIDRAP Viewpoint*, October 21. https://www.cidrap.umn.edu/covid-19/covid-19-cidrap-viewpoint

15. Ayati N, Saiyarsarai P, Nikfar S. (2020) Short and long term impacts of COVID-19 on the pharmaceutical sector. *DARU Journal of Pharmaceutical Sciences* **28**:799–805. https://doi.org/10.1007/s40199-020-00358-5

16. Badreldin HA, Atallah B. (2021) Global drug shortages due to COVID-19: Impact on patient care and mitigation strategies. Research in Social and Administrative Pharmacy, 17:1946-9. https://doi.org/10.1016/j.sapharm.2020.05.017

17. Mehrotra A, Chernew M, Linetsky D, *et al.* (2020) The impact of COVID-19 pandemic on outpatient visits: a rebound emerges. The Commonwealth Fund, May 19. https://www.commonwealthfund.org/publications/2020/apr/impact-covid-19-outpatient-visits

18. Santoli JM, Lindley MC, DeSilva MB, *et al.* (2020) Effects of the COVID-19 pandemic on routine pediatric vaccine ordering and administration — United States, 2020. *Morbidity and Mortality Weekly Report* **69**:591–593. http://dx.doi.org/10.15585/mmwr.mm6919e2

19. Jeffery MM, D'Onofrio G, Paek H, *et al.* (2020) Trends in emergency department visits and hospital admissions in health care systems in 5 states in the first months of the COVID-19 pandemic in the US. *JAMA Internal Medicine* **180**(10):1328–1333. DOI:10.1001/jamainternmed.2020.3288

20. Colclough G, Dash P, Van der Veken L. (2020) Understanding and managing the hidden health crisis of COVID-19 in Europe. McKinsey & Company, June 2. https://www.mckinsey.com/industries/healthcare-systems-and-services/our-insights/understanding-and-managing-the-hidden-health-crisis-of-covid-19-in-europe

21. Pikoulis E, Solomos Z, Riza E, *et al.* (2020) Gathering evidence on the decreased emergency room visits during the coronavirus disease 19 pandemic. *Public Health* **185**:42–43. DOI:10.1016/j.puhe.2020.05.036

22. Santana R, Sousa JS, Soares P, *et al.* (2020) The demand for hospital emergency services: Trends during the first month of COVID-19 response. *Portuguese Journal of Public Health* **38**:30–36. https://doi.org/10.1159/000507764

23. OECD/European Union. (2020) *Health at a Glance: Europe 2020: State of Health in the EU Cycle.* OECD Publishing, Paris. https://ec.europa.eu/health/sites/default/files/state/docs/2020_healthatglance_rep_en_0.pdf

24. Czeisler MÉ, Marynak K, Clarke KE, *et al.* (2020) Delay or avoidance of medical care because of COVID-19–related concerns — United States, June 2020. *Morbidity and Mortality Weekly Report* **69**:1250–1257. http://dx.doi.org/10.15585/mmwr.mm6936a4.

25. Wu K, Smith CR, Lembcke BT, Ferreira TBD. (2020) Elective surgery during the COVID-19 Pandemic. *New England Journal of Medicine* **383**:1787–1790. DOI:10.1056/NEJMclde2028735

26. Hogan AB, Jewell B, Sherrard-smith E, *et al.* (2020) The potential impact of the COVID-19 epidemic on HIV, TB and malaria in low- and middle-income countries. Imperial College London, London. https://spiral.imperial.ac.uk/bitstream/10044/1/78670/2/2020-05-01-COVID19-Report-19.pdf

27. Stop TB Partnership. (nd) The potential impact of the COVID-19 response on tuberculosis in high-burden countries: A modelling analysis. https://stoptb.org/assets/documents/news/Modeling%20Report_1%20May%202020_FINAL.pdf

28. Jenness SM, Le Guillou A, Chandra C, *et al.* (2021) Projected HIV and bacterial sexually transmitted infection incidence following COVID-19-related sexual distancing and clinical service interruption. *The Journal of Infectious Diseases* **223**(6):1019–1028. https://doi.org/10.1093/infdis/jiab051

29. UNICEF. (2020) WHO and UNICEF warn of a decline in vaccinations during COVID-19. Press Release, UNIFCEF, July 16. https://www.unicef.org/eap/press-releases/who-and-unicef-warn-decline-vaccinations-during-covid-19

30. UNICEF (nd) (Immunization coverage estimates data visualization. July 1, 2021 https://data.unicef.org/resources/immunization-coverage-estimates-data-visualization/

31. Azenman N. (2020) How Bad Has The Pandemic Been For Childhood Vaccinations? *Goats and Soda*, National Public Radio, Inc., September 21. https://www.npr.org/sections/goatsandsoda/2020/09/21/913937114/how-bad-has-the-pandemic-been-for-childhood-vaccinations

32. Olsen SJ, Azziz-Baumgartner E, Budd AP, *et al.* (2020) Decreased influenza activity during the COVID-19 pandemic — United States, Australia, Chile, and South Africa, 2020. Morbidity and Mortality Weekly Report **69**:1305–1309. http://dx.doi.org/10.15585/mmwr.mm6937

33. CDC. (nd) Weekly U.S. Influenza Surveillance Report. Centers for Disease Control and Prevention. https://www.cdc.gov/flu/weekly/index.htm. Accessed: May 3, 2021.

34. Jones N. (2020) How COVID-19 is changing the cold and flu season *Nature* **588**:388–390. https://doi.org/10.1038/d41586-020-03519-3

35. Advisory Board. (2021) This year's flu season was virtually nonexistent. That could be bad news for next year. The Advisory Board, March 30. https://www.advisory.com/en/daily-briefing/2021/03/30/flu-season

36. Sepúlveda-Loyola W, Rodríguez-Sánchez I, Pérez-Rodríguez P, *et al.* (2020) Impact of social isolation due to COVID-19 on health in older people: Mental and physical effects and recommendations. *The Journal of Nutrition, Health and Aging*, pp. 1–10. DOI:10.1007/s12603-020-1469-2

37. Vahratian A, Blumberg SJ, Terlizzi EP, Schiller JS. (2021) Symptoms of anxiety or depressive disorder and use of mental health care among adults during the COVID-19 pandemic — United States, August 2020–February 2021. *Morbidity and Mortality Weekly Report* **70**(13):490–494.

38. COVID-19 Mental Disorders Collaborators. (2021) Global prevalence and burden of depressive and anxiety disorders in 204 countries and territories in 2020 due to the COVID-19 pandemic. *Lancet* **398**:1700–12. https://doi.org/10.1016/S0140-6736(21)02143-7

39. Li Y, Scherer N, Felix L, Kuper H. (2021) Prevalence of depression, anxiety and posttraumatic stress disorder in health care workers during the COVID-19 pandemic: A systematic review and meta-analysis. *PLOS One* **16**(3):e0246454. https://doi.org/10.1371/journal.pone.0246454

40. Kisner J. (2021) What the chaos in hospitals is doing to doctors. *The Atlantic*, January/February. https://www.theatlantic.com/magazine/archive/2021/01/covid-ethics-committee/617261/

41. Dzau VJ, Kirch D, Nasca T. (2020) Preventing a parallel pandemic — A national strategy to protect clinicians' well-being. *New England Journal of Medicine* **383**:513–515. DOI:10.1056/NEJMp2011027

42. Lasalvia A, Amaddeo F, Porru S, *et al.* (2020) Levels of burn-out among healthcare workers during the COVID-19 pandemic and their associated factors: A cross-sectional study in a tertiary hospital of a highly burdened area of north-east Italy. *BMJ Open* **11**(1):e045127. http://dx.doi.org/10.1136/bmjopen-2020-045127

43. Khasne RW, Dhakulkar BS, Mahajan HC, Kulkarni AP. (2020) Burnout among healthcare workers during COVID-19 pandemic in India: Results of a questionnaire-based survey. *Indian Journal of Critical Care Medicine* **24**(8):664–671. DOI:10.5005/jp-journals-10071-23518

44. Mehta S, Machado F, Kwizera A, *et al.* (2021) COVID-19: A heavy toll on health-care workers. *Lancet Respiratory Medicine* **9**:226–228.

45. Matsuo T, Kobayashi D, Taki F, *et al.* (2020) Prevalence of health care worker burnout during the coronavirus disease 2019 (COVID-19) pandemic in Japan. *JAMA Network Open* **3**(8):e2017271. DOI:10.1001/jamanetworkopen.2020.1727

46. Ferry AV, Wereski R, Strachan FE, Mills NL. (2021) Predictors of UK healthcare worker burnout during the COVID-19 pandemic. *QJM: An International Journal of Medicine* **114**(6):374–380. https://doi.org/10.1093/qjmed/hcab065

47. Woolf SH, Chapman DA, Sabo RT, Zimmerman EB. (2021) Excess deaths from COVID-19 and other causes in the US, March 1, 2020, to January 2. *JAMA* **325**(17):1786–1789. DOI:10.1001/jama.2021.5199

48. The Economist. (nd) Tracking COVID-19 excess deaths across countries. *The Economist.* https://www.economist.com/graphic-detail/coronavirus-excess-deaths-tracker

49. Giattina C, Ritchie H, Roser (nd) Excess mortality during the Coronavirus pandemic (COVID-19). *Our World in Data.* https://ourworldindata.org/excess-mortality-covid

50. Carrion-Alvarez D, Tijerina-Salina PX. (2020) Fake news in COVID-19: A perspective. *Health Promotion Perspectives* **10**(4):290–291. DOI:10.34172/hpp.2020.44

51. Van der Linden S, Roozenbeek J, Compton J. (2020) Inoculating against fake news about COVID-19. *Frontiers in Psychology*, October 23. https://doi.org/10.3389/fpsyg.2020.566790

52. Fleming N. (2020) Coronavirus misinformation, and how scientists can help fight it. Bogus remedies, myths and fake news about COVID-19 can cost lives. Here's how some scientists are fighting back. *Nature*, June 17. https://www.nature.com/articles/d41586-020-01834-3

53. Hermsen C. (2020) Protecting Americans from COVID-19 scams (written testimony only). Food and Drug Administration (United States), July 21. https://www.fda.gov/news-events/congressional-testimony/protecting-americans-covid-19-scams-written-testimony-only-07212020

54. NYC Consumer and Worker Protection. (nd) COVID-19 scams and safety tips. https://www1.nyc.gov/assets/dca/downloads/pdf/consumers/COVID-19-Scams-and-Safety-Tips-English.pdf

55. Parks M. (2021) The most popular J&J vaccine story on facebook? A conspiracy theorist posted it. National Public Radio, Inc. https://www.npr.org/2021/04/15/987182241/the-most-popular-j-j-vaccine-story-on-facebook-a-conspiracy-theorist-posted-it

56. Saslow E. (2020) What are we so afraid of? *Washington Post*, October 10. https://www.washingtonpost.com/nation/2020/10/10/coronavirus-denier-sick-spreader/?itid=ap_elisaslow

57. WHO. (2021) Fighting misinformation in the time of COVID-19, one click at a time. April 27. https://www.who.int/news-room/feature-stories/detail/fighting-misinformation-in-the-time-of-covid-19-one-click-at-a-time

58. Niburski K, Niburski O. (2020) Impact of Trump's promotion of unproven COVID-19 treatments and subsequent internet trends: Observational study. *Journal of Medical Internet Research* **22**(11):e20044. DOI:10.2196/20044

59. Glatter R. (2020) Calls to poison centers spike after the President's comments about using disinfectants to treat coronavirua. *Forbes*, April. https://www.forbes.com/sites/robertglatter/2020/04/25/calls-to-poison-centers-spike--after-the-presidents-comments-about-using-disinfectants-to-treat-coronavirus/?sh=dbdb50d11574

60. Taylor L. (2021) We are being ignored: Brazil's researchers blame anti-science government for devastating COVID surge. *Nature*, April 27. https://www.nature.com/articles/d41586-021-01031-w

61. Gordon MR, Volz D. (2021) Russian disinformation campaign aims to undermine confidence in Pfizer, other COVID-19 vaccines, US officials say. *Wall Street Journal*, March 7. https://www.wsj.com/articles/russian-disinformation-campaign-aims-to-undermine-confidence-in-pfizer-other-covid-19-vaccines-u-s-officials-say-11615129200

62. Cook S. (2021) Beijing is getting better at disinformation on global social media. *The Diplomat*, March 30. https://thediplomat.com/2021/03/beijing-is-getting-better-at-disinformation-on-global-social-media/

63. Pomeranz JL, Schwid AR. (2021) Governmental actions to address COVID-19 misinformation. *Journal of Public Health Policy* **42**(2):201–210. https://doi.org/10.1057/s41271-020-00270-x

64. Ino H, Nakazawa E, Akabayashi A. (2021) Drug repurposing for COVID-19: Ethical considerations and roadmaps. *Cambridge Quarterly of Healthcare Ethics* **30**(1):51–58. DOI:10.1017/S0963180120000481

65. WHO Solidarity Trial Consortium, Pan H, Peto R, Henao-Restrepo AM, *et al.* (2021) Repurposed antiviral drugs for covid-19 — Interim WHO solidarity trial results. *New England Journal of Medicine* **384**(6):497–511. DOI:10.1056/NEJMoa2023184

66. Harrington DP., Baden, LR, Hogan JW, *et al.* (2021) A large, simple trial leading to complex questions. *New England Journal of Medicine* **384**:576–577. DOI:10.1056/NEJMe2034294

67. Badreldin HA, Atallah B. (2021) Global drug shortages due to COVID-19: Impact on patient care and mitigation strategies. *Research in Social and Administrative Pharmacy* **17**:1946–1949. https://doi.org/10.1016/j.sapharm.2020.05.017

68. Meagher KM, Cummins NW, Bharucha AE, *et al.* (2020) COVID-19 ethics and research. *Mayo Clinic Proceedings*, June. doi.org/10.1016/j.mayocp.2020.04.019

69. Schipper I. (2020) The ethics of clinical trials in times of corona. SOMO, July 8. https://www.somo.nl/the-ethics-of-clinical-trials-in-times-of-corona/

70. Bierer B, White S, Barnes J, *et al.* (2020) Ethical challenges in clinical research during the COVID-19 pandemic. *Bioethical Inquiry* **17**:717–722. https://doi.org/10.1007/s11673-020-10045-4

71. Yan Y, Bayham J, Richter A, *et al.* (2021) Risk compensation and face mask mandates during the COVID-19 pandemic. *Scientific Reports* **11**:3174. https://doi.org/10.1038/s41598-021-82574-w

72. Martinelli L, Kopilaš V, Vidmar M, *et al.* (2021) Face masks during the COVID-19 pandemic: A simple protection tool with many meanings. *Frontiers in Public Health* **8**:606635. DOI:10.3389/fpubh.2020.606635

73. Gostin LO, Cohen IG, Koplan JP. (2020) Universal masking in the United States: The role of mandates, health education, and the CDC. *JAMA* **324**(9):837–838. DOI:10.1001/jama.2020.15271

74. Nderitu D, Kamaara E. (2020) Gambling with COVID-19 makes more sense: Ethical and practical challenges in COVID-19 responses in communalistic resource-limited Africa. *Bioethical Inquiry* **17**:607–611. https://doi.org/10.1007/s11673-020-10002-1

75. Morley G, Grady C, McCarthy J, Ulrich CM. (2020) Covid-19: Ethical challenges for nurses. *Hastings Center Report* **50**(3):35–39. DOI:10.1002/hast.1110

76. Grimm CA. (2020) Hospital experiences responding to the COVID-19 pandemic: Results of a national pulse survey March 23–27. http://oig.hhs.gov/oei/reports/oei-06-20-00300.asp

77. Rosenbaum L. (2020) Facing COVID-19 in Italy — ethics, logistics, and therapeutics on the epidemics front line. *New England Journal of Medicine* **382**:1873–1875. DOI:10.1056/NEJMp2005492

78. WHO. (2020) Shortage of personal protective equipment endangering health workers worldwide. World Health Organization, March 3. https://www.who.int/news/item/03-03-2020-shortage-of-personal-protective-equipment-endangering-health-workers-worldwide

79. CDC. (2021) Strategies for optimizing the supply of isolation gowns. Centers for Disease Control and Prevention, January 21. https://www.cdc.gov/coronavirus/2019-ncov/hcp/ppe-strategy/isolation-gowns.html

80. Peterson A, Largent EA, Karlawish J. (2020) Ethics of reallocating ventilators in the COVID-19 pandemic. *BMJ* **369**:m1828. doi:10.1136/bmj.m1828

81. Bhatt H, Singh S. (2020) The ethical dilemma of ventilator sharing during the COVID-19 pandemic. *Journal of Global Health* **10**(2):020392. DOI:10.7189/jogh.10.020392

82. Feinstein MM, Niforatos JD, Hyun I, *et al.* (2020) Considerations for ventilator triage during the COVID-19 pandemic. *Lancet Respiratory Medicine.* https://doi.org/10.1016/S2213-2600(20)30192-2

83. Martin DE, Parsons JA, Caskey FJ, *et al.* (2020) Ethics of kidney care in the era of COVID-19. *Kidney International* **98**(6):1424–1433. DOI:10.1016/j.kint.2020.09.014

84. Parsons JA, Martin DE. (2020) A call for dialysis-specific resource guidelines during COVID-19. *American Journal of Bioethics* **20**(7):199–201. doi.org/10.1080/15265161.2020.1777346

85. Uchoa P. (2021) Coronavirus: what's behind Latin America's oxygen shortages? *BBC News*, January 30. https://www.bbc.com/news/world-latin-america-55829424

86. Hardy LJ, Weru L, Sadaf N, et al. (2021) Why India needs oxygen more urgently than vaccines. Vox, May 10. https://www.vox.com/22428619/india-covid-oxygen-shortage-supply-tankers-vaccines

87. Melnikow, J, Padovani, A, Miller, M. (2022) Frontline physician burnout during the COVID-19 pandemic: National survey findings. BMC Health Services Research 365. https://doi.org/10.1186/s12913-022-07728-6

88. Davies M, Furneaux R. (2021) Oxygen shortages threaten "total collapse" of dozens of health systems. The Guardian, May 25. https://www.theguardian.com/global-development/2021/may/25/oxygen-shortages-threaten-total-collapse-of-dozens-of-health-systems

89. Supady A, Curtis JR, Abrams D, et al. (2021) Allocating scarce intensive care resources during the COVID-19 pandemic: Practical challenges and theoretical frameworks. Lancet Respiratory Medicine 9:430–434.

90. Mackey K, Ayers CK, Kondo KK, et al. (2021) Racial and Ethnic Disparities in COVID-19-Related Infections, Hospitalizations, and Deaths : A Systematic Review. Ann Intern Med. 2021 Mar; 174(3): 362–373. doi: 10.7326/M20-6306.

91. Mude W, Oguoma VM, Nyanhanda T, Mwanri L, Njue C. (2021) Racial disparities in COVID-19 pandemic cases, hospitalisations, and deaths: A systematic review and meta-analysis. J Glob Health. 2021 Jun 26; 11: 05015. doi: 10.7189/jogh.11.05015.

92. Seligman B, Ferranna M, Bloom DE. (2021) Social determinants of mortality from COVID-19: A simulation study using NHANES. PLOS Medicine 18(1):e1003490. https://doi.org/10.1371/journal.pmed.1003490

93. Arrazola J, Masiello MM, Joshi S, et al. (2020) COVID-19 mortality among American Indian and Alaska native persons — 14 states, January–June 2020. Morbidity and Mortality Weekly Report 69:1853–1856. http://dx.doi.org/10.15585/mmwr.mm6949a3

94. Martins-Filho PR, Araujo BCL, Sposato KB, et al. (2021) Racial disparities in COVID-19 deaths in Brazil: Black lives matter? Journal of Epidemiology 31:239–240. DOI:10.2188/jea.je20200589

95. Yaya S, Yeboah H, Charles CH, et al. (2020) Ethnic and racial disparities in COVID-19-related deaths: Counting the trees, hiding the forest. BMJ Global Health 5:e002913. DOI:10.1136/bmjgh-2020-002913

96. Aljazeera. (2020) Black people in UK four times more likely to die of COVID-19: ONS. Aljazeera, May 7. https://www.aljazeera.com/news/2020/5/7/black-people-in-uk-four-times-more-likely-to-die-of-covid-19-ons

97. Zelner J, Trangucci R, Naraharisetti R, *et al.* (2021) Racial disparities in Coronavirus Disease 2019 (COVID-19) mortality are driven by unequal infection risks. *Clinical Infectious Diseases* 72:e88–e95. DOI:10.1093/cid/ciaa1723

98. Ogedegbe G, Ravenell J, Adhikari S, *et al.* (2020) Assessment of racial/ethnic disparities in hospitalization and mortality in patients with COVID-19 in New York City. *JAMA Network Open* 3(12):e2026881. DOI:10.1001/jamanetworkopen.2020.26881

99. Sze S, Pan D, Nevill CR, *et al.* (2020) Ethnicity and clinical outcomes in COVID-19: A systematic review and meta-analysis. *EClinicalMedicine* 29:100630. https://doi.org/10.1016/j.eclinm.2020.100630

100. Davies M, Keeble E. (2021) The rising tide of COVID-19 infections in our overcrowded prisons. Nuffield Trust, January 19. https://www.nuffieldtrust.org.uk/resource/chart-of-the-week-the-rising-tide-of-covid-19-infections-in-england-and-wales-s-overcrowded-prisons?gclid=EAIaIQobChMIv8r-g52D8QIVrD6tBh02gwAWEAMYAyAAEgJy-_D_BwE

101. The Marshall Project. (nd) A state-by-state look at Coronavirus in prisons. The Marshall Project. https://www.themarshallproject.org/2020/05/01/a-state-by-state-look-at-coronavirus-in-prisons

102. Saloner B, Parish K, Ward JA, *et al.* (2020) COVID-19 cases and deaths in federal and state prisons. *JAMA* 324(6):602–603. DOI:10.1001/jama.2020.12528

103. The Marshall Project. (nd) A state-by-state look at Coronavirus in prisons. The Marshall Project. https://www.themarshallproject.org/2020/05/01/astate-by-state-look-at-coronavirus-in-prisons

104. Nowotny KM, Cloud D, Wurcel Ag, Brinkley-Rubinstein L. (2020) Disparities in COVID-19 related mortality in US prisons and the general population. *medRxiv.* https://doi.org/10.1101/2020.09.17.20183392

105. Patterson EJ. (2010) Incarcerating death: Mortality in US state correctional facilities, 1985–1998. *Demography* 47(3):587–607. DOI:10.1353/dem.0.0123

106. WPB. (2020) International news and guidance on COVID-19 and prisons- 13 March — 30 November. https://www.prisonstudies.org/news/international-news-and-guidance-covid-19-and-prisons-13-march-30-november

107. OECD. (2020) What is the impact of the COVID-19 pandemic on immigrants and their children. Organistion for Economic Co-operation and Development, October 19. https://www.oecd.org/coronavirus/policy-responses/what-is-the-impact-of-the-covid-19-pandemic-on-immigrants-and-their-children-e7cbb7de/

108. Reidy E. (2021) One year on: How the pandemic has affected refugees, asylum seekers and migration. *The New Humanitarian*, March 10. https://www. thenewhumanitarian.org/analysis/2021/3/10/one-year-how-pandemic-has-affected-refugees-asylum-migration

109. Cahan EM. (2021) America's immigration system is a COVID superspreader. *Scientific American*, February 26.

110. Casanova FO, Hamblett A, Brinkley-Rubinstein L, Nowotny KM. (2021) Epidemiology of Coronavirus Disease 2019 in US Immigration and Customs Enforcement Detention Facilities. *JAMA Network Open* **4**(1):e2034409. DOI:10.1001/jamanetworkopen.2020.34409

111. Clark E, Fredricks K, Woc-Colburn L, *et al.* (2020) Disproportionate impact of the COVID-19 pandemic on immigrant communities in the United States. *PLOS Neglected Tropical Diseases* **14**(7):e0008484. DOI:10.1371/journal. pntd.0008484

112. Loweree J, Reichlin-Melnick A, Ewing W. (2020) The impact of COVID-19 on noncitizens and across the U.S. immigration system. American Immigration Council, September 30. https://www.americanimmigrationcouncil. org/research/impact-covid-19-us-immigration-system?gclid=EAIaIQobCh-MIm8PD7cqe8AIVR25vBB3Q6wejEAMYAiAAEgKOSvD_BwE

113. World Health Organization. (2014). Safety of immunization during pregnancy: a review of the evidence: Global Advisory Committee on Vaccine Safety. World Health Organization. https://apps.who.int/iris/handle/10665/340577

114. CDC. (nd). Guidelines for vaccinating pregnant women: ACIP guidelines. Centers for Disease Control and Prevention. https://www.cdc.gov/vaccines/ pregnancy/hcp-toolkit/guidelines.html Updated: August 2016.

115. WHO. (2013) Vaccines and vaccination against yellow fever. WHO Position Paper — June 2013. Weekly Epidemiologic Record, **88**:269–284.

116. The PREVENT Working Group. (2018) *Pregnant Women & Vaccines against Emerging Epidemic Threats (PREVENT). Ethics Guidance for Preparedness, Research, and Response.* The PREVENT Working Group, Baltimore, September. https://static1.squarespace.com/static/574503059f72665be88193e9/t/5c-082429c2241ba2553ee1f5/1544037418944/PREVENT-Web.pdf

117. WHO. (2021) WHO Strategic Advisory Group of Experts (SAGE) on Immunization has issued Interim recommendations for use of the Moderna mRNA-1273 vaccine against COVID-19: The Moderna COVID-19 (mRNA-1273) vaccine: what you need to know 26 January 2021. https://www.who.int/news-room/

feature-stories/detail/the-moderna-covid-19-mrna-1273-vaccine-what-you-need-to-know

118. CDC. (nd) Information about COVID-19 Vaccines for People who Are Pregnant or Breastfeeding. Centers for Disease Control and Prevention. https://www.cdc.gov/coronavirus/2019-ncov/vaccines/recommendations/pregnancy.html. Updated: April 28, 2021.

119. CDC. (2021) V-safe COVID-19 vaccine pregnancy registry. Centers for Disease Control and Prevention, May 3. https://www.cdc.gov/coronavirus/2019-ncov/vaccines/safety/vsafepregnancyregistry.html

120. Pfizer. (2021) Pfizer and BionTech commence global clinical trial to evaluate covid-19 vaccines in pregnant women. Pfizer, February 18. https://www.pfizer.com/news/press-release/press-release-detail/pfizer-and-biontech-commence-global-clinical-trial-evaluate

121. WHO. (2021) Considerations regarding proof of COVID-19 vaccination for international travelers. Interim Position Paper. World Health Organization, February 5. https://www.who.int/news-room/articles-detail/interim-position-paper-considerations-regarding-proof-of-covid-19-vaccination-for-international-travellers

122. AMA. (2021) Vaccine passports: Benefits, challenges and ethical concerns. American Medical Association Featured Topic. April 22. https://www.ama-assn.org/delivering-care/public-health/vaccine-passports-benefits-challenges-and-ethical-concerns

123. Parker K. (2021) Skipping the vaccine line is not only unethical — it may undermine trust in the rollout. *The Conversation*, March 11. https://theconversation.com/skipping-the-vaccine-line-is-not-only-unethical-it-may-undermine-trust-in-the-rollout-155277.

124. Weiner S. (2021) Is it ever okay to jump to the front of the vaccine line? An ethics expert weighs in. *AAMCNews*, March 23. https://www.aamc.org/news-insights/it-ever-okay-jump-front-vaccine-line-ethics-expert-weighs

125. Finnegan G. (2017) Mandatory vaccination: Does it work in Europe? *Vaccine Today*, November 27. https://www.vaccinestoday.eu/stories/mandatory-vaccination-work-europe/comment-page-1/

126. Miller AC, Ross RW. (2010) Mandated influenza vaccines and health care workers' autonomy. *AMA Journal of Ethics* **12**(9):706–710. DOI:10.1001/virtualmentor.2010.12.9.ccas2-1009

127. Gostin LD, Salmon DA, Larson HG. (2021) Mandating COVID-19 vaccines. *JAMA* **325**:532–533.

128. Mashal M, Yee V. (2021) The newest diplomatic currency: COVID-19 vaccines. *NY Times*, February 11. https://www.nytimes.com/2021/02/11/world/asia/vaccine-diplomacy-india-china.html

129. Dyer O. (2021) Chinese vaccines may need changes to improve efficacy, admits official. *BMJ* **373**:n969. DOI:10.1136/bmjn969

130. Bloomberg. (2021) Low efficacy of Chinese shots sows concern on global rollout. Bloomberg News, April 12. https://www.bloomberg.com/news/articles/2021-04-11/sinovac-shot-cuts-risk-of-symptomatic-covid-in-half-in-key-study

131. Londono E, Andreoni M, Casado L. (2021) Brazilian researchers find a Chinese vaccine once hailed as a triumph is far less effective than thought. New York Times Coronavirus Briefing, January 12. https://www.nytimes.com/2021/03/03/world/americas/brazil-covid-variant.html

132. Gettleman J, Schmall E, Mashal M. (2021) India cuts back on vaccine exports as infections surge at home. *NY Times*, April 22. https://www.nytimes.com/2021/03/25/world/asia/india-covid-vaccine-astrazeneca.html

133. Thakur D. (2021) India is suffering immensely under the weight of Covid. Now its failures are threatening much of the world. *STAT*, May 5. https://www.statnews.com/2021/05/05/india-vaccine-heist-shoddy-regulatory-oversight-imperil-global-vaccine-access/

134. Litvinova D. (2021) Russian scores points with vaccine diplomacy, but snags arise. *AP News*, March 6. https://apnews.com/article/europe-global-trade-middle-east-diplomacy-moscow-e61ebd3c8fe746c60f5ec-c1ec323c99a

135. UN. (2020) Policy brief: Education during COVID-19 and beyond. United Nations. https://www.un.org/development/desa/dspd/wp-content/uploads/sites/22/2020/08/sg_policy_brief_covid-19_and_education_august_2020.pdf

136. Pokhrel S, Chhetri R. (2021) A literature review on impact of COVID-19 pandemic on teaching and learning. *Higher Education for the Future* **8**(1):133–141.

137. Murgatrotd S. (2020). *COVID-19 and Online Learning*. Alberta, Canada. DOI:10.13140/RG.2.2.31132.8512

138. Kamenetz A. (2020) Lessons from Europe, where cases are rising but schools are open. National Public Radio, Inc., November 13. https://www.npr.org/2020/11/13/934153674/lessons-from-europe-where-cases-are-rising-but-schools-are-open

139. Rice KL, Miller GF, Coronado F, Meltzer MI. (2020) Estimated resource costs for implementation of CDC's recommended COVID-19 mitigation strategies

in pre-kindergarten through grade 12 public schools — United States, 2020–21 school year. *Morbidity and Mortality Weekly Report*, December 11. https://www.cdc.gov/mmwr/volumes/69/wr/pdfs/mm6950e1-H.pdf

140. The New York Times. (2020) Kenya's radical school solution. New York Times Coronavirus Briefing, August 5. https://www.nytimes.com/2020/08/05/world/africa/Kenya-cancels-school-year-coronavirus.html

141. Green EL. (2020) New data show some children aren't falling as far behind as predicted. *NY Times*, December 2. https://www.nytimes.com/2020/08/05/world/africa/Kenya-cancels-school-year-coronavirus.html

142. Spinelli M, Lionetti F, Pastore M, Fasolo M. (2020) Parents' stress and children's psychological problems in families facing the COVID-19 outbreak in Italy. *Frontiers in Psychology*, July 3. https://doi.org/10.3389/fpsyg.2020.01713

143. Bateman N, Ross M. (2020) Why has COVID-19 been especially harmful for working women? Brookings-Series on Gender Equality, October. The Brooking Institution, October. https://www.brookings.edu/essay/why-has-covid-19-been-especially-harmful-for-working-women/

144. WHO. (nd) Key criteria for the ethical acceptability of COVID-19 human challenge studies. World Health Organization, May 6. https://apps.who.int/iris/bitstream/handle/10665/331976/WHO-2019-nCoV-Ethics_criteria-2020.1-eng.pdf

145. Jamrozik J, Selgelid MJ. (2020) COVID-19 human challenge studies: Ethical issues. *Lancet* **20**:E198–E203. https://doi.org/10.1016/S1473-3099(20)30438-2

146. Zeiger H. (2020) Coronavirus vaccine ethics. The Center for Bioethics and Human Dignity, Trinity International University, December 8. https://cbhd.org/content/coronavirus-vaccine-ethics

147. Wibawa T. (2021) COVID-19 vaccine research and development: ethical issues. *Tropical Medicine & International Health* **26**(1):14–19. DOI:10.1111/tmi.13503

7 Origin Story

"Every new beginning comes from some other beginning's end."

"Closing Time"
Semisonic
American rock band
formed in Minneapolis, Minnesota, in 1995

Contents

1. What is an Infectious Disease?
2. What is an Emerging Infectious Disease (EID)?
3. When and Where did COVID-19 Become an EID?
4. What was the Source of SARS-CoV-2?
5. Why are Bats the Likely Animal Long-term Host for SARS-CoV-2?
6. Is there an Intermediate Host for SARS-CoV-2?
7. How does COVID-19 Compare with Other Coronavirus-caused Infections?
8. Does the Recent Appearance of More Lethal Coronaviruses Globally Suggest that these Viruses have the Ability to Evolve Rapidly?
9. Is there any Possible Explanation for How a Coronavirus can Suddenly Appear in the Human Population and Cause Disease?
10. Are these Three New Coronavirus-caused EID (COVID-19, MERS, SARS) Isolated Events, or Are they Part of a Larger Global Phenomenon?
11. What Risk Factors can Play a Role Increasing the Likelihood of an EID Event?
    a. Transition to an agricultural society
    b. City size
    c. War
    d. Famine
    e. Slavery

    f. Colonization

    g. Ignorance = Undiscovered

    h. Climate change

12. Summary

1. What is an Infectious Disease?

An infectious disease is a disease caused by a microorganism that can be transmitted from the environment or an animal host (to include humans) and cause disease in a new host.

2. What is an Emerging Infectious Disease (EID)?

The Centers for Disease Control (CDC) and Prevention began publishing the journal called *Emerging Infectious Diseases* in 1995. Their definition of an emerging infectious disease (EID) was one whose incidence in humans had increased in the past two decades or threatened to increase in the near future.[1] In this chapter, we will look at COVID-19 as an EID and compare it with other emerging coronaviruses and other historically important EIDs to determine how COVID-19 is similar and different.

3. When and Where did COVID-19 Become an EID?

COVID-19 first emerged in Wuhan, China, somewhere between November 17 and December 14, 2019, and was first reported to the WHO on December 31, 2019.[2-4] On February 11, 2020, the WHO named the disease COVID-19, and on March 11, the WHO declared it a pandemic.[4] In March 2020, the International Committee on Taxonomy of Viruses determined that the virus causing COVID-19 should be named SARS-CoV-2 Wuhan-Hu-1 or SARS-CoV-2 for short, a genetic subspecies of the Severe Acute Respiratory Syndrome (SARS)-related coronavirus, which causes SARS in humans.[5]

4. What was the Source of SARS-CoV-2?

To understand where SARS-CoV-2 came from, one must first understand the importance of animal hosts for coronaviruses. All viruses, including

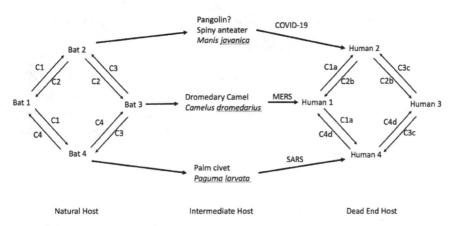

Figure 7.69. Ecology of coronaviruses causing severe disease in humans. Bats are the natural host, and different coronavirus strains (C1–C4) circulate between different species of bats (Bat 1 – Bat 4). Transmission can occur from a bat to an intermediate host (pangolin, dromedary camel, or palm civet). Finally, transmission can occur from the intermediate host to humans with resultant COVID-19, MERS, or SARS infection. Once coronaviruses are transmitted to humans, continued mutation occurs with the formation of new coronavirus strains (C1a–C4d) that differ from the strains in bats (C1–C4) and even those found within intermediate hosts.

coronaviruses, require living inside a cell to survive, and coronaviruses prefer living inside the cells of animals, including humans. Coronaviruses live in a wide range of animal species, including pig, cat, dog, rabbit, mouse, rat, cattle, antelope, deer, llama, buffalo, horse, chicken, turkey, giraffe, palm civet, raccoon dog, bird, bat, pangolin (spiny anteater), dromedary camel, and humans.[6,7] Over the last 50 years, it has become increasingly clear that coronaviruses have a life cycle that allows classifying these different animal species into three types of hosts: primordial or natural host (their long-term ecological niche), intermediate host (where the virus undergoes further genetic evolution), and dead-end host (where the organism is either cleared by the immune system or the host dies) as shown in Figure 7.69.[6,8] Although humans are generally thought to be dead-end hosts for coronaviruses, it is clear that humans can transmit SARS-CoV-2 to animals, including humans, minks, cats and dogs.[6,9] Thus, for a human to become infected, a virus must go from its long-term host animal, either to an intermediate host animal and then to a human or directly to a human. It remains to be determined whether there was an intermediate host involved in initiating the SARS-CoV-2 pandemic.

5. Why are Bats the Likely Animal Long-term Host for SARS-CoV-2?

Ten SARS-CoV-2 isolates from nine patients in Wuhan, China, were 98–99% related to each other, 88% related to two bat coronavirus strains, 79% related to SARS-CoV, and 50% related to MERS (Middle East Respiratory Syndrome)-CoV, suggesting bat strains were more closely related to SARS-CoV-2 than SARS-CoV or MERS-CoV strains.[10] Another study in China found that SARS-CoV-2 shared a 79.5% sequence with SARS-CoV, but 96% overlap with a bat coronavirus strain.[11] These are small numbers of strains. What other evidence exists?

A 2007 study compared SARS coronavirus RNA sequences obtained from humans and animals in China with published RNA sequences from bats and other animals and concluded that bats are likely the natural long-term hosts for all presently known coronavirus lineages.[12] A 2017 publication evaluated a multicontinent, systematic sampling of global coronavirus strain diversity and found 100 different viral strains (species), 91 of which were found in bats, and the different coronavirus species correlated with different bat species.[13] Said another way, coronaviruses have adapted to bats, such that different species of bats have different species of coronavirus; this suggests that the overwhelming majority of global coronavirus diversity (>90%) can be attributed to coronavirus bat adaptation. The magnitude of coronavirus diversity is likely 10-fold greater than this study demonstrated because bats make up 20% of mammalian species with more than 1,400 bat species, second only to rodents, and bats host more virus species per bat than rodents or any other mammal.[14–16]

What makes bats so unique as viral reservoirs? When bats are infected by viruses, they show minimal evidence of disease, even with high viral loads (up to 10^7 virus particles per gram of tissue).[17,18] Recent studies have demonstrated that bats have evolved their ability for their primary immune response to be dampened in comparison to humans and mice, which show brisk inflammatory responses when infected with similar viruses.[17] This immune tolerance likely facilitates the long-term persistence of viruses in bats without the bats becoming sick or dying.[18,19] Under certain circumstances, such as nutritional stress or pregnancy, bats can shed higher quantities of virus, which likely facilitate viral spillover into other animal species.[20,21] Given that bats can live from 20 to 40 years, much longer than other mammals of similar size, be persistently colonized by viruses, and have occasional viral blooms (increased viral secretion) permitting transmission to other species, they are uniquely suited for causing intermittent outbreaks, such as has been seen with SARS, MERS and COVID-19.[20]

Questions to be addressed:

1. Since the global bat diversity appears to be increasing, coronavirus strains seem to be unique to the bat species they colonize, and evidence increasingly suggests that coronaviruses, bats, and their intermediate hosts have co-evolved.[13–15,22–30] What implications does this have for future coronavirus pandemics?

2. What is the importance of the bat, intermediate host, and human immune systems in this co-evolutionary process?[17–19,31]

6. Is there an Intermediate Host for SARS-CoV-2?

Early in the COVID-19 outbreak in China, an analysis of five Malayan pangolins (spiny anteaters) tissue samples obtained in an anti-smuggling operation found that they had coronavirus infection with 85.5% to 92.4% similarity to SARS-CoV-2 RNA.[32] Additional studies comparing bat, pangolin, and human strains of coronavirus have found that bat and pangolin strains were quite similar (>90% similarity) to the human SARS-CoV-2 strains isolated from COVID-19 patients in Wuhan.[7,32,33] Superficially, these studies are consistent with Figure 1.1, that a bat CoV strain (SARS-CoV-2) moved to pangolins and then to humans.

If a pangolin is the source of SARS-CoV-2, where did humans get exposed to these animals? In one of the initial descriptions of the COVID-19 outbreak in Wuhan, China, it was noted that 49% of 99 COVID-19 patients had exposure to a seafood market where live animals were also for sale, a so-called "wet market".[34] Until shortly after the outbreak began in Wuhan, pangolins could be purchased at such wet markets, but after the linkage to the pandemic was suspected, the wet markets were closed by the Chinese government, only to be reopened a short time later.[35,36] Pangolins come from various locations in Asia and Africa and are valued in the Chinese culture for meat, traditional medicine, and a number of other uses.[37,38] Pangolins are thought by many to be the most trafficked non-human mammal in the world, and not surprisingly, the species is currently critically endangered.[38,39] Another location where pangolins originate is wildlife farms within China.[40] A recent study by the WHO suggests that animals from such farms are likely the source of COVID-19. Notably, in February 2020, China shut down many such farms as one of their interventions.[40] Furthermore, there are significant data suggesting that SARS-CoV and MERS-CoV were also likely transmitted through wet markets.[41,42] At present, there are no good data supporting the popular hypothesis that SARS-CoV-2 came from a research laboratory in Wuhan.[43]

Genomic data have been used to study the evolution of SARS-CoV and SARS-CoV-2 by Boni and colleagues, looking at the relationship between different coronavirus isolates from various animals, especially bats.[44] Using a molecular clock approach (see Section 10 below) that allows an estimation of when different coronavirus strains came into existence, they determined that SARS-CoV diverged from its bat origin between 1952 and 1970 and SARS-CoV-2 diverged from its bat strain origin between 1948 and 1982. They further estimated that the time of divergence from the closest SARS-CoV-2 strain isolated from a pangolin was between 1851 and 1877. This latter finding casts some doubt on pangolins being the intermediate host for SARS-CoV-2. An additional study published by Li and colleagues in 2020 has provided further evidence that the pangolin is unlikely to be the intermediate host.[45] Given the first appearance of SARS-CoV and SARS-CoV-2 roughly half a century ago, why did it take so long to become a problem for humanity?

Questions to be addressed:

1. At present, we are not certain of the precise route of transmission of SARS-CoV-2, whether it is from bats directly to humans or from bats to an intermediate host and then to humans;[1-4] this must be determined definitively in order to precisely design future interventions that interrupt transmission.

2. Given data suggesting that SARS-CoV and MERS-CoV were transmitted from wet markets and SARS-CoV-2 might be transmitted through wet

markets,[40–42,46–48] shouldn't we eliminate wet markets as recommended by the WHO?[49]

7. How does COVID-19 Compare with Other Coronavirus-caused Infections?

Coronaviruses were first identified in 1965 as a cause of human cold-like illnesses and chicken bronchitis.[6,7] It was not until SARS appeared in November 2002 in Guangdong, China, and MERS appeared in 2012 in Saudi Arabia — both causing atypical pneumonia — that we knew that coronaviruses could cause more severe infections in humans with intact immune systems.[50–52] Similarities between all coronaviruses infecting humans seem to be the requirement for both a long-term natural animal host and an intermediate animal host prior to human infection (Figure 7.69). Low virulence coronaviruses, i.e., those that cause colds, have at least three identified sequences of transmission: mouse → cow → human (strain HCoV-OC43), bat → camel → human (HCoV-229E) or bat → alpaca → human (HCoV-229E).[6] Considering SARS-CoV-2's genetic cousin and namesake, SARS-CoV, at least two studies in China have shown that SARS-CoV can be found in bats in the nearby environment.[53,54] Further work demonstrated that a virus nearly identical to SARS-CoV existed in palm civets and raccoon dogs being sold at wet markets near the center of the original Guangdong, China outbreak, likely candidates for intermediate hosts.[46,47] In a study looking at SARS-CoV transmission, it was found that a waitress and a customer likely acquired SARS-CoV from palm civets housed in cages inside a restaurant, suggesting transmission from the palm civet to humans was feasible.[55] Further studies by a number of Chinese groups increasingly suggest that bat coronavirus strains are relatively bat species specific and quite mobile, since bats can migrate thousands of miles.[8,56,57] In the case of MERS-CoV, a more distant relative of SARS-CoV-2 and SARS-CoV, there are data demonstrating that MERS-CoV strains from camels and humans in Saudi Arabia are virtually identical, and MERS-CoV in bats is similar enough to be the likely starting point.[6,8,58–61] These data collectively suggest the following chains of transmission for the three more virulent human coronavirus strains: SARS-CoV (bat → palm civet or raccoon dog → human), MERS (bat → camel → human), and SARS-CoV-2 (bat → pangolin (?) → human), as shown in Figure 7.69.[6,7]

The biggest differences between SARS, MERS and COVID-19 are in mortality and their ability to be transmitted and cause outbreaks. As to mortality, SARS resulted in 8,422 known cases with a 11% mortality rate.[52] SARS would also be considered an EID using the CDC definition above, but notably it disappeared in the second half of 2004. In 2012, MERS appeared in Saudi Arabia, ultimately causing 2,494 cases with a 34% mortality rate, a second coronavirus EID.[52] MERS remains active. COVID-19 has a lower mortality (1–3%) than SARS and MERS; however, in aggregate, it was responsible for many more deaths due to the much greater number of people infected during the pandemic. The explanation for its ability to be transmitted and cause a pandemic will be discussed in Chapter 8.

8. Does the Recent Appearance of More Lethal Coronaviruses Globally Suggest that these Viruses have the Ability to Evolve Rapidly?

An analysis of coronavirus isolates from humans and palm civets from the original 2002 Guangzhou SARS outbreak found them to be nearly identical, but a comparison of coronavirus isolates from palm civets and humans a year later in Guangzhou found that the new isolates were significantly different from the previous isolates but still quite similar to each other.[62] This suggests that coronavirus evolution occurs rapidly (less than a 1-year period).

What might accelerate such evolution? A factor that may be quite important in accelerating evolution is for different coronavirus strains to be exposed to each other, such as what might happen in a cave housing different bat species carrying different coronavirus species. Such a cave has been identified in Yunnan Province, China, where samples taken from four different bat species yielded 11 different strains of SARS-CoV with strong evidence of recombination (exchange of RNA fragments) between various strains.[63] Their findings have further demonstrated that SARS-CoV evolution is strongly correlated with geographic location, yet another variable in Coronavirus evolution.[63]

Recent estimates of coronavirus evolutionary rates show that SARS-CoV, MERS-CoV and SARS-CoV-2 evolutionary rates are all approximately

10^{-3} substitutions/site/year, similar to the evolutionary rate for HIV and influenza (Chapter 4), viruses well known to rapidly evolve.[64,65] Thus, for SARS-CoV, MERS-CoV and SARS-CoV-2, there are continuous mutation and recombination events going on that change their ability to infect animals and humans.[8] These evolutionary findings are very important because they suggest that coronavirus pandemics may resemble influenza A pandemics, which occur due to the constant evolution of influenza virus strains as they move between pigs and chickens (see Chapter 8). Thus, it is quite possible that a new coronavirus strain will appear in the near future that would have evolved sufficiently in bats and/or intermediate hosts so that humans will not be immune and, theoretically, another pandemic could occur.[66] If true, this suggests that the vaccines under development, like current influenza vaccines, may not protect against such future strains.

9. Is there any Possible Explanation for How a Coronavirus can Suddenly Appear in the Human Population and Cause Disease?

Increasingly, it is thought that coronavirus transmission to humans may represent a spillover event (spillover = transmission) from an animal host to humans. It has been demonstrated for other bat viruses such as Nipah, Hendra, Ebola, and Marburg that spillover events can occur when the amount of virus in bat secretions suddenly increases.[67,68] For Marburg, in particular, it has been shown that there is a biannual spike in the prevalence of Marburg-positive bats that correlates with an increased incidence of spillover to humans with resultant infections.[68] Other studies suggest that the same may be true for Nipah, Hendra and Ebola viruses.[67,68] A recent 4-year longitudinal study in the bat cave mentioned above found that SARS-like coronaviruses vary 5-fold in bat fecal concentration in different months (i.e., July, September and October are greater than April and May).[69] While there is no linkage yet between increased fecal bat coronavirus levels and human transmission, it raises the possibility that this same spillover phenomenon might occur, which might explain the sudden appearance of previously unknown viruses such as SARS-CoV, MERS-CoV or

SARS-CoV-2.[70,71] Additional ecological studies with bats and viral spillover events have shown that human population density is the biggest single risk factor for such events, implying that the more humans there are in a given area, the greater is the risk of bat exposure.[15]

10. Are these Three New Coronavirus-caused EID (COVID-19, MERS, SARS) Isolated Events, or Are they Part of a Larger Global Phenomenon?

Jones and colleagues published a paper in 2008 entitled "Global trends in emerging infectious diseases".[72] They analyzed 335 EID events between 1940 and 2004 and concluded that EID events during that period of time were increasing, reaching a peak in the 1980s, thought largely due to HIV/AIDS-related infectious diseases. The increase in EID events during the 1940–2004 period held true, even when controlling for better reporting or surveillance of infectious diseases. The majority of EID events (60%) were caused by zoonotic (nonhuman animal source) pathogens, and 72% of the zoonotic events had a wildlife origin. COVID-19 would be viewed as a zoonotic virus. The second-largest group, vector-borne (vectors being mosquitos, ticks, lice, flies, etc.) infectious diseases caused 22.8% of the EID events. Human population density was found to be a significant independent predictor of EID events in both major subgroup categories (zoonotic, vector-borne). Geographic analysis demonstrated that there is a mismatch between hotspots for EID, which are concentrated in lower latitudes (tropical Africa, Latin America, Asia), and EID surveillance, which is more robust in the richer, developed countries in Europe, North America, Australia, and parts of Asia. They were unable to address the role of climate change in EID events, although they noted that it almost certainly played a role. They also noted that efforts to conserve areas rich in wildlife diversity may have the added value of decreasing the risk of zoonotic disease emergence.

Not all EIDs are equally impactful globally. After reviewing the 335 EID events mentioned above occurring between 1940 and 2004, the authors (RJS, JSA) chose 15 historically important EIDs — 12 before and 3 after

Table 7.20. Historically important emerging infectious diseases: 1940 to 2020.

EID Date	Organism	Disease
1954	Dengue virus (reemergence, originally 800 YA)	Dengue
1959	Human immunodeficiency virus 1	AIDS
1960	Methicillin resistant *Staphylococcus aureus*	MRSA infection
1962	*Borrelia burdorferi*	Lyme disease
1967	Marburg virus	Hemorrhagic fever
1968	Norwalk virus	Gastroenteritis
1973	*Clostridium difficile*	Colitis
1976	*Legionella pneumophila*	Pneumonia
1976	Ebola virus	Hemorrhagic fever
1977	Zika virus	Zika
1999	West Nile virus	Encephalitis
2002	SARS-CoV	SARS
2009	H1N1 Influenza A virus	Influenza pandemic
2012	MERS-CoV	MERS
2019	SARS-CoV-2	Coronavirus pandemic

EIDs from 1940–2004 were selected by this book's authors from reference 37. EIDs that happened after 2004 were selected by the authors of this book.

2004 that were globally impactful enough to be reported frequently in the lay press and had easily recognizable clinical syndromes (Table 7.20), for further analysis. Also, the time frame considered above (1940–2020) is only a tiny fraction of human history. To gain a broader perspective, it is worth looking back at historically important infectious diseases that became EIDs prior to 1940. Since the Germ Theory (the theory that microorganisms cause infectious diseases) only came to be accepted in the late 1800s,[73] we can only consider those infectious diseases with easily recognizable clinical syndromes. RJS and JSA chose 23 historically important emerging infectious diseases with easily recognizable clinical syndromes that had EID events prior to 1940 (Table 7.21), with their date of appearance based on papers employing molecular clock technology (the average rate at which a species genome accumulates mutations) or historical records (if no molecular clock estimate is available, this applied to polio only).[74,75]

Table 7.21. Historically important emerging infectious diseases: Pre-1940.

EID Date[49-72,120,147]	Discovery Date*	Organism	Disease	Animal Reservoir[69,73-81]
300 MYA	1879	Streptococcus pyogenes	Scarlet fever	Horse, dog?
150 MYA	1909	Rickettsia prowazekii	Epidemic typhus	Rodents
10 MYA	1873	Mycobacterium leprae	Leprosy	Armadillo, primates
>3 MYA	1884	Clostridium tetani	Tetanus	Cattle, sheep?
>3 MYA	1884	Corynebacterium diphtheriae	Diphtheria	Domestic herbivores
70,000 YA	1882	Mycobacterium tuberculosis	Tuberculosis	Cattle
43,000 YA	1880	Salmonella typhi	Typhoid fever	Swine, primates?
35,000 YA	1897	Shigella dysenteriae	Dysentery	Primates, cattle?
16,000 YA	1906	Variola virus	Smallpox	Cattle, Swine
10,000 YA	1880	Plasmodium falciparium	Malaria	Primates, birds
8,000 YA	1954	Varicella zoster virus	Chickenpox	Primates
5,000 YA	1905	Treponema pallidum	Syphilis	Primates?
5,000 YA	1894	Yersinia pestis	Plague	Rodents
2,000 YA	1931	Influenza virus	Influenza	Birds, swine
1,500 YA	1885	Rabies virus	Rabies	Canines, bats
1,500 YA	1927	Yellow fever virus	Yellow fever	Primates
800 YA	1954	Measles morbillivirus	Measles	Cattle
500 YA	1906	Bordetella pertussis	Whooping cough	Mammals
200 YA	1854	Vibrio cholera	Cholera	Birds, copepods
200 YA	1887	Neisseria meningitidis	Epidemic meningitis	Primates
150 YA	1962	Rubella virus	Congenital rubella	Horse?
145 YA	1934	Mumps virus	Mumps, orchitis	Swine
130 YA	1908	Poliovirus	Epidemic polio	Swine

*Estimated date of initial appearance (based on molecular clock technology, except polio), discovery date, genus species name, and possible animal reservoir. MYA = million years ago, YA = years ago. Primates = nonhuman primates.

In Figure 7.70, 10 of 38 organisms appeared on or before 10,000 years ago, whereas 28 of 38 organisms appeared in the last 10,000 years.[76-99,147] Significantly, the likelihood of an easily diagnosable historical infectious disease appearing in the last 10,000 years was over 800 times greater than in the 3,000,000 years prior (28/10,000 versus 10/3,000,000).

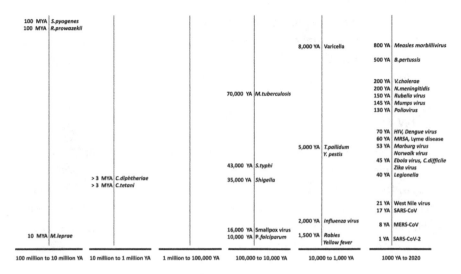

Figure 7.70. Historically important infectious diseases. Their rate of occurrence is accelerating. 100 million years ago (MYA) to 2020 CE. YA = years ago. Data taken from Tables 20 and 21 and displayed in this semi-logarithmic fashion. Figure courtesy of R. Sherertz.

These findings suggest that in the last 10,000 years, changes have occurred that increased the risk of EID events. We will now explore what some of those changes might be and whether this idea is plausible.

11. What Risk Factors can Play a Role Increasing the Likelihood of an EID Event?

a. Transition to an agricultural society

Approximately 10,000 BCE, humanity transitioned from hunter-gatherers (Pleistocene Period) to an agricultural society (Neolithic Period) and began residing in settlements, ultimately cities.[100,101] Agricultural societies domesticated animals to assist with farming and to be used for food.[100,101] Increased time of humans around animals led to increased exposure to animal microorganisms. Ecologic and genetic studies suggest 100% of the 23 organisms shown in Table 7.21 may have originated in animals, even though some have evolved to be virtually human species specific.[78,102–111,147] Animal exposure alone would not be sufficient to cause or sustain infection outbreaks, since many people were not around animals. So what other factors are important?

b. City size

Research has shown that human settlements became larger at the start of the Neolithic period.[112] It has been speculated, based on an analysis of city size, that larger cities would increase the risk of human infections.[113] While no data exist, co-variates of increasing city size, such as the increasing likelihood of water supplies being contaminated by human waste, and close human-to-human proximity, were likely involved.

c. War

In 541, Roman Emperor Justinian attempted to attack Persia but was thwarted by the appearance of the Plague (*Y. pestis*) from Asia,[113,114] the first Plague pandemic, which killed an estimated 25 million people with a 25% mortality rate.[113] In 1525, Pope Clement VII, Francis I (King of France), and Henry VIII (King of England) fought against Charles V (King of Spain) and ultimately surrounded Charles V's army in Naples.[115] There, epidemic typhus (*R. prowazekii*) caused 35,000 deaths in the French army within a month, and they sued for peace.[116] In 1812, Napoleon invaded Russia, starting with 680,000 soldiers and returning home with less than 100,000 men; more than half of his losses were thought to be due to typhus.[117] Between 1853 and 1856, the Crimean War was fought by the Ottoman Empire, France, Britain, and Sardinia against Russia.[118] Florence Nightingale's records showed that 21% of the British casualties were the result of battle while 79% were due to infectious diseases like malaria (*P. falciparum*), typhoid fever (*S. typhi*), epidemic typhus (*R.prowazekii*), and dysentery (*S. dysenteriae*).[118] These four examples of war-related infection mortality were the tip of the iceberg. In Wikipedia's list of wars by date, there were 148 wars in the 1500s, 158 in the 1600s, 169 in the 1700s, and 535 in the 1800s.[119] This is likely an underestimate, so the potential for wars contributing to human pestilence was extraordinary.

d. Famine

In 1739, the Great Frost hit Europe with subsequent failure of the Irish potato crop and 10–20% Irish mortality, largely due to famine and infectious diseases outbreaks.[120] In 1847, a potato blight caused the second great Irish Famine.[120] It is estimated that one million people died — half from infectious diseases (typhus, dysentery, smallpox, and others). Another million emigrated from Ireland, overall reducing Ireland's population by 20–25%.

Wikipedia also lists famines; 17 in the 1500s, 26 in the 1600s, 27 in the 1700s, and 33 in the 1800s.[121] Since the 1700s, it has been estimated that 14 famines had mortality greater than one million each, and six famines had greater than ten million deaths each. As demonstrated in the Irish famines and others, at least half of the famine mortality was due to infectious diseases, suggesting famines play a significant role in facilitating human pestilence.[120,122]

e. Slavery

Slaves from Africa and elsewhere were both victims and vectors of infectious diseases. Smallpox transmission via the Royal African Company slave trade led the British Government in 1721 to pass the Quarantine Act and the Royal Society to recommend that the Royal African Company shift their focus from slave trading to selling ivory.[123] The slave trade was thought to have transmitted yellow fever, malaria, tuberculosis, schistosomiasis and other infectious diseases to the Americas.[124–127]

Steckel and Jensen found that during slave ship loading in Africa in the 1700s, the slave mortality rate was 4,530/100,000 (58.7% due to infections, two-thirds of which were gastrointestinal illnesses) and crew mortality rate was 23,800/100,000 (86% infections, 79% of which were due to febrile illnesses — probably malaria or yellow fever).[128] During the Middle Passage across the Atlantic, the slave mortality rate was 11,570/100,000 (63.5% due to infections, and again approximately two-thirds were gastrointestinal illnesses) and crew mortality rate was 20,740/100,000 (71% due to infections, 63% febrile illnesses).[128] Since the crew likely had better living conditions than the slaves, this suggests the crew might be more susceptible to infections than the slaves.

Slave mortality due to infectious diseases acquired while working could also be quite high. Ian Read found in Recife, Brazil, between 1856 and 1870 that tetanus mortality among freeborn people decreased from 5.6% to 3.4% as a percentage of the total; whereas, among slaves, it increased from 14% to nearly 17%.[129]

f. Colonization

After Cortes's invasion of Mexico, it has been estimated that 8,000,000 people died of smallpox.[130] Smallpox similarly devastated North American Indians and Australian Aborigines.[131,132] Diamond thought it likely that infectious diseases spread by explorers were more important than guns in the conquest of native peoples in the global colonization efforts that took place between 1500 and 1800.[133]

It has been shown that measles was poorly transmitted from Australia to the Fiji Islands via slow travel by clipper ship because all passengers were infected and recovered by the end of the voyage. Measles transmission became feasible when travel changed to steamships, which have shorter travel times, such that some passengers still had active infection at the time of arrival.[134,135] In Iceland, with its small population, they demonstrated that measles died out without frequent travelers.[134] With cholera, they speculated that improved travel across oceans facilitated the global pandemics of the 1800s.[134]

g. Ignorance = Undiscovered

Until the second half of the 1800s, the concept of infection due to microorganisms was undiscovered. For over 2,000 years, medical thinking about "infectious" diseases was dominated by two Greek theories[136,137] — Aristotle's Theory of Spontaneous Generation (living creatures arise from nonliving matter)[136] and Galen's Miasma Theory (diseases such as cholera, smallpox, and the plague spread due to bad air or night air emanating from rotting organic matter).[137,138] Miasma Theory's intrinsic problem was that it posited that disease transmission could not be prevented. To make progress toward an understanding of infectious diseases and how to prevent and treat them, microorganisms needed to be discovered, their transmission understood, and both of these theories had to be overturned.

By the late 1800s, enough research had been done by historical giants, to include Dr. Edward Jenner (smallpox vaccination), Dr. Louis Pasteur (first proposer of the Germ Theory), Dr. Robert Koch (father of medical microbiology and discover of *M. tuberculosis*), and Dr. Joseph Lister (father of surgical antisepsis), and supported by many others, including Dr. John Snow (father of epidemiology and public health interventions for cholera), Dr. Ignac Semmelweis (proved the efficacy of handwashing), and countless others, that a "Gladwell tipping point" had been reached.[139-146] This means that from that point in history on, no one would doubt that infectious diseases were caused by microorganisms. Perhaps the best overview of the rapid pace of change during this time period is provided by the Germ Theory Timeline, an online database put together by Dr. William Campbell (Nobel Laureate for Ivermectin) as part of a course he taught.[146]

h. Climate change

Increasingly evidence suggests that new EIDs are facilitated by climate change.[148-153] This will be discussed in detail in Chapter 8.

12. Summary

It is very clear that our current coronavirus (SARS-CoV-2) pandemic represents an EID event that is one of many EID events that are occurring at an increasingly rapid pace. It is likely that all EID events have a multifactorial etiology. Some predisposing factors are largely of historical interest, such as the pre-Germ Theory ignorance, colonization or slavery. Other predisposing factors, such as war or famine, will be germane in any time period. Certain factors, such as population growth, increasing city size, rapid global transportation, climate change are likely of increasing significance and will be discussed in more detail in the next chapter as to their importance in causing pandemics.

Key Points:
1. SARS-CoV-2 is a new viral microorganism (≤71 years old) that naturally resides in bats and was likely transmitted to humans through an as yet undetermined intermediate host, possibly a spiny anteater that was raised in Chinese wildlife farms and sold in Chinese wet markets.
2. Similar to other RNA viruses, it mutates rapidly, at a rate not dissimilar to Influenza and HIV.
3. SARS-CoV-2 was likely transmitted to the intermediate host and then on to humans through an as yet unidentified spillover event, similar to that which occurs with other bat viruses (Nipah, Hendra, Ebola, Marburg).
4. SARS-CoV-2 causes the infectious disease COVID-19, which meets the definition of an emerging infectious disease (EID), like its coronavirus cousins, SARS and MERS.
5. As an EID, it is part of a global phenomenon that is occurring with increasing frequency during the last 10,000 years, and especially the last 200 years (Figure 7.70).
6. Factors that facilitate SARS-CoV-2's appearance as an EID include the farming activities ushered in by the Neolithic period, increasing city size, wars, famines, slavery, colonization, and the pre-Germ Theory.
7. It is likely that other factors are currently more important, such as population growth and global transportation (see Chapter 8).

References

1. CDC. (nd) EID journal background and goals. Centers for Disease Control and Prevention. https://wwwnc.cdc.gov/eid/page/background-goals
2. SCMP. (2020) Coronavirus: China's first confirmed Covid-19 case traced back. *South China Morning Post*, March 13. https://www.scmp.com/news/china/society/article/3074991/coronavirus-chinas-first-confirmed-covid-19-case-traced-back
3. Wu Z, McGoogan J. (2020) Characteristics of and important lessons from the Coronavirus Disease 2019 (COVID-19) outbreak in China. Summary of a report of 72,314 cases from the Chinese Center for Disease Control and Prevention. *JAMA* **323**(13):1239–1242. DOI:10.1001/jama.2020.2648

4. WHO. (nd) WHO receives first report. World Health Organization. https://www.who.int/emergencies/diseases/novel-coronavirus-2019/events-as-they-happen

5. Coronaviridae Study Group of the International Committee on Taxonomy of Viruses. (2020) The species Severe acute respiratory syndrome-related coronavirus: Classifying 2019-nCoV and naming it SARS-CoV-2. *Nature Microbiology* **5**:536–544.

6. Corman VM, Muth D, Niemeyer D, Drosten C. (2018) Hosts and sources of endemic coronaviruses. *Advances in Virus Research* **100**:163–188.

7. Andersen KG, Rambaut A, Lipkin WI, *et al.* (2020) The proximal origin of SARS-CoV-2. *Nature Medicine* **26**:450–452. https://doi.org/10.1038/s41591-020-0820-9

8. Cui J, Li F, Shi Z-L. (2019) Origin and evolution of pathogenic coronaviruses. *Nature Reviews Microbiology* **17**:181–192.

9. Oreshkova N, Molenaar RJ, Vreman S, *et al.* (2020) SARS-CoV-2 infection in farmed minks, the Netherlands, April and May 2020. *Eurosurveillance* **25**(23). https://www.doi.org/10.2807/1560-7917.ES.2020.25.23.2001005

10. Lu R, Zhao X, Li J, *et al.* (2020) Genomic characterization and epidemiology of 2019 novel coronavirus: implications for virus origins and receptor binding. *Lancet* **395**:565–74.

11. Zhou P, Yang X-L, Wang X-G, *et al.* (2020) Discovery of a novel coronavirus associated with the recent pneumonia outbreak in 2 humans and its potential bat origin. *bioRxiv*. https://doi.org/10.1101/2020.01.22.914952

12. Vijaykrishna D, Smith GJ, Zhang JX, *et al.* (2007) Evolutionary insights into the ecology of coronaviruses. *Journal of Virology* **81**(8):4012–4020. DOI:10.1128/JVI.02605-06

13. Anthony SJ, Johnson CK; PREDICT Consortium, *et al.* (2017) Global patterns in coronavirus diversity. *Virus Evolution* **3**(1):vex012. DOI:10.1093/ve/vex012

14. Luis AD, Hayman DTS, O'Shea TJ, *et al.* (2013) A comparison of bats and rodents as reservoirs of zoonotic viruses: are bats special? *Proceedings of the Royal Society B* **280**:20122753. http://dx.doi.org/10.1098/rspb.2012.2753

15. Brierly L, Vonhof MJ, Olival KJ, *et al.* (2016) Quantifying global drivers of zoonotic bat viruses: A process-based perspective. *The American Naturalist* **187**:E53–E64.

16. Brook CE, Dobson AP. (2015) Bats as "special" reservoirs for emerging zoonotic pathogens. *Trends in Microbiology* **23**:172–180. http://dx.doi.org/10.1016/j.tim.2014.12.004

17. Ahn M, Anderson DE, Zhang Q, *et al.* (2019) Dampened NLRP3-mediated inflammation in bats and implications for a special viral reservoir host. *Nature Microbiology* **4**(5):789–799. DOI:10.1038/s41564-019-0371-3

18. Subudhi S, Rapin N, Misra V. (2019) Immune system modulation and viral persistence in bats: Understanding viral spillover. *Viruses* **11**(2):192. DOI:10.3390/v11020192

19. Banerjee A, Subudhi S, Rapin N, *et al.* (2020) Selection of viral variants during persistent infection of insectivorous bat cells with Middle East respiratory syndrome coronavirus. *Scientific Reports* **10**:7257. https://doi.org/10.1038/s41598-020-64264-1

20. Gorbunova V, Seluanov A, Kennedy BK. (2020) The world goes bats: Living longer and tolerating viruses. *Cell Metabolism* **32**(1):31–43. DOI:10.1016/j.cmet.2020.06.013

21. Plowright RK, Eby P, Hudson PJ, *et al.* (2015) Ecological dynamics of emerging bat virus spillover. *Proceedings of the Royal Society B: Biological Sciences* **282**(1798):20142124. DOI:10.1098/rspb.2014.2124

22. Beyer RM, Manica A, Mora C. (2021) Shifts in global bat diversity suggest a possible role of climate change in the emergence of SARS-CoV-1 and SARS-CoV- 2. *Science of the Total Environment* **767**:145413. https://doi.org/10.1016/j.scitotenv.2021.145413

23. Liang J, Zhu C, Zhang L (2021). Cospeciation of coronavirus and paramyxovirus with their bat hosts in the same geographical areas. *BMC Ecology and Evolution* **21**:148. https://doi.org/10.1186/s12862-021-01878-7

24. Joffrin L, Goodman SM, Wilkinson DA, *et al.* (2020) Bat coronavirus phylogeography in the Western Indian Ocean. *Scientific Reports* **10**:6873. https://doi.org/10.1038/s41598-020-63799-7

25. Cui J, Han N, Streicker D, *et al.* (2007) Evolutionary relationships between bat coronaviruses and their hosts. *Emerging Infectious Diseases* **13**(10):1526–1532. DOI:10.3201/eid1310.070448

26. Guo H, Hu BJ, Yang XL, *et al.* (2020) Evolutionary arms race between virus and host drives genetic diversity in bat severe acute respiratory syndrome-related coronavirus spike genes. *Journal of Virology* **94**(20):e00902-20. DOI:10.1128/JVI.00902-20

27. MacLean OA, Lytras S, Weaver S, *et al.* (2021) Natural selection in the evolution of SARS-CoV-2 in bats created a generalist virus and highly capable human pathogen. *PLOS Biology*, March 12. https://doi.org/10.1371/journal.pbio.3001115

28. Liu K, Tan S, Niu S, *et al.* (2021) Cross-species recognition of SARS-CoV-2 to bat ACE2. *Proceedings of the National Academy of Sciences* **118**(1):e2020216118. https://doi.org/10.1073/pnas.2020216118

29. El-Sayed A, Kamel M. (2021) Coronaviruses in humans and animals: the role of bats in viral evolution. *Environmental Science and Pollution Research* **28**(16):19589–19600. https://doi.org/10.1007/s11356-021-12553-1

30. Campos FS, Lourenco-de-Moraes R. (2020) Ecological fever: The evolutionary history of coronavirus in human-wildlife relationships. *Frontiers in Ecology and Evolution*, October 15. https://doi.org/10.3389/fevo.2020.575286

31. Wynne JW, Wang LF. (2013) Bats and viruses: Friend or foe? *PLOS Pathogens* **9**(10):e1003651. DOI:10.1371/journal.ppat.1003651

32. Lam TT-Y, Shum MH-H, Zhu H-C, *et al.* (2020) Identifying SARS-CoV-2 related coronaviruses in Malayan pangolins. *Nature* **583**:282–285. https://doi.org/10.1038/s41586-020-2169-0

33. Zhang T, Wu Q, Zhang A. (2020) Probable pangolin origin of SARS-CoV-2 associated with the COVID-19 outbreak. *Current Biology* **30**:1346–1351.

34. Chen N, Zhou M, Dong X, *et al.* (2020) Epidemiological and clinical characteristics of 99 cases of 2019 novel coronavirus pneumonia in Wuhan, China: A descriptive study. *Lancet* **395**:507-513.

35. Standaert M. (2020) Illegal wildlife trade goes online as China shuts down markets. *Aljazeera*, March 24. https://www.aljazeera.com/economy/2020/03/24/illegal-wildlife-trade-goes-online-as-china-shuts-down-markets

36. Samuel S. (2020) The coronavirus likely came from China's wet markets. They're reopening anyway. https://www.vox.com/future-perfect/2020/4/15/21219222/coronavirus-china-ban-wet-markets-reopening

37. Nijman V, Zhang MX, Shepherd CR. (2016) Pangolin trade in the Mong La wildlife market and the role of Myanmar in the smuggling of pangolins into China. *Global Ecology Conservation* **5**:118-126.

38. National Geographic. (nd) Pangolins. https://www.nationalgeographic.com/animals/mammals/group/pangolins/

39. Zhang F, Wu S, Cen P. (2022) The past present and future of the pangolin in mainland China. *Global Ecology Conservation* e01995. https://doi.org/10.1016/j.gecco.2021.e01995

40. Doucleff M. (2021) WHO points to wildlife farms in southern China as a likely source of pandemic. Goats and Soda, National Public Radio, Inc, March 15. https://www.npr.org/sections/goatsandsoda/2021/03/15/977527808/who-points-to-wildlife-farms-in-southwest-china-as-likely-source-of-pandemic

41. Webster RG. (2004) Wet markets — A continuing source of severe acute respiratory syndrome and influenza? *Lancet* **363**(9404):234–236. DOI:10.1016/S0140-6736(03)15329-9

42. Hemida MG, Elmoslemany A, Al-Hizab F, *et al.* (2017) Dromedary camels and the transmission of Middle East Respiratory Syndrome Coronavirus. *Transboundary and Emerging Diseases* **64**:344–353. DOI:10.1111/tbed.12401

43. Maxmen A, Mallapaty S. (2021) The COVID lab-leak hypothesis: what scientists do and don't know. *Nature*, June 8. https://www.nature.com/articles/d41586-021-01529-3

44. Boni MF, Lemey P, Jiang X, *et al.* (2020) Evolutionary origins of the SARS-CoV-2 sarbecovirus lineage responsible for the COVID-19 pandemic. *Nature Microbiology* **5**:1408–1417. https://doi.org/10.1038/s41564-020-0771-4

45. Li X, Giorgi EE, Marichann MH, *et al.* (2020) Emergence of SARS-CoV-2 through recombination and strong purifying selection. *Science Advances* **6**(27):eabb9153. DOI:10.1126/sciadv.abb9153

46. Guan Y, Zheng BJ, He YQ, *et al.* (2003) Isolation and characterization of viruses related to the SARS coronavirus from animals in southern China. *Science* **302**:276–278.

47. Kan B, Wang M, Jing H, *et al.* (2005) Molecular evolution analysis and geographic investigation of Severe Acute Respiratory Syndrome coronavirus-like virus in palm civets at an animal market and on farms. *Journal of Virology* **79**:11892–11900.

48. Naguib MM, Li R, Ling J, *et al.* (2021) Live and wet markets: Food access versus the risk of disease emergence. *Trends in Microbiology* **29**(7):573–581. https://doi.org/10.1016/j.tim.2021.02.007

49. UN. (2021) WHO and partners urge countries to halt sales of wild mammals at food markets. *UN News*, April 13. https://news.un.org/en/story/2021/04/1089622

50. Kahn JS, McIntosh K. (2005) History and recent advances in coronavirus discovery. *Pediatric Infectious Disease Journal* **24**:S223–S227.

51. Institute of Medicine. (2004) *Learning from SARS: Preparing for the Next Disease Outbreak: Workshop Summary.* The National Academies Press, Washington, DC. https://doi.org/10.17226/10915

52. Park M, Thwaites RS, Openshaw PJM. (2020) COVID-19 Lessons from SARS and MERS. *European Journal of Immunology* **50**:308–316.

53. Lau SK, Woo PC, Li KS, *et al.* (2005) Severe acute respiratory syndrome coronavirus-like virus in Chinese horseshoe bats. *Proceedings of the National Academy of Sciences of the United States of America* **102**:14040–14045.

54. Li W, Shi Z, Yu M, *et al.* (2005) Bats are natural reservoirs of SARS-like coro-naviruses. *Science* **310**:676–679.

55. Wang M, Yan M, Xu H, *et al.* (2005) SARS-CoV infection in a restaurant from palm civet. *Emerging Infectious Diseases* **11**:1860–1865.

56. Wang L-F, Shi Z, Zhang S, *et al.* (2006) Review of bats and SARS. *Emerging Infectious Diseases* **12**:1834–1840.

57. Cui J, Han N, Streicker D, *et al.* (2007) Evolutionary relationships between bat coronaviruses and their hosts. *Emerging Infectious Diseases* **13**:1526–1532.

58. Memish ZA, Mishra N, Olival KJ, *et al.* (2013) Middle East respiratory syn-drome coronavirus in bats, Saudi Arabia. *Emerging Infectious Diseases* **19**:1819–1823.

59. Anthony SJ, Gilardi K, Menachery VD, *et al.* (2017) Further evidence for bats as the evolutionary source of Middle East Respiratory Syndrome Coronavi-rus. *MBio* **8**(2):e00373-17.

60. Chastel C. (2014) Middle East respiratory syndrome (MERS): Bats or drome-dary, which of them is responsible? *Le Bulletin de la Société de Pathologie Exotique* **107**:69–73.

61. Widagdo W, Begeman L, Schipper D, *et al.* (2017) Tissue distribution of the MERS-coronavirus receptor in bats. *Scientific Reports* **7**:1193.

62. Song H-D, Tu C-C, Zhang G-W, *et al.* (2005) Cross-host evolution of severe acute respiratory syndrome coronavirus in palm civet and human. *Proceed-ings of the National Academy of Sciences* **102**:2430–2435.

63. Hu B, Zeng L-P, Yang X-L, *et al.* (2017) Discovery of a rich gene pool of bat SARS-related coronaviruses provides new insights into the origin of SARS coronavirus. *PLOS Pathogens* **13**(11):e1006698. https://doi.org/10.1371/journal.ppat.1006698

64. Taiaroa G, Rawlinson D, Featherstone L, *et al.* (2020) Direct RNA sequenc-ing and early evolution of SARS-CoV-2. *bioRxiv*, April 3. https://doi.org/10.1101/2020.03.05.976167

65. Lu H, Zhao Y, Zhang J, *et al.* (2004) Date of origin of the SARS coronavirus strains. *BMC Infectious Diseases* **4**,3. http://www.biomedcentral.com/1471-2334/4/3

66. Taubenberger JK, Kash J. (2010) Influenza virus evolution, host adaptation and pandemic formation. *Cell Host & Microbe* **7**:440–451.

67. Plowright RK, Peel AJ, Streicker DG, *et al.* (2016) Transmission of within-host dynamics driving pulses of zoonotic viruses in reservoir-host populations. *PLOS Neglected Tropical Diseases* **10**(8):e0004796. DOI:10.1371/journal.pntd.0004796

68. Amman BR, Carroll SA, Reed ZD, *et al.* (2012) Seasonal pulses of Marburg virus circulation in juvenile Rousettus aegyptiacus bats coincide with periods of increased risk of human infection. *PLOS Pathogens* **8**:e1002877.

69. Wang M-N, Zhang W, Gao Y-T, *et al.* (2016) Longitudinal surveillance of SARS-like coronaviruses in bats by real-time PCR. *Virological Sinica* **31**:78–80.

70. Banerjee A, Kulcsar K, Misra V, *et al.* (2019) Bats and coronaviruses. *Viruses* **11**(1):41.

71. Olival KJ, Hosseini PR, Zambrana-Torrelio C, *et al.* (2017) Host and viral traits predict zoonotic spillover from mammals. *Nature* 546:646–650.

72. Jones KE, Patel NG, Levy MA, *et al.* (2008) Global trends in emerging infectious diseases. *Nature* **451**:990–994.

73. The Climate Change and Public Health Law Site. (nd) Pasteurs' papers on the germ theory. Historic Public Health Articles. https://biotech.law.lsu.edu/cphl/history/articles/pasteur.htm

74. Kumar S. (2005) Molecular clocks: Four decades of evolution. *Nature Reviews Genetics* **6**:654–662.

75. Simon Y, Ho W, Duchene S. (2014) Molecular-clock methods for estimating evolutionary rates and timescales. *Molecular Ecology* **23**:5947–5965.

76. Battistuzzi FU, Feijao A, Hedges SB. (2004) A genomic timescale of prokaryote evolution: Insights in the origin of methanogenesis, phototrophy, and the colonization of land. *BMC Evolutionary Biology* **4**:1–14.

77. Weinert LA, Werren JH, Aebi A, *et al.* (2009) Evolution and diversity of Rickettsia bacteria. *BMC Biology* **7**:1741.

78. Han XY, Silva FJ. (2014) On the age of Leprosy. *PLOS Neglected Tropical Diseases* **8**:1–8.

79. Kunisawa T. (2015) Evolutionary relationships of completely sequenced Clostridia species and close relatives. *International Journal of Systematic and Evolutionary Microbiology* **65**:4276–4283.

80. Nishio Y, Nakamura Y, Usuda Y, *et al.* (2004) Evolutionary process of amino acid biosynthesis in Corynebacterium at the whole genome level. *Molecular Biology Evolution* **21**:1683–1691.

81. Letek M, Ordonez E, Fernandez-Natal I, *et al.* (2006). Indentification of the emerging skin pathogen Corynebacterium amycolatum using PCR-amplification of the essential divIVA gene as a target. *FEMS Microbiology Letters* **265**:256–263.

82. Comas I, Coscolla M, Luo T, *et al.* (2013) Out-of-Africa migration and Neolithic co-expansion of Mycobacterium tuberculosis with modern humans. *Nature Genetics* **45**:1176–1182.

83. Otto TD, Gilabert A, Crellen T, *et al.* (2018) Genomes of all known members of Plasmodium subgenus reveal paths to virulent human Malaria. *Nature Microbiology* **3**:687–697.

84. Pupo GM, Lan R, Reeves PR. (2000) Multiple independent origins of Shigella clones of Escherichia coli and convergent evolution of many of their characteristics. *Proceedings of the National Academy of Sciences* **97**:10567–10572.

85. Roumagnac P, Weill F-X, Dolecek C, *et al.* (2006) Evolutionary history of Salmonella typhi. *Science* **314**:1301–1304.

86. De Melo F, De Melo JCM, Fraga AM, *et al.* (2010) Syphilis at the crossroad of phylogenetics and paleopathology. *PLOS Neglected Tropical Diseases* **4**:e575.

87. Suzuki Y, Nei M. (2002) Origin and evolution of influenza virus hemagglutinin genes. *Molecular Biology and Evolution* **19**:501–509.

88. Bourhy H, Reynes J-M, Dunham EJ, *et al.* (2008). The origin and phylogeography of dog rabies virus. *Journal of General Virology* **89**:2673–2681.

89. Sall AA, Faye O, Diallo M, *et al.* (2010) Yellow fever virus exhibits slower evolutionary dynamics than dengue virus. *Journal of Virology* **84**:765–772.

90. Bryant JE, Holmes EC, Barrett ADT. (2007) Out of Africa: A molecular perspective on the introduction of yellow fever virus into the Americas. *PLOS Pathogens* **3**:0668–0673.

91. Rascovan N, Sjogren K-G, Kristiansen K, *et al.* (2019) Emergence and spread of basal lineages of Yersinia pestis during the Neolithic Decline. *Cell* **176**:295–306.

92. Furuse Y, Suzuki A, Oshitani H. (2010) Origin of measles virus: divergence from Rinderpest virus between the 11th and 12th centuries. *Virology Journal* **7**:52.

93. Bart MJ, Harris SR, Advani A, *et al.* (2014) Global population structure and evolution of Bordetella pertussis and their relationship with vaccination. *mBio* **5**:e01074-14.

94. Duggan AT, Perdomo MF, Piombino-Mascali D, *et al.* (2016). 17th century Variola virus reveals the recent history of smallpox. *Current Biology* **26**:3407–3412.

95. Hu Dalong, Liu B, Feng L, *et al.* (2016) Origins of the current seventh cholera pandemic. *Proceedings of the National Academy of Sciences* **113**(48):E7730–E7739. https://doi.org/10.1073/pnas.1608732113

96. Schoen C, Blom J, Claus H, *et al.* (2008) Whole-genome comparison of disease and carriage strains provides insights into virulence evolution in

Neisseria meningitidis. *Proceedings of the National Academy of Sciences* **105**:3473–3478.

97. Padhi A, Ma L. (2014) Molecular evolutionary and epidemiological dynamics of genotyes 1G and 2B of Rubella virus. *PLOS One* **9**:e110082.

98. Pomeroy LW, Bjornstad ON, Holmes EC. (2008) The evolutionary and epidemiological dynamics of the Paramyxoviridae. *Journal of Molecular Evolution* **66**:98–106.

99. Sass EJ, Gottfried G, Sorem A, eds. (1996). <u>Polio's Legacy: An Oral History</u>. University Press of America, Washington, D.C.

100. Lewin R. (2009) *The Origin of Agriculture and the First Villagers. Human Evolution: An Illustrated Introduction.* John Wiley & Sons, Hoboken NJ.

101. Barker G. (2009) *The Agricultural Revolution In Prehistory: Why Did Foragers Become Farmers?* Oxford University Press, Oxford, England.

102. Weiss RA. (2001). The Leeuwenhoek Lecture, 2001. Animal origins of human infectious disease. *Philosophical Transactions of the Royal Society B* **356**:957–977.

103. Diamond J. (2002). Evolution, consequences and future of plant and animal domestication. *Nature* **418**:700–707.

104. Pearce-Duvet JMC. (2006). The origin of human pathogens: Evaluating the role of agriculture and domestic animals in the evolution of human disease. *Biological Reviews* **81**:369-382.

105. Wolfe ND, Dunavan CP, Diamond J. (2012). *Origins of Major Human Infectious Diseases. Improving Food Safety Through a One Health Approach: Workshop Summary.* The National Academies Press, Washington, DC.

106. Lefebure T, Richards, VP, Lang P, *et al.* (2012) Gene repertoire evolution of streptococcus pyogenes inferred from phylogenomic analysis with streptococcus canis and streptococcus dysgalactiae. *PLOS One* **7**:e37607. DOI:10.1371/journal.pone.0037607

107. Harper KN, Ocampo PS, Steiner BM, *et al.* (2008) On the origin of the treponematoses: A phylogenetic approach. *PLOS Neglected Tropical Diseases* **2**:e148. DOI:10.1371/journal.pntd.0000148

108. Weyand NJ, Wertheimer AM, Hobbs TR, *et al.* (2013) Neisseria infection of rhesus macaques as a model to study colonization, transmission, persistence, and horizontal gene transfer. *Proceedings of the National Academy of Sciences* **110**:3059–3064.

109. Combelas N, Holmblat B, Joffret M-L, *et al.* (2011) Recombination between poliovirus and Coxsackie A viruses of species C: A model of viral genetic plasticity and emergence. *Viruses* **3**:1460–1484. DOI:10.3390/v3081460

110. Gulberg M, Tolf C, Jonsson N, *et al*. (2010) Characterization of a putative ancestor of Coxsackievirus B5. *Journal of Virology* **84**:9695–9708.
111. Chandler T, Fox G. (1974) *3000 Years of Urban Growth*. Academic Press, New York.
112. Dobson AP, Carper ER. (1996) Infectious diseases and human population history. Throughout history the establishment of disease has been a side effect of the growth of civilization. *BioScience* **45**:115–126.
113. Procopius. (1914) *History of the Wars*, 7 Vols, trans. Dewing HB. Harvard University Press. **1**:451–473.
114. Harbeck M, Seifert L, Hansch S. (2013) Yersinia pestis DNA from skeletal remains from the 6th century AD reveals insights into Justinianic Plague. *PLOS Pathogens* **9**:E1003349.
115. Mallett M, Shaw C. (2012) *The Italian Wars, 1494–1559: War, State and Society In Early Modern Europe*. Pearson Education Limited, Harlow, England.
116. Seaman RM, ed. (2018) *Epidemics and War: The Impact of Disease on Major Conflicts in History*. ABC-CLIO, Santa Barbara CA, Chapter 5.
117. Talty S. (2009) *The Illustrious Dead. The Terrifying Story of How Typhus Killed Napoleon's Greatest Army*. Crown Publishing Group, New York City.
118. Gill CJ, Gill GC. (2005) Nightingale in Scutari: Her legacy reexamined. *Clinical Infectious Diseases* **40**:1799–1805.
119. Wikiepedia. (nd) List of wars by date. https://en.wikipedia.org/wiki/Category:Lists_of_wars_by_date
120. Schellekens J. (1996) Irish famines and English mortality in the eighteenth century. *Journal of Interdisciplinary History* **27**:29–42.
121. Wikipedia. (nd) List of famines by date. https://en.wikipedia.org/wiki/List_of_famines.
122. Mokyr J, Gráda CO. (1999) Famine disease and famine mortality: Lessons from the Irish experience. University College Dublin Centre for Economic Research Working Paper.
123. Stewart L. (1985) The edge of utility: Slaves and smallpox in the early eighteenth century. *Medical History* **29**:54–70.
124. Rodrigues PT, Valdivia HO, de Oliveira TC, *et al*. (2018). Human migration and the spread of malaria parasites to the new world. *Scientific Reports* **8**:1993.
125. Yalcindag E, Elguero E, Arnathau C, *et al*. (2012) Multiple independent introductions of Plasmodium falciparum in South America. *Proceedings of the National Academy of Sciences* **109**:511–516.

126. Jaeger LH, de Souza SMFM, Dias OF, Iniguez AM. (2013) Mycobacterium tuberculosis complex in remains of 18th–19th century slaves, Brazil. *Emerging Infectious Diseases* **19**:837–839.

127. Crellen T, Allan F, David S, *et al.* (2016) Whole genome resequencing of the human parasite Schistosoma mansoni reveals population history and effects of selection. *Scientific Reports* **6**:20954.

128. Steckel RH, Jensen RA. (1986) Determinants of slave and crew mortality in the Atlantic slave trade. *Journal of Economic History* **46**:57–77.

129. Read I. (2012) A triumphant decline? Tetanus among slaves and freeborn in Brazil. *History, Science, Health, Manguinhos, Rio de Janeiro* **19**:107–132.

130. Acuna-Soto R, Stahle DW, Cleaveland MK, Therrell MD. (2002). Mega-drought and megadeath in 16th century Mexico. *Emerging Infectious Diseases* **8**:360–362.

131. Robertson RG. (2001). *Rotting Face: Smallpox and the American Indian*, Caxton Press, Caldwell, Idaho.

132. Bennett FC, ed. (1968) The story of the aboriginal people of the central coast of New South Wales. Brisbane Water Historical Society, Brisbane, Australia.

133. Diamond J. (1999) *Guns, Germs, And Steel*. WW Norton & Company, New York City.

134. Cliff AD, Haggett P, Smallman-Raynor MR. (2000) *Island Epidemics*. Oxford University Press, Oxford England.

135. Cliff A, Haggett P. (2004) Time, travel and infection. *British Medical Bulletin* **69**:87–99.

136. Farley J. (1977) *The Spontaneous Generation Controversy From Descartes to Oparin*. Johns Hopkins University Press, Baltimore MD.

137. Sterner CS. (2007) A brief history of the miasmic theory. *Bulletin History Medicine* **22**:747.

138. Halliday S. (2001) Death and miasma in Victorian London: An obstinate belief. *BMJ* **323**:1469–1471.

139. Gladwell M. (2000) *The Tipping Point*. Little, Brown and Company, New York City.

140. Behbehani AM. (1983) The smallpox story: Life and death of an old disease. *Microbiological Reviews* **47**:455–509.

141. Debre P. (1994) *Louis Pasteur*, tran. E. Forster. The Johns Hopkins University Press, Baltimore & London.

142. Gradmann C. (2009) *Laboratory Disease, Robert Koch's Medical Bacteriology*, tran. E. Forster, Johns Hopkins University Press, Baltimore MD.

143. Fitzharris L. (2017) *The Butchering Art, Joseph Lister's Quest to Transform the Grisly World of Victorian Medicine.* Scientific American, Farrar, Straus and Giroux, New York.

144. Snow J. (1855) *On the Mode of Communication of Cholera.* John Churchill, London.

145. Semmelweis I. (1981) *The Etiology of Childbed Fever*, trans. Murphy F, eds. Nuland SB, Gyorgyey FA. The Classics of Medicine Library, Birmingham, AL.

146. Campbell WC (nd) The Germ Theory Timeline. http://germtheorytimeline. info/intro

147. Pontremoli C, Forni D, Clerici M, *et al.* (2020) Possible European origin of circulating Varicella zoster virus strains. *Journal of Infectious Diseases* **221**:1286–1294.

148. Polgreen PM, Polgreen EL. (2018) Infectious Diseases, Weather, and Climate. *Clin Infect Dis.* Mar 5; **66**(6):815–817. doi: 10.1093/cid/cix1105.

149. Thomas MB (2020) Epidemics on themove: Climate change and infectious disease. *PLoS Biol* **18**(11):e3001013. https://doi.org/10.1371/journal. pbio.3001013

150. Rohr JR, Cohen JM (2020) Understanding how temperature shifts could impact infectious disease. *PLoS Biol* **18**(11):e3000938. https://doi. org/10.1371/journal.pbio.3000938

151. Byers JE (2020) Effects of climate change on parasites and disease in estuarine and nearshore environments. *PLoS Biol* **18**(11):e3000743. https://doi. org/10.1371/journal.pbio.3000743

152. Burdon JJ, Zhan J (2020) Climate change and disease in plant communities. *PLoS Biol* **18**(11):e3000949. https://doi.org/10.1371/journal.pbio.3000949

153. Lowe R, Ryan SJ, Mahon R, Van Meerbeeck CJ, Trotman AR, Boodram L-LG, *et al.* (2020) Building resilience to mosquito-borne diseases in the Caribbean. *PLoS Biol* **18**(11):e3000791. https://doi.org/10.1371/journal. pbio.3000791

8 Pantheon of Plagues

"The plague marked the end of the Middle Ages and the start of a great cultural renewal. Could the coronavirus, for all its destruction, offer a similar opportunity for radical change?"

Lawrence Wright
"How Pandemics Wreak Havoc — and Open Minds"
The New Yorker, July 7, 2020

Contents

1. Epidemiology Definitions
   a. What defines an outbreak, an epidemic or a pandemic?
2. Outbreaks
3. Epidemics
4. Pandemics
5. Superspreaders
6. Global Trends
7. Summary of Factors Leading to Pandemics

1. Epidemiology Definitions

To understand pandemics, it is necessary to understand a few things about outbreaks, epidemics and pandemics, expanding upon what was already discussed in Chapter 1. We will begin by considering the definitions necessary to describe an outbreak, epidemic and pandemic.

a. What defines an outbreak, an epidemic or a pandemic?

An outbreak refers to an increase, often sudden, in the number of cases of a disease above what is normally expected in that population in a defined geographic area.[1] An epidemic carries the same definition as an outbreak, but it is often used for a more expanded geographic area. A pandemic refers to an epidemic that has spread over several countries or continents, usually affecting a larger number of people.[1] Thus, "outbreak", "epidemic" and "pandemic" are words that describe the relative number of clustered infections associated with a given organism. "Outbreak" and "epidemic" are sometimes used interchangeably, as there is no universally accepted definition for their relative size. An approximation might be as follows: Outbreak, <100 people; Epidemic, 100 to <1,000,000 people; Pandemic > a million people and usually involving several countries or continents.

> Key Point: "Outbreak", "Epidemic" and "Pandemic" are words that roughly describe the numbers of cases caused by an infectious agent.

How do you know for sure if you have an outbreak?

To decide if you have an outbreak, those carrying out the investigation must first verify that there is indeed a problem. This involves interviewing, examining, and testing the patients who may be part of the outbreak. This must be done very carefully, as the investigators are sometimes themselves at risk of acquiring and even dying from the infection, for example, Ebola. Thus, the interviews are sometimes done wearing personal protective equipment (PPE) or over the phone. Once it has been verified that the cases are valid, then a case definition for the possible outbreak cases must be developed.[2] A case definition is a standard set of criteria for deciding whether an individual should be classified as having the health condition of interest. The case definition can have a dramatic effect on the estimates of outbreak size.[3] For example, between January 15 and March 3, 2020, the National Health Commission in China changed the COVID-19 case definition seven times. If the fifth version of the case definition had been used throughout the early outbreak, which included radiographic evidence of pneumonia for the first and only time, the number of confirmed cases would have been 232,000, rather than the 55,508 confirmed cases reported in this time interval. Also, changing the definition in the middle of the outbreak can have an effect on graphs designed to show trends in whether the number of cases is increasing or decreasing and whether interventions are having the desired effect. The graph most commonly used to show changes in

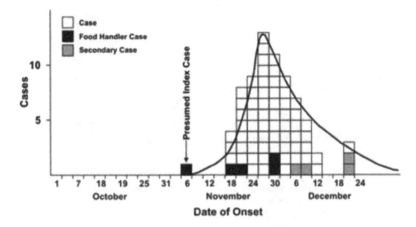

Figure 8.71. Point-source outbreak. Hepatitis A epidemic curve (histogram) shows the presumed index (first) case, followed four days later by a steep increase in cases, which taper off to 0. Cases who were food handlers and secondary cases are also shown. CDC, unpublished data.[6]

the outbreak over time is called an epidemic curve (epi curve). Epi curves depict when people became ill by day, week or month.[4] An example of an epi curve depicting hepatitis A cases is shown in Figure 8.71.[5]

The simplest kind of outbreak is a point-source outbreak.[1] In such an outbreak, persons are exposed over a brief time to the same source, such as a single individual, meal or event. Everyone who becomes ill does so within one incubation period. The incubation period is the range of time from the shortest to the longest that it takes people to become ill following exposure to the source. Typically, the epidemic curve for such outbreaks has a steep upslope and a more gradual decline (Figure 8.71).[1] If a microorganism can be transmitted person-to-person, then a point-source outbreak can transform into a propagated outbreak (Figure 8.72).[1,6] In propagated outbreaks, cases occur over more than one incubation period (Figure 8.72).[6]

In propagated outbreaks, the likelihood of person-to-person transmission is expressed by R_0, spoken of as "R naught", previously called the basic reproduction number.[7] The importance of R_0 related to transmission is shown in Figure 1.3 (Chapter 1); simply put, R_0 is the average number of people that can be infected by one person. If R_0 is greater than one, the outbreak will continue; if less than one, it will end. R_0 is nearly always estimated retrospectively using laboratory data, such as blood antibodies, which indicate prior infection, or PCR (polymerase chain reaction looking for RNA or DNA,

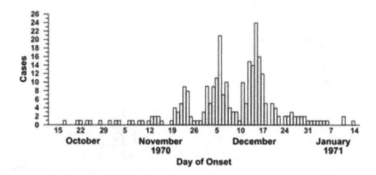

Figure 8.72. Propagated outbreak. Measles cases by the date of onset, October 15, 1970, to January 16, 1971. The peaks occur about 11 days apart, consistent with the incubation period for measles. CDC, unpublished data.[6]

such as the RNA PCR testing used for COVID-19 testing), or mathematical models.[7,8] It may change as a result of outbreak interventions. It is more complex when a vector is involved, such as mosquitos transmitting malaria.[7] It can also be used to determine what proportion of the population needs to be immunized to achieve herd immunity (Figure 1.4). Herd immunity is the proportion of the population that needs to be immune to prevent a propagated outbreak. For example, if the R_0 is near 2, like that estimated for the coronavirus pandemic (Tables 1.2, 8.24), the proportion of the population needing to be immune to prevent propagation is approximately 50%; whereas, if the R_0 is 10, like for measles (Table 8.23), then 90% of the population needs to be immune (Figure 1.4).[9]

> Key Point: R_0, or the basic reproduction number, is an outbreak data-derived number that gives us the average number of people that can be infected by one person (Figure 1.3). It can be used to make decisions about what percentage of the population needs vaccinating to stop the outbreak (Figure 1.4).

We will now explore the factors, both microorganism-related and others (those that are the drivers behind outbreaks), and why some remain small and self-limited, while others go on to cause epidemics or even pandemics.

2. Outbreaks

What infectious diseases cause self-limited outbreaks and why?

Table 8.22 lists nine infectious diseases chosen from Tables 7.20 and 7.21 in Chapter 7 that cause self-limited outbreaks. The explanation why five of these diseases (tetanus, Lyme disease, legionellosis, West Nile fever, rabies) have minimal ability to cause outbreaks has to do with absolute or near-absolute lack of person-to-person transmission.

Tetanus, a.k.a. lockjaw, is an infectious disease caused by *Clostridium tetani* that can cause spasms and death if an infection occurs in a nonimmune host (one without preexisting antibodies to tetanus toxin).[42] However, to cause an outbreak, it requires multiple people to have both open wounds and an exposure to soil. This can happen, but only in association with mass casualty events, such as wars, earthquakes and tsunamis, and is not sustainable, because person-to-person transmission does not

Table 8.22.   Infectious diseases that cause self-limited outbreaks.[18-52]

Transmission Route	Source	Infection Name[10-34]	R_0[35-39]	Mortality[40-47] Rx, No Rx	% with No Symptoms[48-52]	Other
Vector-borne	Ticks	Lyme disease	0	0, 0%	7%	Deer reservoir, seasonal
	Mosquito	West Nile encephalitis	0	N/A, 14%	80%	Bird reservoir
Environment	Soil	Tetanus	0	81, 10%	0	Trauma, nonimmune
	Water	Legionellosis	0	1–32%, N/A	50%	Potable water, aerosols
	Animals	Rabies	1.2	0, 99%	0	Animal bites
Person-to-Person	Feces	*C.difficile* colitis	0.6–2.0	1–9%, N/A	0–50%	Hospitals, antibiotics
		Typhoid Fever	1.2	2.5, 17%	2–5%	50% from carriers
	Skin	Leprosy	1.4–4	N/A, N/A	0	Lepromatous > other
	Nose	MRSA BSI	1.5–3	16–37%, N/A	0	Hospitals, antibiotics

—Transmission route = how the organism is transmitted

—Source = transmission route details

—R_0 = basic reproduction number, the likelihood of person-to-person transmission. Those with zeros are not thought to have significant person-to-person transmission

—Mortality: Rx = treated and/or vaccinated; no Rx = not treated

—Other = what factors facilitated the outbreak occurring

—MRSA = methicillin-resistant *Staphylococcus aureus*.

occur.[10,11] With the advent of tetanus antitoxin use in the First World War, the risk of death due to tetanus during the war dropped greater than 10-fold, and even further after a vaccine became available in 1926.[11]

Lyme disease, a.k.a. the great imitator, is a nonlethal, tick-borne infection caused by *Borrelia burgdorferi*, which has been steadily increasing in the United States (US) since its discovery in 1981, so it meets the definition of an outbreak, but person-to-person transmission does not occur, so a propagated outbreak is not possible.[12,40] It has been speculated that this increase relates to global warming, increased forestation, and other factors, but thus far, proof of these speculations is lacking.

Legionellosis, a.k.a. Legionnaire's disease, caused by *Legionella pneumophila*, was first described when a point source outbreak occurred in 1976 in a hotel in Philadelphia, Pennsylvania, US, associated with a Legionnaire's conference. It causes pneumonia with significant mortality.[43] Subsequently, this organism has been shown to cause outbreaks all over the world.[13,14] It is typically transmitted via drinking water or aerosolized water. It is difficult to eradicate in the environment because of its long-term persistence in free-living amoebae, but it cannot be transmitted person-to-person.[15]

West Nile Fever, a.k.a. West Nile neuroinvasive disease, caused by the *West Nile virus*, spread throughout the Mediterranean, Europe and the US in the 1990s.[16] It can cause severe neurologic infections with long-term complications, and can be fatal (Table 8.22).[41] Its reservoir is birds, and it is transmitted to humans by mosquitoes, and rarely, from human to human via transfusion. Fortunately, 80% of its infections are asymptomatic (Table 8.22).

Rabies, a.k.a. "mad dog disease" or hydrophobia, caused by the *Rabies virus*, is transmitted most commonly from bats or various omnivores, such as dogs, raccoons, or skunks, to other animals, including humans, by biting with resultant occasional outbreaks.[17,35] It is nearly 100% fatal unless there is pre-existing immunity due to vaccination or post-exposure prophylaxis (Table 8.22); asymptomatic infection in humans is not known to occur. Person-to-person transmission of rabies is extremely uncommon. Thus, all five organisms above can cause outbreaks, but these are not sustainable due to their limited person-to-person transmission, so their R_0 is essentially zero.

> Key Point: An outbreak of infections can occur without person-to-person transmission, but it is not sustainable.

The other four infections in Table 8.22 can be transmitted from person-to-person but only cause sustained outbreaks under well-defined circumstances. They can be divided into two groups based on their route of transmission: (1) fecal-oral, or (2) direct contact. Two infections in Table 8.22 are transmitted by the fecal-oral route — Typhoid fever and C. difficile colitis — and two by direct contact — MRSA infection and Leprosy.

Typhoid Fever, a.k.a. night-soil fever, is caused by Salmonella Typhi, and can be fatal (Table 8.22).[45] There is no environmental reservoir for S. Typhi, so all outbreaks must originate from an infected or colonized human carrier, either directly through food preparation, or indirectly through ingestion of fecally contaminated water downstream.[18] As a result typhoid fever is a disease that affects countries that do not have reliable water treatment systems, primarily in Asia, Africa, and Central and South America.[19,20] At least 50% of typhoid fever outbreaks are associated with chronic carriers, individuals who shed the organism asymptomatically in their stool due either to gallbladder colonization or schistosomiasis parasite colonization by S. Typhi.[18,21,22] In South America, Africa and Asia, where schistosomal parasites reside in the human intestines or the bladder, the intestinal tract of the schistosomal parasite can become colonized by S. Typhi, making it difficult to get rid of without first eliminating the schistosomal worms.[22] Fortunately, such carriers are uncommon (2–5% of those infected by S. Typhi, Table 8.22). The most notable historical example of such a carrier was Mary Mallon, a.k.a. "Typhoid Mary", who caused a series of typhoid fever outbreaks in the New York City area in the early 1900s while serving as a cook for wealthy families, largely because the Public Health System had no surveillance system in place and could not track her movements.[21] She ultimately was arrested and died while incarcerated. With the advent of public health surveillance systems and improvement in water treatment (chlorination, waste treatment, etc.), there has been a steady decline in typhoid fever globally during the last hundred years, but there are still many cases occurring in developing countries.[19,20,23-25]

C. difficile colitis, a.k.a. C. diff., caused by Clostridium difficile, is the other fecal-oral transmitted infection that can cause a typically self-limited outbreak. Outbreaks occur almost exclusively in hospitals because the most important risk factor for C.difficile-related colitis is receiving antibiotics, and greater than 50% of hospitalized patients are on antibiotics; antibiotic use in the community is substantially less common.[26,27] It causes significant mortality, if not diagnosed and treated early in its course.[44]

Infections that cause limited outbreaks and are transmitted by close contact include an ancient disease, Leprosy, and a newer one, MRSA infection. Leprosy, a.k.a. Hansen's disease, is caused by *Mycobacterium leprae*, a cousin of *Mycobacterium tuberculosis*. It is more likely to be transmitted if the index (first) case in a group of people has lepromatous leprosy (many *M. leprae* organisms seen in skin microscopic analysis), rather than tuberculoid leprosy (few organisms seen).[28] The introduction of multidrug leprosy therapy in 1982 has led to a dramatic decline in leprosy transmission and the number of global cases, resulting in the WHO proposing 'Towards Zero Leprosy'.[29]

Staphylococcus aureus infection, a.k.a. Staph, is thought to be primarily transmitted by direct contact, although it occasionally occurs as a point source outbreak with associated airborne transmission due to a viral upper respiratory tract infection.[30,31] MRSA infections are more common in hospitalized patients receiving antibiotics in intensive care units (ICUs, hospital-acquired) or healthcare-associated patients (nursing homes, home healthcare) than in outpatients, and can be fatal.[32,47] The risk of developing MRSA infection in the ICU can be reduced by active surveillance for MRSA, isolation, and/or decolonization (nasal treatment, daily antiseptic bathing).[33,34]

Key Point: Self-limited outbreaks that are transmitted person-to-person only occur in unique risk groups (for example, those receiving antibiotics: *C. difficile*, MRSA) or where transmission is either slow (leprosy) or requires contaminated food or water (typhoid fever).

---

3. Epidemics

What infectious diseases cause epidemics and why?

Table 8.23 is a list of 20 infectious diseases chosen from Tables 7.20 and 7.21 in Chapter 7 because they all have the capability of causing epidemics (large regional outbreaks). They can be divided into four categories based on their routes of transmission: (1) vector-borne, (2) fecal-oral, (3) via body fluids, and (4) airborne and/or droplet.

Table 8.23. Infectious diseases that cause epidemics.[53–178]

Transmission Route	Source	Infection Name[53–123]	R_0[55,124–137]	Mortality[138–153] Rx, No Rx	% with No Symptoms[154–178]	Other
Vector borne	Lice	Epidemic Typhus	~2.0	<5, 30–60%	Rare	War, prison
	Mosquito	Zika	3.02	N/A, 0%, 8%[A]	46%	Tropics
Person-to-person Adults/children	Feces	Dysentery	<1.5–2.2	<1, 9–17%	14%	War, refugees
		Norovirus	1.6–4.0	N/A, 7% (elderly)	12%	Cruise ships
		Polio	10–15	N/A, 5–24% (polio)	>99%	Vaccine status
	Body fluids	Syphilis	1.3–1.5	0, 0.15%	38–80%	STD
		Ebola	1.3–1.8	35%, 50%	3%	Grieving, HCWs
		Marburg	1.3–1.8	N/A, 23–90%	0%	Grieving, HCWs
	Droplet, airborne	Tuberculosis	<1–3.0	5%, 70%	40–80%	Infrastructure
		SARS	<1 (0.5–8.0)	N/A, 11%	Rare – 7.5%	Bats, Civets
		MERS	1.1 (0.4–2.4)	N/A, 34%	0.06%	Bats, Camels
		Influenza	1.28	Half, 0.05%	65–85%	Unvaccinated
Children	Droplet, airborne	Meningitis	1.3	<10%, 75–80%	5–15%[B]	Unvaccinated
		Rubella	3.3–5.0	<0.01%, 0.04%	24–50%	Unvaccinated
		Chickenpox	3.7–5.0	<0.01%, <0.01%	Rare	Unvaccinated
		Mumps	3.8–5.7	<0.01%, 0.02%	0–27%	Unvaccinated
		Diphtheria	4.9	<1%, 8.7–40%	20–24%	Unvaccinated
		Scarlet fever	5.4	<1%, 2.3–50%	5–25%	No vaccine
		Measles	8.3–40	<1%, 5–10%	16–25%	Unvaccinated
		Pertussis	11.4–17	<0.01%, 0.5–2%	>75%	Unvaccinated

— Transmission route = how the organism is transmitted

— Source = transmission route details

— Droplet => 5 micron respiratory tract derived particles in the air with transmission over less than six-foot distances

— Airborne =< 5 micron respiratory tract derived particles in the air with transmission over greater than six-foot distances

— R_0 = basic reproduction number, likelihood of person-to-person transmission

— Mortality: Rx = treated, vaccinated or both; no Rx = not treated

— Other = what factors facilitated the outbreak occurring

— A = mortality for microcephaly

— B = nasopharyngeal carriage

— No vaccine = no vaccine available

Two of the infections are vector-borne, Epidemic Typhus and Zika. Epidemic Typhus, a.k.a. gaol fever, jail fever, camp fever, or ship fever, caused by *Rickettsia prowazekii*, is perhaps the most dramatic example of an organism that causes large-scale regional outbreaks. It is transmitted by lice and thus requires the very close human contact that occurs in the settings of large-scale human strife, such as wars, famines, jails, and refugee camps.[53-58] Historically, it has been responsible for deaths on an almost unimaginable scale, with mortality rates as high as 30–60% (Table 8.23).[137] For example, it has been estimated that epidemic typhus was responsible for killing over half of Napoleon's army in his campaign against Russia, with millions more dying during the First and Second World Wars (in the trenches, prisoner of war camps, or concentration camps), and Ireland's potato famines.[53-56] Epidemic typhus still remains a problem in large refugee camps and jails and it has a chronic form called Brill-Zinsser disease, which allows it to persist until favorable conditions allow it to be transmitted.[57-59] R_0 values are likely to be at least 2 in the heavily crowded circumstances described above.[55]

Zika virus infection, a.k.a. Zika, caused by the Zika virus, is another vector-borne infection that causes epidemics. It is transmitted by mosquitoes (*Aedes aegypti*, the same mosquito that transmits yellow fever, dengue and chikungunya). Zika is moderately infectious, having an R_0 of 3.0 (Table 8.23). It has caused large epidemics that affected multiple continents in 2015 and 2016.[60] In an isolated population, such as an island, with the vector present, it has been capable of infecting about 75% of the population; whereas without the appropriate vector, the risk of infection is essentially zero.[60] Its overall mortality is low (<1%), with 80% of cases being asymptomatic, but it causes microcephaly (small head with incomplete brain development) in 3–15/10,000 live births when acquired during pregnancy and microcephaly is associated with a nearly 10% mortality rate.[60-62] Thus, it is a pandemic by case numbers, an epidemic by mortality. No treatment or vaccine is currently available.

Key Points: Epidemic typhus has killed millions associated with wars, incarceration and famines. Zika is important because it can cause microcephaly in developing fetuses.

Three of the infectious agents causing epidemics are fecal-oral transmitted — Norovirus, Shigella and Poliovirus. Norovirus infection, a.k.a. winter vomiting disease, is considered by the CDC to be the most common cause of gastroenteritis epidemics worldwide.[63] It causes outbreaks in a wide variety of settings, including long-term care and other healthcare facilities, restaurants, cruise ships, and schools.[63] While it is thought to be transmitted predominantly person-to-person, it can survive on surfaces and remain infectious for greater than three weeks in the absence of adequate disinfection, so transmission by contact with surfaces may also be quite important.[63] Although each outbreak has the potential to infect hundreds of people, its associated mortality is low — 1.8% in older adults and much lower in younger people.[64]

In contrast, *Shigella dysenteriae* gastroenteritis, a.k.a. dysentery, can cause mortality rates that range up to 12% and is considered to be one of the most important global causes of gastrointestinal infection mortality.[65–68] Shigella epidemics occur largely in developing countries with underlying problems with crowding, water purification, and waste disposal.[65,66] The organism is highly infectious, requiring as few as ten organisms to be ingested to cause infection.[69] Control mechanisms for Shigella outbreaks are ideally multifaceted to include isolation, hand hygiene, school closure, antibiotics, and water disinfection, which are difficult to achieve in most, if not all, developing countries.[68]

Poliovirus infection, a.k.a. polio, is perhaps the most unique infectious agent in the fecal-oral group. It is the most infectious of the three, with an R_0 of 10–15 (Table 8.23), but has the lowest overall mortality, approximately 0.15%, because only about 1–2% of all those infected actually develop paralytic polio.[38,70] In spite of the low mortality, the ~85% of those with paralytic polio that survive are left with substantial lifelong morbidity and the possibility of spending the rest of their lives living with a respiratory assist device (iron lung, ventilator, etc.). Polio remains endemic in only two countries. The incidence of polio has markedly decreased worldwide during the past six decades and currently most cases of paralytic polio are related to the type 2 strain in the oral polio vaccine.[71]

Key Point: Of the three fecal-oral transmitted organisms that cause epidemics (*norovirus*, *Shigella*, and *poliovirus*), only *Shigella* is an important global cause of mortality.

Three organisms — *Treponema pallidium*, *Marburg virus* and *Ebola virus* — that cause epidemics are transmitted person-to-person by body fluids. A fourth organism, HIV, is also transmitted by body fluids, but will be covered as a pandemic organism in the section below. Syphilis, a.k.a. the Great Pox (to distinguish it from smallpox), caused by *T. pallidum*, is transmitted sexually. It is thought to have first become a problem in Europe in the 1500s (see the Pandemic section later in this chapter) and continues to be a problem through the present. No historical R_0 values are available, but in the early 1900s, nearly 10% of the UK population was infected, and it carried a 1–2% mortality rate that disappeared with the use of penicillin beginning in the 1940s.[72,73] In the penicillin era, its R_0 is low, about 1.3 (Table 8.23). A big problem with syphilis control is that up to 80% of those with active infection are asymptomatic (Table 8.23).

Marburg hemorrhagic fever and Ebola hemorrhagic fever, a.k.a. Marburg and Ebola, caused by the *Marburg virus* and *Ebola virus*, respectively, cause hemorrhagic fevers in Africa, and both cause significant epidemics with high mortality (Table 8.23).[74–77] Both are thought to have a bat reservoir, but it is unclear how they move from bats to humans.[78,79] The majority of transmissions occur because family members, friends or healthcare workers are exposed to body fluids (vomitus, stool, blood) as an infected patient worsens. No treatments or vaccines are available for Marburg hemorrhagic fever, but effective treatment and a vaccine are now available for Ebola hemorrhagic fever.[80,81] All three agents transmitted by body fluids have low R_0s (1.28–1.8, Table 8.23).

Key Points: Body fluid exposure can lead to epidemics of syphilis, Marburg and Ebola, either through sexual exposure (syphilis) or exposure to body fluids, including blood, vomitus, or stool (Marburg, Ebola).

The remaining 12 infectious diseases that cause epidemics are all transmitted through respiratory droplets (>5-micron size) and/or smaller airborne particles (<5-micron size, transmissible over a longer distance). The two infections — Severe Acute Respiratory Syndrome (SARS) and Middle East Respiratory Syndrome (MERS) — with the lowest average R_0s transmitted by droplet/airborne particles are caused by two recently discovered coronaviruses (SARS-CoV, MERS-CoV).[82] Both have average R_0s only slightly greater than 1.0 (Table 8.23). Bats are their primary hosts, but they have different intermediate hosts (Chapter 7). As discussed in Chapter 7, both SARS and MERS cause lower respiratory tract infections with high mortalities (11% and 34%, respectively).[82] In spite of their lower average R_0 values than the other infectious agents in this group, they have both caused thousands of cases (SARS, 8,422 cases; MERS, greater than 2,494 cases) since their initial appearance; the explanation for the high numbers with a low R_0 is not clear.[82] No treatment or vaccine is available for either agent.

The next two airborne transmissible agents — *Mycobacterium tuberculosis* and *Influenza virus* — are of great importance, historically and currently. Tuberculosis, the infection caused by *M. tuberculosis*, has been known by many names over the centuries because of the profound effects it can have on the infected patient over many years. Examples include phthisis (ancient Greece), king's evil (middle ages), consumption (the 1700s), "The White Plague" (Dr. Oliver Wendell Holmes), and *Masque of the Red Death* (written by Edgar Allan Poe, inspired by the death of his wife and mother from tuberculosis).[83,84] Tuberculosis was once responsible for many millions of deaths per year globally (Figure 8.73) and is still responsible for greater than a million deaths per year, making it the current greatest global cause of infectious disease mortality.[85]

The tuberculosis R_0 ranges from 3 in areas of poverty (Table 8.24), likely due to the lack of infrastructure necessary to trace contacts of active cases and to make sure treatment is given, to less than 1 in industrialized countries (Table 8.23). Mortality is on a steep decline (Figure 8.73). Tuberculosis outbreaks are commonly associated with delays in diagnosis, treatment nonadherence, homeless populations, jails, prisons, nursing homes, substance abuse, AIDS, multidrug resistance, and a lack of public health infrastructure.[86–88] A vaccine exists (BCG) and has been shown to decrease the risk of progression from initial infection to active disease in children.[89] Multidrug treatment has been available for many years and has had a major effect on reducing mortality. The WHO recently estimated that treatment has saved 22 million lives.[90]

Key Points: The WHO continues to report that tuberculosis is the leading global cause of infectious disease mortality. It is on a steady decline in industrialized countries but still remains a very important problem in developing countries.

Nonpandemic (Seasonal) Influenza, a.k.a. Flu, caused by *influenza A and B virus*, is responsible yearly for epidemics worldwide. In the United States (US) it has caused an estimated average mortality per year of 6,309 or 2.4 per 100,000 from 1976 to 2007 and 6,515 or 2.0 per 100,000 for 2017.[91-93] The WHO estimates the global influenza mortality in nonpandemic years at 389,000 (range: 294,000 to 518,000) or approximately 2.1 per 100,000.[94] This is in comparison to an estimated greater than 2,500 per 100,000 for the 1918 influenza pandemic.[95] Influenza vaccination can reduce mortality by an estimated 50% in individuals over 65.[96,97] Timely antiviral treatment is available and has been shown to reduce mortality by

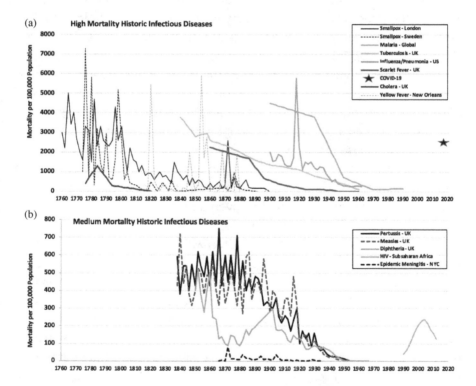

Figure 8.73. A comparison of mortality per 100,000 population for 12 historic infectious diseases seen in the last 260 years. A. High Mortality Historic Infectious Diseases, 1760–2020. Created by estimating the data points from published graphs and creating an original graph from mortality and population data (Yellow fever). B. Medium Mortality Historic Infectious Diseases, 1838–2020. Created by estimating and graphing the data points from published graphs and creating an original graph from data from the World Bank (HIV).[478-491]

Table 8.24. [A] Infectious diseases that cause pandemics.[179-402,431-477]

Transmission Route	Source	Infection Name[179-402]	R_0[431-440]	Mortality[441-461] Rx, No Rx	Mortality Modifiers Other	% with No Symptoms[462-477] (Infectious)
Vector borne	Mosquito	YF (1800s)	1.1–7.0	N/A, 25–73% N/A, 1–14%		55%
		YF (2000s)		N/A, 40% N/A, <1%	No vaccine Vaccine	
		Dengue	2.7–5.4	N/A, 0.07–19%	No Vaccine	7–84%
		Malaria (falciparum)	2.0 – >1000	< 1%, 100%	No Vaccine	23%
	Flea	Plague (14th century)	5–7	10–60% >60%	Less 40 years old Greater 40 years old	7–45
		Plague (2008–2016)		26%, N/A		
Environment	Water	Cholera (1853)	1.9–551	N/A, 54–68%		40–80%
		Cholera (2010)		<1%, N/A	Flooding Earthquakes	
Person-to-person	Body fluids	Syphilis (1500s)	N/A	N/A, 20–40%	South Africa	38–80%
		HIV	1.2–11.3	17%, 99%		

(Continued)

Table 8.24. (Continued)

Transmission Route	Source	Infection Name[179-402]	R_0[431-440]	Mortality[441-461] Rx, No Rx	Mortality Modifiers Other	% with No Symptoms[462-477] (Infectious)
Airborne or Droplet		COVID-19	1.2–6.5	15%, 99%	North America	14% (undiagnosed)
				5%, 99%	Europe	62% (asymptomatic)
				2% (.5–10%)		18–40%
		Influenza (1918)	1.8	2.5%		59%
		Influenza (1957)	1.65	0.02%		
		Influenza (1968)	1.80	0.01%		
		Influenza (2009)	1.46	0.02%		6–55%
		TB (1900)	3.0	17%/70%	HIV negative	0%
				13%/83%	HIV positive	2%
		Smallpox	3.5–6.0	30%, N/A		10–27%

Table 2 Expanded^A — first five columns are the same.
- Transmission route = how the organism is transmitted
- Source = transmission route details
- Droplet => 5 micron respiratory tract derived particles in the air with transmission over less than six-foot distances
- Airborne =< 5 micron respiratory tract derived particles in the air with transmission over greater than six-foot distances
- R_0 = basic reproduction number, likelihood of person-to-person transmission
- Mortality: Rx = treated; no Rx = not treated
% with No Symptoms = how likely is it for an infectious person to be without symptoms

50% in the overall Influenza-infected population and by 31% in patients requiring ICU care.[98,99] Seasonal Influenza has a low R_0 (1.28, Table 8.23), likely related to partial immunity due to previous strains of Influenza virus, or vaccine use. Control of outbreaks is often difficult due to the high frequency of asymptomatic infection, especially in children (65–85%, Table 8.23).

Key Point: The WHO data suggest that seasonal influenza may be the second most common global infectious disease cause of mortality.

The last eight droplet/airborne transmissible agents (*Neisseria meningitidis, Rubella virus, Varicella zoster virus, Mumps virus, Corynebacterium diphtheriae, Streptococcus pyogenes, Measles morbillivirus, Bordetella pertussis*) are predominantly childhood infections. The most feared of these eight infections is meningococcal infection, including spinal meningitis, caused by *N. meningitidis*. At its worst, this infection can cause death in less than 24 hours despite treatment.[100] In a country with all currently available medical resources, the mortality of meningococcal meningitis ranges from 5 to 7% for children and adults.[101,102] Untreated, its mortality approaches 75–80% (Table 8.23).[152] Global mortality per 100,000 population has declined almost 50% since 1999.[103] A vaccine exists that has been shown to reduce mortality both in Europe and Subsaharan Africa.[104,105] It is the least infectious of the eight airborne transmitted infectious diseases in Table 8.23, having an R_0 of 1.3, and 5–15% (or greater) of people can carry the organism asymptomatically.

The remaining seven infectious diseases (rubella, chickenpox, mumps, diphtheria, scarlet fever, measles, and pertussis) are among the most easily transmitted infectious diseases known to humanity, with R_0s ranging from 3.3 to 15 (Table 8.23). Rubella, a.k.a. German measles, caused by the Rubella virus, is very infectious (R_0: 3.3–5, Table 8.23). It has very low mortality (<0.01%, Table 8.23), but it causes severe congenital malformations when females acquire the infection during their first trimester of pregnancy.[106] Fortunately, a very effective vaccine is available. Improved global rubella vaccination has led to dramatic reductions in the number of congenital rubella syndrome cases.[106]

Chickenpox infection, a.k.a. chickenpox, caused by the *Varicella zoster virus*, is similarly infectious to rubella (R_0: 3.3–5, Table 8.23) and with similarly low mortality (<0.01%). For many years, it was largely considered a childhood nuisance, such that some parents arranged for chickenpox parties so they could get their children all infected at once, perhaps when they were off from school so they could be done with it. A vaccine was developed for chickenpox to prevent the uncommon severe complications in children and the 30% or greater frequency of developing "shingles" in adults.[107] Shingles is a manifestation of varicella infection that represents reactivation of the virus from its reservoir in a nerve, such that the virus recurs in the distribution of that nerve and can thereafter cause chronic, debilitating pain.[107]

Mumps infection, a.k.a. epidemic parotitis, is another quite infectious childhood disease (R_0 = 3.8–5.7) with very low mortality (<0.02%, Table 8.23).[108] A vaccine was developed for this infection due to the 20–30% incidence of orchitis (testicular infection) in post-pubertal males, with 30–50% of this group developing testicular atrophy and possible infertility.[109] Up to 27% of the individuals infected with mumps are asymptomatic, making outbreak control more difficult. A vaccine is available, but its effect wanes in individuals over the age of 20.[108,109]

> Key Points: Some infectious diseases have had vaccines developed, not due to mortality but very specific morbidities. Examples include rubella (congenital infection), chickenpox (shingles), and mumps (orchitis).

The last four childhood infections (diphtheria, scarlet fever, measles, and pertussis) are not only quite infectious (R_0 = 3.8–11, Table 8.23), but caused significant mortality prior to the advent of vaccines, antisera and antibiotics (Table 8.23, Figure 8.73). Diphtheria, a.k.a. bull neck disease or the strangling angel of children, is caused by *Corynebacterium diphtheriae*. Scarlet fever, a.k.a. scarlatina, is caused by *Streptococcus pyogenes*. Measles, a.k.a. red measles, is caused by *Measles morbillivirus*. Pertussis, a.k.a. whooping cough, is caused by *Bordetella pertussis*. All four infections had a periodicity to their outbreaks in the prevaccine, pre-antibiotic era that related to enough nonimmune children having accumulated to support the next outbreak.[110] The outbreaks/epidemics typically occurred every 2–4 years and their magnitude, and mortality were dramatically muted with the advent of vaccines.[42,110,111] For the two most infectious agents (*Measles virus* and

B. pertussis), the average age of infection was younger (4–7) than the other two (7–14).[110] Under outbreak settings, the R_0 may be significantly higher (pertussis, 17; measles, 40).[7,111] The extraordinary infectivity of pertussis under outbreak circumstances has led epidemiologists to calculate the speed and distance an epidemic wave can spread. In the UK, it has been estimated that pertussis can spread at a rate of 110–320 km/month.[112,113]

The mortality of these four infections in the prevaccine, pre-antibiotic era was substantial, ranging from 0.5 to 8.7% (Table 8.23, Figure 8.73), but could be much higher in an outbreak setting. In children less than 1 year of age, reported mortalities in Glasgow, Scotland, between 1916 and 1945 ranged from 9.2% for scarlet fever, 13.7% for measles, 19% for pertussis, to 23.6% for diphtheria.[114] For diphtheria, in the absence of an antitoxin, vaccine and antibiotic availability, and especially during outbreaks, the rates can be even higher (>40%).[115] With scarlet fever, outbreak fatality rates in the 1800s have been reported to be as high as 50% in children.[116] These four infectious agents were considered important enough that health departments would publish relevant statistics in newspapers and notify the public about any outbreaks.[117–119] With the development of antitoxins, vaccines and antibiotics, all four of these infectious diseases declined steadily in the 1800s and early 1900s (Table 8.23, Figure 8.73).[120–123]

Key Points: The four most historically important childhood infections — diphtheria, scarlet fever, measles, and pertussis — have had dramatic reductions in mortality (from 2–10% down to less than 1%) due to the development of vaccines, antibiotics, antitoxins, and education.

---

4. Pandemics

Which infectious diseases have caused pandemics?

In the last two millennia, the world has experienced pandemics caused by at least 11 infectious diseases — Plague, smallpox, yellow fever, dengue, malaria, cholera, syphilis, HIV, COVID-19, influenza, and tuberculosis (Table 8.24). All 11 of these pandemic organisms were originally zoonoses (Chapter 7, animal source: plague — rodents, smallpox — cattle, yellow fever — primates, malaria — primates, cholera — birds and fish, syphilis —

primates, HIV — primates, influenza — birds and pigs, tuberculosis — cattle and primates, COVID-19 – bats), many of which ultimately became totally adapted to humans. Two of the infectious diseases that cause pandemics, plague (*Yersinia pestis*) and smallpox (*Variola virus*), have come and gone as causes of pandemics. Three of the infectious diseases — yellow fever (*Yellow fever virus*), dengue (*Dengue virus*), and malaria (*Plasmodium falciparum* and others) — are mosquito-borne and still present. Two of the infectious diseases are sexually transmitted — syphilis (*Treponema pallidum*) and HIV (*Human immunodeficiency virus*) — and both are still present. Only one infection, cholera (*Vibrio cholerae*), is transmitted by contaminated water, and it is still very much present. Finally, three of the infectious diseases are airborne transmitted — tuberculosis (*Mycobacterium tuberculosis*), influenza (*Influenza virus*), and COVID-19 (SARS-CoV-2) — and all three remain global problems. We will go over each of these infectious agents as to what factors predisposed to them causing pandemics.

Plague, a.k.a. bubonic plague or the Black Death, is caused by *Yersinia pestis*. The Greek physician Galen may have been the first to use the word "plague" to describe an outbreak of infection (circa 200 CE).[179] Since then, many outbreaks/epidemics have been called "plagues", but since the middle-ages, the word "plague" has most commonly been used to represent an outbreak, epidemic or pandemic, caused by *Y. pestis*. *Y. pestis* is a bacteria, which has its reservoir in rodents and other animals. Unless previously infected with survival or vaccinated, there is no evidence humans are immune to this organism, so essentially all of humanity was likely susceptible to being infected at the time of the previous pandemics.[180] Initial infection most commonly involves a skin bite from a flea or louse, which inoculates the organism into the skin.[181] Thereafter, the organism spreads to the closest lymph node where it causes a painful, swollen, infected lymph node (lymphadenitis), which came to be known as a buboe during the second pandemic and led to the term "bubonic plague". As the infection spreads, it can reach the bloodstream and spread to other parts of the body, particularly the lungs. Once in the lungs, it causes pneumonia and then can be airborne, dispersed with a high R_0 (5–7, Table 8.24), which greatly enhances the potential spread of the organism.

It first emerged as a cause of infection approximately 5,000 years ago (Chapter 7) and was responsible for three pandemics.[182] The first pandemic was the Plague of Justinian (541–544 CE), centered around Constantinople

(Istanbul).[183] The second was the Black Death in Europe (1347–1351), with successive waves that extended all the way into the 18th century.[183] The third began in China in 1894 and continued into the early 20th century.[183] At its worst, the plague was capable of causing greater than 60% mortality and still may be as high as 26% today (Table 8.24). It has been estimated that the first pandemic caused as many as 25 million deaths, and the second pandemic (the Black Death) may have resulted in the death of 30–50% of the population in Europe.[184,185] Historically, it has been taught that the pandemics occurred because Y. pestis was spread from rats to humans via fleas or lice only, but more recent data and epidemic modeling suggest that it is more likely that ectoparasites (fleas, lice) transmitted the organism from person-to-person with the additional contribution of airborne spread once bubonic plague progressed to pneumonic plague, especially in high-density urban areas.[186,187] Geographic spread was likely along trade routes, both by land and by water.[187–189]

Factors contributing to the plague's ability to cause pandemics include ignorance of its cause and route of transmission, lack of immunity, a high degree of infectivity (R_0), no available treatment or vaccine, and the inability to control the vectors that spread the infection. The importance of ignorance cannot be overstated and can be summarized as follows: (1) the Germ Theory was not accepted until the late 1800s (Chapter 7), with the consequence being that Y. pestis was not discovered until 1894, the year the third pandemic began, (2) rats were not appreciated as a potential reservoir until 1903, (3) fleas were not recognized as vectors until 1908, (4) the first vaccine was not developed until 1895, and (5) the first treatment (streptomycin) did not become available until 1944.[120–123,190,191] Simply put, it is impossible to control something that you do not understand, cannot treat, and cannot prevent. In current times, it no longer causes pandemics, and mortality is less than half of what it used to be in the middle ages. This is attributable to a better understanding of the organism, its transmission with associated vector control, and better medical care, to include antibiotics (Chapter 7).

> Key Points: The Plague caused pandemics because of pre-Germ Theory ignorance, a high degree of infectivity (R_0), transmission along trade routes, and a lack of human immunity, antibiotics, and other current medical support capabilities.

Smallpox, a.k.a. smallpox to distinguish it from "the Great Pox" (syphilis), is the only historically important pandemic that is now eradicated from the planet. The causative organism, *Variola virus*, first appeared approximately 16,000 years ago, likely coming from swine or cattle (Chapter 7). It was known in India and China for at least several thousand years.[192] We may never know when the first smallpox pandemic occurred, but we do know that smallpox pandemics occurred beginning in the 1500s and continued into the early 1900s, involving Europe, Africa, India, China, and North America.[192,193] Thus, the majority of the pandemics were pre-Germ Theory, again making ignorance a major factor.

Smallpox virus causes a blistering rash with a unique clinical course.[194] It was quite infectious, with historical data showing it to have an R_0 of 3.5–6 (Table 8.24). Historically, it carried a mortality of greater than 30%; in children, mortality can be as high as 60% (Table 8.24). In larger cities, infection was endemic; whereas, in smaller cities, outbreaks had a periodicity of approximately every 5–10 years, representing the time it took for a new group of susceptible children to appear (Figure 8.74) and someone from outside the city to reintroduce the organism.[195] A major factor affecting its transmission early on was the transportation of infected slaves (Chapter 7).

Everything changed in the late 1700s when William Jenner realized that the cowpox virus could be used to variolate (vaccinate) and give people lifelong immunity, without the risk of mortality associated with variolation with the Variola virus (2%).[196] Within 10–15 years, smallpox vaccination was being used globally with a steady decline in smallpox cases and mortality (Figures 8.73 and 8.74).[196,197,503] In 1980, the WHO declared the eradication of smallpox.[198] The first available drug active against smallpox was not discovered until after it was eradicated.[122,123] The impact of smallpox globally has been profound. It affected so many countries that country-specific quarantine acts with mandatory vaccination were enacted.[192,199,200] After eradication, the side effects of the vaccine were felt to outweigh the benefits, and global vaccination efforts were terminated with the only known residual Variola virus residing in freezers in the US and Russia.[192,198,201] Recently, historical outbreak data has been analyzed by a number of investigators and mathematically modeled to gain a better understanding of how smallpox outbreaks occur and propagate and how this can be used to handle future similar outbreaks.[195,202,203] A final interesting note is that the enormous

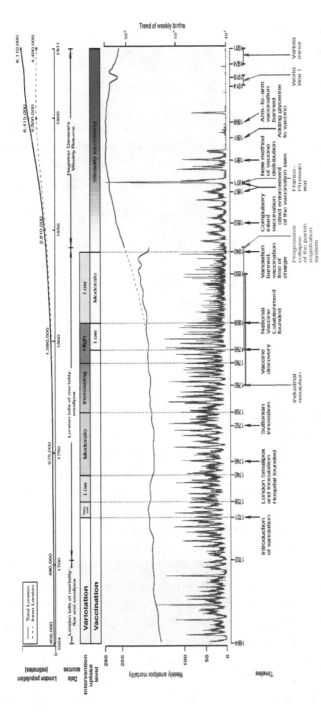

Figure 8.74. Patterns of smallpox mortality in London, England, over three centuries.[503] The decline after the introduction of Jenner's small-pox vaccine in the early 1800s is evident. With permission.[503]

evolutionary pressure on humans provided by smallpox in Europe during its last 500 years has recently been proposed as the possible explanation for the 10% prevalence of the CCR5-delta32 deletion allele in the human genome that confers resistance to HIV-1 infection.[204]

Key Points: Factors contributing to smallpox's ability to cause pandemics include pre-Germ Theory ignorance, the slave trade and global exploration, a lack of sustained herd immunity, a high degree of infectivity (R_0 = 3.5–6), no available vaccine until approximately 1800, and no available treatment until after it was eradicated.

Yellow Fever, a.k.a. yellow jack, yellow plague, or bronze john, was first noted to cause outbreaks in 1648, although the *Yellow Fever virus* is thought to have made its appearance 1,500 years ago (Chapter 7).[205] For centuries, it has been a cause of epidemics/pandemics in Africa, and the current R_0 of greater than 6 still exists in certain areas.[205–209] Colonialism and slave trade introduced the organism into the Americas with devastating consequences.[210–214] As an example, yellow fever and malaria by themselves were the likely explanation for the French failing to build the Panama Canal, with greater than 30,000 worker mortalities.[214]

Yellow fever is a mosquito-borne infection that causes a spectrum of illnesses. Fifty-five percent are asymptomatic, 33% have a mild infection of the liver (hepatitis), and 12% develop severe disease (hemorrhagic fever), with 20–40% overall mortality (Table 8.24).[209,215,216] Natural infection produces lifelong immunity.[217] Evolutionary exposure to yellow fever in Africa has conferred a level of innate immunity, for example, non-Caucasians are 6.8 times less likely to die from yellow fever than Caucasians.[218] No treatment exists, but there is an effective vaccine.[219] Use of the vaccine in the late 1900s led to a global reduction in the number of yellow fever outbreaks (Figure 8.73).[205] It has been thought by some that the global control of yellow fever can be achieved if greater than 80–90% vaccine-derived immunity can be achieved in at-risk areas; however, this is very difficult with many parts of Africa still having less than 80% vaccine coverage as of 2016.[216,220,221] Pertinent to this consideration, multiple areas of Africa have seen a resurgence in yellow fever between 2010 and 2020.[222] The WHO feels that a single dose of the existing vaccine is adequate for lifelong immunity, but others think that a booster dose is necessary every ten years.[220,221,223,224] This debate is not trivial, given the recent global resurgence; thus, the reason for this surge must be determined in order for control to be achieved.[205,214,225]

A variety of evidence suggests that the reason for the resurgence of yellow fever is multifactorial and likely is at least in part due to evolving changes affecting the yellow fever vector, mosquitoes. Yellow fever is transmitted by the same mosquito, *Aedes aegypti*, that transmits dengue, Zika and chikugunya with the associated finding that the global distribution of dengue and yellow fever substantially overlap (Figure 8.75).[226,499–501] Aedes mosquitoes are day-time feeders and reproduce in urban areas in tires, pots

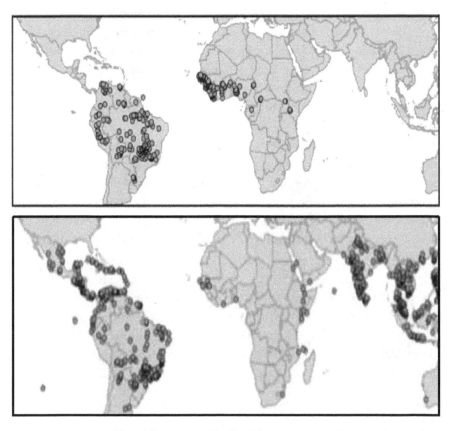

Figure 8.75. Similar global distribution of yellow fever (top, 1960–2005) and dengue (bottom, 1960–2005). This reflects their sharing of a common mosquito vector, *Aedes aegypti*. With permission.[499]

and ditches containing rainwater.[213,214,226] Factors that affect the mosquitoes can have a dramatic effect on the risk of infection for humans.[227]

Appreciation for the complexity of how mosquitoes transmit the *yellow fever virus* can be partially gained by understanding that this virus has three different transmission cycles: (1) Sylvatic — nonhuman primate to nonhuman primate via sylvatic *Aedes* mosquitoes, (2) Intermediate — humans to nonhuman primates via peridomestic *Aedes* species, and (3) Urban — human to human via *Aedes aegypti* mosquitoes.[209] This is complex enough, but studies examining the rapidly changing global landscape both at the local level and via satellite suggest that these three transmission cycles are being affected in ways that will actually further increase the risk of transmission, particularly due to increased international sea and air traffic.[205,227,228]

"In recent decades, an extremely novel method for controlling Dengue, the release of Wolbachia-infected A. aegypti mosquitoes, has been trialed on many continents. Wolbachia is an obligate intracellular bacterium, that confers resistance to the transmission of infection by A. aegypti with Dengue for sure, and likely other infections requiring A. aegypti for transmission, such as Yellow Fever, Chikungunya and Zika.[249A–249C] Wolbachia inhibit intracellular viral replication and are passed on to each new generation of mosquito by the female. In a field trial of this intervention, the frequency of symptomatic Dengue disease was reduced by 77%.[249A] So far there has been no significant downside to this approach, but only time will tell whether the targeted arboviruses will evolve resistance to this intervention, such as that already discovered in insect-specific flaviviruses.[249D]

Key Points: Factors contributing to yellow fever's ongoing ability to cause pandemics include a difficulty in achieving adequate herd immunity through vaccination with associated hot spots of transmission ($R_0 > 6$), a resurgence of mosquitoes related to increased international travel (land and sea), and no available treatment. However, hope does exist, as Wolbachia-infected A. aegypti show great promise in reducing global Dengue infection.

Dengue, a.k.a. breakbone fever, outbreaks are harder to pinpoint historically because their appearance is not quite as distinctive as some of the other infections being discussed. The earliest known outbreak consistent

with dengue, occurred in China in 992 CE, and then a whole series of outbreaks were reported in the Americas beginning in 1635 in Martinique and
Guadeloupe, and 1699 in Panama.[229,230] The earliest documented dengue
virus outbreak in Africa was in 1823 in Zanzibar.[231] From then until the 20th
century, the reporting of dengue outbreaks has been inconsistent. After
the 1940s and the founding of the WHO (1948), there has been a steady
increase in the global reporting of dengue outbreaks.[232] While some part
of the increase in disease cases may have been an artifact of improved
reporting, the overall increase in global dengue infections is felt to be real.[232]

Dengue is an infection caused by the *dengue virus* and transmitted
primarily by the *A. aegypti* mosquito, the same virus that transmits yellow
fever, Zika, and chikungunya, and less commonly, by *Aedes albopictus*.[233,234]
There are four serotypes of the *dengue virus*.[234,235] The first time an individual
is infected by the *dengue virus*, the individual has a mild infection with a
fever and myalgias (muscle aches), and develops immunity to the serotype
that infected them.[234,235] The second infection may result in a more severe
antibody-dependent, hemorrhagic-fever-like presentation, likely driven
by a cytokine storm.[235,236] While in any given part of the world, the relative
proportion of mild versus severe presentations will depend upon the prior
history of dengue infections in the area; an estimate of the ratio can be
approximated as three mild cases to one severe.[236] A vaccine has existed
since 2015 that is effective, but the vaccine can lead to a more severe
infection in previously dengue naïve individuals, making it unclear how
best to use the vaccine.[237,238] No antiviral treatment is currently available.

The likelihood of the dengue virus causing a pandemic is tightly linked
to its transmission by *A. aegypti*. *A. aegypti* can transmit the dengue virus
from one infected individual (asymptomatic or symptomatic) to multiple
individuals with a high R_0 of up to 5+ (Table 8.24). In a household setting, the
transmission rate can be even higher (greater than 20 in one instance).[239,240]
Factors that increase the numbers of *A. aegypti* mosquitoes are likely to
have a strong influence on the likelihood of continued transmission in a
geographic area. Increased global rates of dengue infection appear to
be related to increased global air travel.[241,242] This would imply that there
has been a simultaneous increase in the presence of *A. aegypti* in the
same distribution geographically, and this has been documented.[243,505,506]
Based on projected climate changes and population changes, as well as
the growing expansion of the mosquito vectors, mathematical modeling

by several groups has projected that over the next 60 years, this trend in dengue expansion will continue, with associated increases in yellow fever, Zika and chikungunya.[244–246] An interesting and related question is whether *A. aegypti* can simultaneously transmit two or more of these infectious agents; vector competency studies suggest this is currently not likely.[247–249]

Key Points: Factors contributing to dengue's ongoing ability to cause pandemics include the global expansion of the *A. aegypti* mosquito vector due to travel and trade, no effective vaccine without significant associated risk, and no available treatment.

Malaria, a.k.a. ague or jungle fever, is the third infection transmitted by mosquitoes that has caused pandemics. For the purpose of this discussion, the focus will be exclusively on malaria caused by *Plasmodium falciparum* since it causes greater than 99% of malaria-related mortality. Evolutionary studies suggest malaria originated in Africa by transmission from primates to humans approximately 10,000 years ago (Chapter 7), and then spread to the rest of the world.[250–252] It is documented in Chinese records as far back as 5,000 years ago, in the Middle East 3,500 to 4,000 years ago, in India between 2,800 and 3,500 years ago, and in Europe approximately 2,000 years ago.[251] It appears to have come to the Americas in the 15th century C.E. with explorers and slave traders and has been present globally since that time.[253,254] As recently as the 20th century, *P. falciparum* was thought to have caused between 150 and 300 million fatalities.[250,251]

Malaria caused by *P. falciparum* is a disease whereby the parasite is transmitted to humans as the mosquito feeds on human blood, and then inside humans, the parasite attaches to red blood cells where it is internalized and replicates.[255] As part of a complex life cycle, the parasite subsequently causes red blood cell lysis (destruction) and then infects new red blood cells until either the patient is treated or the patient dies.[255] Mortality is greatest in nonimmune, untreated individuals where it likely approaches 100%.[256] In areas endemic for *P. falciparum*, the mortality is greatest in young children having their first infection.

Two innate immune factors decrease the risk of mortality due to *P. falciparum* infection. The first is prior infection, which leads to partial immunity, that increases with subsequent infections, and decreases the risk of mortality.[255,257] The second innate factor affecting mortality in individuals of African descent is the immunity provided by the sickle cell trait (if the individual is heterozygous, having only one copy of the abnormal hemoglobin gene, they are asymptomatic; if homozygous with two abnormal gene copies, they manifest sickle cell anemia), which reduces the risk of mortality by approximately 90%.[258] Human genome studies suggest that sickle-cell hemoglobin first appeared less than 10,000 years ago, shortly after the evolutionary pressure provided by the first appearance of epidemic *P. falciparum* malaria.[259] Even with these immunologic protective mechanisms, overall mortality in Africa was extremely high (greater than 50%) through the early 1800s.

The first available treatment was the mid-19th-century discovery that cinchona bark (active ingredient — quinine) could effectively treat malaria, leading to a sharp drop in mortality rates (Figure 8.73).[251] At present, with early diagnosis and treatment, mortality is less than 1% (Table 8.24); after pre-existing immunity, early diagnosis is the current most important outcome variable. The WHO still reports 600,000 falciparum-related deaths per year, 90% in Africa, an overall greater than 90% global mortality reduction since 1900 (Figure 8.74).[255] *P. falciparum* malaria is still highly infectious in Africa, with calculated R_0s ranging up to 1,000 in hyperendemic areas (Table 8.24). As of 2021 there is now a malarial vaccine against *P. falciparum* that can reduce mortality by 45% and has been recommended for use by the WHO.

Like other mosquito-borne infections, factors affecting the *P. falciparum* mosquito vector, *Anopheles*, affect human mortality. Unlike the rapidly expanding global distribution of the Aedes mosquitoes that transmit yellow fever, dengue, Zika, and chikungunya, the global distribution of the *Anopheles* mosquito vectors of *P. falciparum* has changed relatively little in the last 100 years.[259] Anopheles are night-feeding mosquitoes that reproduce near the water's surface of ponds, rivers, swamps or in rainwater around houses.[214]

Little progress occurred in reducing global malaria-related mortality until Major William Gorgas took the circa 1900 discovery by Dr. Walter Reed and Carlos Finlay in Cuba that *Aedes aegypti* mosquitoes transmit yellow fever and systematically eliminated the mosquito breeding sites adjacent to the Panama Canal, with the resultant reduction of yellow fever and malaria mortality.[214] Armed with this understanding, there followed intensive global efforts to control mosquito breeding areas, with associated reductions in global malaria mortality (Figure 8.73).

The next important, and most controversial intervention, was the use of dichlorodiphenyltrichloroethane (DDT) beginning in the 1940s. Its promise for the control of malaria-carrying mosquitoes led to Paul Hermann Muller being awarded the Nobel Prize in 1948.[261] Temporally, the early intensive use of DDT corresponded to further reduction in global malaria mortality (Figure 8.73). However, its widespread use led to environmental havoc (widespread global decline in bird and aquatic species) and a public backlash, so its use declined but did not disappear.[262-264] Data analyses in the late 1990s suggested that in areas where DDT use had declined significantly, the incidence of malaria was steadily increasing.[264,265] Such findings led the WHO in 2006 to recommend indoor spraying of DDT for the control of malaria.[266]

A more recent malaria intervention is the use of mosquito nets for sleeping, which have been shown to reduce mortality in Africa (10% of African village residents using nets equals 5–12% mortality reduction), but have also been hard to implement on a large scale.[260] Recent computer modeling has suggested it would be more cost effective to use insecticide-treated bed nets and environmental management rather than continued DDT spraying.[267] It is quite clear that the best approach for the control of malaria has not yet been determined and further advances would be necessary for anything close to eradication to occur.[268]

Key Points: Factors contributing to malaria's ongoing ability to cause pandemics include the heroic efforts required to control the *Anopheles* mosquito vector and the lack of a high efficacy vaccine.

Syphilis, a.k.a. the Great Pox, has been estimated by molecular clock techniques to have come into existence approximately 5,000 years ago (Table 7.23, Chapter 7).[269-270] The first clear documentation of syphilis in humans is thought to have been in about 1500 and was associated with a pandemic that started in Naples, Italy, and spread via troop movements throughout Europe.[269,270] A number of publications have suggested that the early mortality in this pandemic approached 20–40%, spawning infectious disease hospitals and the use of quarantine, but soon thereafter, mortality declined substantially.[271-273] By the early 20th century, mortality had fallen to 15 per 100,000 and then to zero, with the advent of penicillin.[73]

Syphilis is a sexually transmitted disease that has three phases; (1) primary — with initial skin or mucosal lesions, (2) secondary — with systemic symptoms, including fever, weight loss and manifestations in internal organs, and (3) tertiary — dementia or other neurologic symptoms, aortitis (inflammation of the aorta with associated aneurysms), or gummas (masses of inflammatory tissue due to *T. pallidum* anywhere in the body). It has low infectivity (R_0 = 1.3, Chapter 7) but is successful in transmission because of a long, silent incubation phase (up to 90 days or more, during which time it is transmissible to others), maintaining global prevalence rates in some populations of 10–30% up until the early 1900s.[274,275] In 1910, syphilis serology (Wasserman test) was discovered, and the drug arsphenamine (Salvarsan) was found to have activity against *T. pallidum*. Although penicillin treatment led to a global decline in syphilis prevalence, the WHO has estimated that there was still a global prevalence of at least 7 million cases of syphilis in 2020, substantially related to men who have sex with men.[276]

Key Points: Factors contributing to Syphilis's ability to cause a pandemic include a long silent incubation period and pre-Germ Theory ignorance, with these factors partially negated by the widespread use of penicillin.

Human immunodeficiency virus, a.k.a. HIV, likely emerged from primates in Africa in approximately 1959 (Chapter 7) and was first recognized as a unique human infection in 1981.[277,278] By 1983, the causative virus was identified, and by 1984, a diagnostic test was created.[278] Effective three-drug therapy was not available until 1995.[278] In spite of diagnostic testing and treatment availability, HIV went on to cause a global pandemic for which we were unable to reduce global mortality until 2005 (Figure 8.73).[279] Since there is no cure, although this may change utilizing CRISPR (clustered regularly interspaced short palindromic repeats) gene therapy, or available vaccine yet, there continues to be a steadily increasing number of people living with HIV/AIDS, reaching 38.8 million in 2016.[279]

HIV is transmitted by blood and body fluids, most commonly through sexual activity and intravenous drug use.[279] Most cases still occur in sub-Saharan Africa, remarkably in areas of high socioeconomic status due to risky sexual behavior.[280,281] It has an extraordinary range of clinical manifestations, including unusual infections and cancers, associated with the near-total destruction of cell-mediated immunity.[278,282,283] Even though sexually transmitted, it can have a R_0 as high as 11 (Table 8.24) due to its long, largely asymptomatic incubation period (approximately 8 years) before AIDS is diagnosed.[278] The risk of spread is further augmented by global travel.[284] These factors make contact tracing difficult and would have made control of the HIV pandemic extremely difficult if it had not been for the development of the three-drug therapy for HIV infection, which not only arrests the progression of the infection but essentially restores immunity in most patients and renders them noninfectious.[278,285] Since 2005, the escalating global use of the three-drug therapy has increasingly turned HIV infection into more of a chronic disease with HIV-infected persons living a relatively healthy life.[279]

> Key Points: Factors contributing to HIV's ability to cause a pandemic include an extremely long silent incubation period, ease of transmission through intravenous drug use or sexual activity, the initial lack of a diagnostic test, as well as going 14 years without an effective treatment. There still is no vaccine or cure.

Cholera, caused by *Vibrio cholerae*, a.k.a. the Blue Death, blue terror, or dog death, likely existed in India for thousands of years but first caused pandemics in the 1800s.[286] Between 1817 and 2020, cholera caused seven pandemics.[286,287] In the pre-Germ Theory period, its mortality rate was as high as 70% in symptomatic individuals and is thought to have caused millions of deaths during the 1800s (Table 8.24, Figure 8.73). The last pandemic occurred in 1961, but epidemics continue to occur, particularly in endemic countries, especially in Africa.[288] The global burden of cholera is particularly difficult to determine, because the majority of cases are not reported, but a spatial modelling technique has recently estimated (2015), that globally there are 2.9 million cases per year and 95,000 deaths per year (range: 21,000–143,000) in 69 endemic countries.[288,289]

Cholera is the only organism causing pandemics that is transmitted through the fecal-oral route.[290] In symptomatic individuals, it causes death by dehydration due to large volume diarrhea (greater than 20 liters in a 24-hour period).[290] It has a short incubation period (1.4 days) and can become hyperinfective (see superspreaders later in the chapter) with R_0s of up to 551 (Table 8.24) within the first few days after infection, making explosive outbreaks possible.[291–293] Close to half of the people infected are asymptomatic, making silent person-to-person transmission possible (Table 8.24). Its mortality has been declining since the discovery of oral rehydration salts and the development of a vaccine.[290]

A remaining mystery for cholera: What causes the organism to suddenly reappear and cause outbreaks, epidemics or pandemics? It is a halophilic (salt-loving) Vibrio that thrives in estuaries where fresh and saltwater meet and is known to colonize a number of creatures that live in that environment and may be important in its transmission.[294] These include waterfowl, fish, crustaceans, and more microscopic creatures such as plankton.[295–297] Birds can fly, fish can swim with the currents, and crustaceans could potentially transmit cholera by being uploaded in the ballast water of ships and then dumped out at the ship's destination, contaminating a new ecosphere.[298,299] It has even been suggested recently that El Niño plays a role in cholera transmission, raising the possibility that evolving global warming will have an effect as well.[300] The other obvious possibility is that the organism could be transmitted by asymptomatically colonized people through international travel, especially airplanes, as was demonstrated in the 2010 Cholera epidemic in Haiti.[301,302]

Key Points: Factors contributing to cholera's ability to cause a pandemic include hyperinfectivity, a very short incubation period, short-term asymptomatic carriers, global travel and trade, mobile vectors, and pre-Germ Theory ignorance.

Tuberculosis, a.k.a. the White Plague, the red death, and perhaps the most powerful literary description of all: "The captain of all these Men of Death ... was the consumption" (The Life and Death of Mr. Badman by John Bunyan), is caused by Mycobacterium tuberculosis.[83,303,304] During the 1700s and 1800s, tuberculosis reached pandemic proportions and was thought to have killed millions in Europe, leading to it being named the "White Plague".[303] In the last 200 years, tuberculosis-related mortality has declined (Figure 8.73) but still is significant in Africa and Asia for multiple reasons, including HIV coinfection.[305–307] As noted earlier in the chapter, tuberculosis remains the leading infectious cause of global mortality.

M. tuberculosis is transmitted through the air and can be highly contagious (R_0 = 3, Table 8.24). Factors that increase the risk of transmission include pre-Germ Theory ignorance, an undiagnosed patient, recirculated air (submarine, ship, airplane), closed space, coughing or singing, longer duration of exposure, cavitary pulmonary disease, HIV co-infection, having a more virulent organism, or combinations (travel, closed space).[308-319] In a recent replication of a famous 1950s study the infectiousness of air exhausted from tuberculosis patient rooms through guinea pig cages was examined, and multivariate analysis demonstrated that the only independent predictor of airborne transmission to guinea pigs was multidrug-resistant (MDR) organism status.[316-318] Sputum smear-positive MDR-negative patients had a 3% risk of transmission, smear-negative MDR-positive patients or smear-positive MDR-negative had an 18% risk of transmission, and smear-positive MDR-positive patients had a 59% risk of transmission. Transmission risk can be reduced by treating patients with antibiotics, getting them to wear masks, and employing air filtration or treatment of the air via UV lights.[316-318]

The ability of tuberculosis to cause a pandemic began to decline before the causative bacterium was discovered in 1880 by Dr. Robert Koch, likely influenced by the Public Health movement that began in approximately 1850, and then by the resultant declining numbers of human contacts.[320-323] Thereafter, its decline continued, especially after the discovery of antituberculous treatment in the mid-1900s and the more recent use of directly observed therapy.[316-318,324-326] Other factors that have influenced the decline of tuberculosis include the BCG vaccine, contact tracing in communities, and comprehensive infection control programs in hospitals, which included placing masks on patients.[327-330] The WHO has targeted tuberculosis reduction as a major focus, especially in Asia and Africa, where poverty and HIV infection continue to be strongly associated with the spread of tuberculosis.[305,331-333]

Key Points: Factors contributing to tuberculosis's ability to cause a pandemic include pre-Germ Theory ignorance, undiagnosed patients, global transportation, airborne transmission, and HIV coinfection. Its pandemic ability has lessened substantially due to antibiotics (especially with directly observed therapy), public health interventions, the BCG vaccine, and the use of masks.

Influenza A, a.k.a. flu, causes pandemics and is thought to have first appeared about 2,000 years ago (Chapter 7). The first recorded pandemic likely occurred about 500 years ago in 1510.[334] Subsequently, there have been at least 14 more Influenza pandemics.[334,335] The 1918 pandemic is considered the worst, killing an estimated 50–100 million people.[336,337] Of note, it is thought that all of the pandemic influenza A viruses since 1918 are descendants of the 1918 strain because they all have genes present in the 1918 virus.[335] Perhaps the most unique thing about influenza A pandemics is that they only occur when a new strain or "variant" emerges that is different enough from previous strains and that there is inadequate preexisting immunity within humans to prevent infection.[335]

Influenza A has a unique ecology, moving interchangeably between mammals, birds and humans. The host range for mammals and birds includes pigs, horses, dogs, minks, ferrets, civets, cats, seals, muskrats, bats, whales, wild birds (ducks, geese), and chickens.[335,338–343] As it moves back and forth between these different species, it acquires new genetic material, and evolves.[335,344] With a wider and wider host range being identified, this favors reticulate evolution (intercrossing between many species that is simultaneously both convergent and divergent) and perhaps a greater risk of new strain formation and greater risk of pandemics.[344,345] Pandemics previously had a periodicity of roughly 20 years, but in recent years, evidence suggests that the rate of appearance of new influenza A strains is accelerating, which could lead to the appearance of pandemics at a more rapid rate.[345]

Influenza causes a characteristic illness manifested by high fevers for up to a week, cough, severe muscle aches, loss of appetite, and prostration.[346] Factors facilitating pandemics include its short incubation period (1–2 days), transmission by asymptomatic individuals (>50% of infected young children are asymptomatic), and airborne transmissibility for distances up to and likely greater than 6 feet with very high R_0s (as high as 6 early in an outbreak, up to 8 on ships, as high as 16 with young children, and 38 associated with an airplane outbreak).[133,347–354] The flu sufferer becomes essentially noninfectious when the fever resolves.[346] Extraordinary mortality was seen with the 1918 pandemic, where 90% of the deaths were due to secondary bacterial pneumonia at a time when neither antibiotics, antivirals, nor intensive care units existed, and mortality was 100 times greater than that seen with the 2009 pandemic (2.5% versus

0.02%, Table 8.24) when such resources were all available.[336,337,355] The other major factor augmenting the 1918 pandemic was the First World War with its global troop movements, close quarters in trenches, and the stress of war on bodily health.[337]

Influenza has continued to cause pandemics for two main reasons: (1) The scientific community has been unable to develop a single vaccine that offers long-lasting protection.[346] Once identified as a pandemic, it takes approximately one year to mass-produce a new vaccine. (2) It has an extraordinary ability to globally disseminate due to the combination of short incubation period (1–4 days), airborne spread, and increasing global airplane travel (see below).[356]

Increasingly, a better scientific understanding of influenza A has led to the identification of interventions that can mitigate the impact of influenza A pandemics. These include early identification of pandemics through global syndromic/internet surveillance, wearing of masks (both surgical and N95), social distancing, household isolation, the closing of schools, aggressive use of vaccines, neuraminidase inhibitors (antiviral medications for treatment/prevention of flu), and the willingness to implement public health interventions.[357–368] A particularly powerful tool for understanding pandemic interventions has been mathematical modeling.[364–368] Further work needs to be done internationally to determine the optimum combination of these interventions to mitigate mortality without collapsing the global economy.

Key Points: Factors contributing to influenza A's ability to cause a pandemic include a short incubation period, the ability to transmit while asymptomatic, airborne transmission with a high R_0 in closed spaces, the lack of an effective, long-acting vaccine, and airplane and ship travel with the rapid dissemination of a pandemic strain. Effective interventions exist, including vaccination, masks, antiviral drugs, social distancing, and household isolation.

The 2020 coronavirus pandemic first began in late 2019 in Wuhan, China, and was declared a pandemic in March 2020.[369–371] It is caused by SARS-CoV-2, a newly described coronavirus, and globally caused more than 500,000,000 cases and 6,000,000 deaths in the first two years after being declared a pandemic, both significant underestimates of the real number of cases.[372] It is transmitted through the air, by both small and large droplets, over distances greater than ten feet, especially indoors, and likely through direct contact with contaminated surfaces.[373-379] Its incubation period averages 5.1 days (95% CI 4.5–5.8) in symptomatic cases, but a significant proportion of those infected are asymptomatic (17.9–45%), and transmission can occur equally well (Chapter 4) from these asymptomatic people.[380-387] Although it is felt by many experts, including the US CDC, that viral shedding (infectiousness) occurs largely between Days 2 and 14 of illness, viral shedding with the ability to infect cell cultures may go on for as long as 30 days with more severe COVID-19 illnesses or in infected immunocompromised hosts.[388,389] PCR tests can be positive as long as 60 days, and symptoms can persist greater than six months (long haulers, Chapter 4).[390,391] As discussed in earlier chapters, it has an average R_0 of 2–3, but under unusual indoor circumstances, such as restaurants or a choir practice (see the superspreader discussion to follow), the R_0 can be much higher (individual R_0s of 9 and 53, respectively).[392,393]

The reported case fatality rate depends upon the accuracy with which the number of symptomatic and asymptomatic cases are determined, the ability of hospitals to handle the volume of cases being admitted, proven therapeutic options being used by clinicians at the time of diagnosis, and the use of vaccines. A review of publications through July 11, 2020, found a range of infection fatality rates (IFR) from 0% to 1.63%, with median corrected IFRs ranging from 0.1% to 0.9%.[394] As discussed in Chapter 4 (Table 4.9), there is one treatment modality with proven mortality benefit and at least five medications with randomized trial data supporting likely efficacy in hospitalized patients (anticoagulation, high titer convalescent plasma, remdesivir, monoclonal antibodies against the spike protein, and anti-IL-6 monoclonal antibodies).[395-400] Clinicians are commonly using two or more of these treatments to try and improve mortality over and above using steroids alone (see Chapter 10 for updated treatment efficacy). At the time of this book's completion, there are six vaccines actively in use (3 in the US, 1 in Europe and elsewhere, 1 in Russia, and 1 in China) and over 200 vaccine candidates in various stages of investigation (Chapter 5). Data from the US in mid-2021 suggests that 99% of the current mortality is in unvaccinated individuals.

Factors that favored COVID-19 causing a pandemic included airborne transmission, the lack of global appreciation that it was spreading for over a month (Chapters 2 and 3), transmission via airplane and ship travel, an unwillingness to be aggressive about societal control measures (Chapters 2 and 3), and ignoring the recommendations of experts (Chapters 2 and 3). Interventions that proved successful during the outbreak to date have included the wearing of masks, aggressive contact tracing, sheltering in place, and closing schools and workplaces (Chapters 2 and 3). Mathematical modeling has been used to examine interventions that might flatten the curve and reduce mortality. Current unknowns, such as whether SARS-CoV-2 infection results in long-lasting immunity, limit the accuracy with which predictions can be made.[401,402]

> Key points: Factors contributing to SARS-CoV-2's ability to cause a pandemic include airborne transmission with high Ro's indoors, prolonged infectiousness (at least 10 days), airplane travel, politics, unwillingness to embrace societal controls (social distancing, sheltering in place, closing schools and businesses, wearing masks), and vaccine hesitancy.

5. Superspreaders

In the last 20 years, the concept of superspreaders has been introduced as a mechanism that likely plays an important role in causing outbreaks, epidemics and pandemics. Superspreaders are individuals more capable of transmitting infectious diseases than other infected individuals.[403–413] It has been shown that there is heterogeneity in infectiousness, and it has been estimated that for many infectious diseases, 80% of infections are transmitted by less than 20% of those initially infected (see below).[404,405] When this occurs, it results in so-called superspreader events.[404,405]

Unrecognized or misdiagnosed infectious diseases are the most common cause of superspreader events, followed by airborne transmission in confined spaces, high contact rates, and co-infections that aid transmission.[405] Superspreader events have occurred with many types of infection: bacterial (sexually transmitted diseases, *Streptococcus pyogenes*, *Staphylococcus aureus*, pneumonic plague, mycoplasma, *Salmonella typhi*), mycobacterial (*M. tuberculosis*), viral (HIV, smallpox, influenza, monkeypox, measles, rubella, hantavirus, Ebola, Lassa fever, SARS, MERS, COVID-19), and parasitic (schistosomiasis, malaria, leishmaniasis).[19,403–413] For example, in the SARS outbreaks in Singapore and Beijing, 80–90% of secondary cases could be attributed to 20% of the cases.[403,414] In particular, in Beijing, one case led to

33 second-generation cases, 31 third-generation cases, and 12 fourth-generation cases.[403] The Beijing SARS superspreader events that occurred in the hospital were associated with fatal infection, delayed diagnosis, large numbers of close contacts, and the lack of early administrative controls.[403] Similarly, in the MERS outbreak in Korea, five superspreaders resulted in 92% of the other cases.[403] Days in the hospital without the patient under isolation was the only factor that distinguished the superspreaders from the usual spreaders.[403] These two examples support the lack of diagnosis and isolation as the main reason for superspreader events, especially before the outbreak, epidemic or pandemic, has been recognized.

Other superspreader events suggest that individual variation in the risk of transmission is an important additional cause of such events. Perhaps the best overall analysis of this possibility was done by Lloyd-Smith and colleagues.[405] They analyzed data from eight directly transmitted (person-to-person) infectious diseases and demonstrated that the distribution of R_0 for individuals is highly skewed, as a few individuals have much higher R_0s (up to >100) than the rest of the infected population. They further demonstrated that outbreaks containing such high R_0 individuals are more explosive, albeit more likely to extinguish, and that models that take such individuals into consideration are more predictive. In particular, they demonstrated through mathematical modeling that individual-specific control measures outperform population-wide measures. For example, contact tracing with isolation is more effective than population-wide isolation. Galvani and May confirmed the importance of highly infectious individuals in outbreaks but acknowledged the great difficulty associated with identifying such individuals in a way that allows real-time interventions.[404]

An additional phenomenon that likely plays a role in superspreader events is that highly infectious agents introduced into highly susceptible populations will follow mathematically predictable transmission rates that mimic wildfires.[415,416] This has been shown clearly by Roy and colleagues for cholera, where in epidemic circumstances, R_0s can be as high as 17, compared to the R_0s of endemic cholera, which are in the 1–2 range.[415] They modeled data from 15 cholera outbreaks, both contemporary and historic in India and Africa, and showed that all of them strikingly mimicked the super-critical phase of a wildfire. Finkenstadt and colleagues showed that mathematical modeling predicts that with unlimited numbers of susceptible individuals (such as in a large city or large forest), the introduction of a highly infectious agent, such as measles, will lead to a sustained outbreak (or wildfire), whereas for a small localized area of susceptibles (small city or small forest), it will lead to a self-extinguishing event.[415–417]

Perhaps the biggest missing link in understanding superspreader events is the role that host and organism factors play in the phenomenon. One of the first descriptions of superspreader events was a publication about so-called "cloud babies" who, when nasally colonized with *S. aureus* and co-infected with a respiratory virus, exhaled *S. aureus* into the air and were capable of causing outbreaks.[418] Subsequently, it was shown that "cloud adults" also exist, and that these individuals were able to airborne disperse *S. aureus*, in association with a viral respiratory infection, and cause an outbreak.[31] Of note, the outbreak source also had allergic rhinitis. In subsequent volunteer studies, it was shown that the crucial factor for airborne dispersal was not the rhinovirus infection but the presence of respiratory allergies (allergic rhinitis and/or asthma).[419] Volunteers with a history of allergy had a 17-fold greater likelihood of airborne dispersal of *S. aureus* associated with sneezing, which can also greatly increase the distance of *S. aureus* transmission.[420] The likelihood of *S. aureus* nasal carriage without allergic rhinitis is approximately 30%, whereas, with allergic rhinitis, it increases to almost 90%.[419,421] Allergic rhinitis in the general population may affect up to 30% of adults, so it is quite common.[421] What role allergic nasal inflammation might play in the superspreader process is not understood but deserves further investigation, given the increasing appreciation that superspreader events occur with a wide range of different infectious diseases, especially those that are airborne transmitted from the respiratory tract (measles, influenza, rubella, smallpox, SARS, MERS, and COVID-19). Given that aging is an inflammatory state, and COVID-19 affects those who are older or with inflammatory states (obesity, diabetes, hypertension, heart failure, COPD), baseline respiratory inflammation might be important in the pathogenesis of SARS-CoV-2 transmission.[422,423]

Pertinent to the coronavirus pandemic, there have been multiple documented COVID-19 superspreader events.[393,424–428] Perhaps the best-studied event was in association with a choir practice.[393] In this investigation, it was determined that a secondary attack rate associated with exposure to a single member of the choir was likely to be as high as 87% among 60 individuals exposed during a 2.5-hour practice.[393] It was speculated that the index case was a super-emitter, which has been described in association with using a loud voice, singing, or sneezing.[420,428,429] An analysis of transmission dynamics involving a number of superspreader events found they had several things in common — they largely occurred indoors, in crowded places, and without wearing masks.[428] They calculated the odds ratio of having a superspreader event transmitted indoors to be 33-fold greater than outdoors.[428] Others have looked at the impact of including superspreaders in models examining mitigation and found that the models are much more accurate when superspreaders are included.[430]

Key Points: Many outbreaks have documented superspreaders that account for greater than 80% of the transmission coming from less than 20% of the cases. Some superspreaders represent only an undiagnosed case, but other superspreaders actually have an increased ability to spread the organism. Further research is necessary to understand the mechanism(s) for superspreaders and how to detect and minimize superspreader events.

---

6. Global Trends

Finally, we must consider the impact of evolving global trends on the risk of pandemics. In Chapter 7 and this chapter, it was noted that global travel and the rapidity of global travel impact the risk of global organism transmission. Since the mid-20th century, the amount of ship traffic has increased greater than 6-fold.[478] For even infectious diseases with longer incubation periods, the rapidity of ship travel would be enough to increase the global risk of organism transmission. However, the amount of air traffic has increased greater than 1,000-fold since 1950 (Figure 8.76).[479] For short incubation infectious diseases, especially those that can be transmitted asymptomatically (such as COVID-19 and influenza A), this dramatically increases the risk of global transmission.

Two other increasingly apparent global trends that may be quite important related to the risk of pandemics are global warming and land use. While there is still active political debate, scientifically, there is no question that the planet is warming rapidly (Figure 8.77), even more so if ocean temperatures are considered.[480,481] A related consideration is the rapid increase in land use for grazing and cropland during the last 2,000

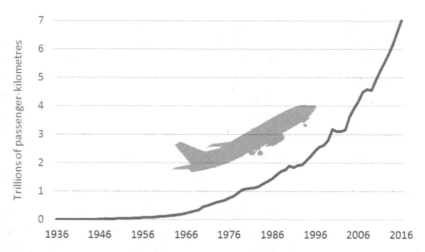

Figure 8.76.   Increasing global air travel in the last 80 years (1936–2016), trillions of passenger-kilometres per year.[479] With permission.

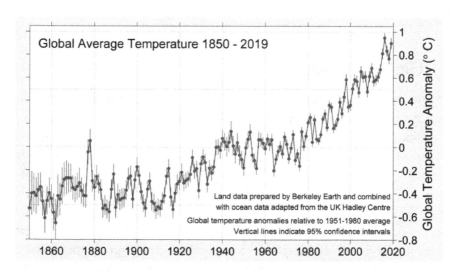

Figure 8.77.   Global warming from 1850 to 2020.[480] With permission.

years (Figure 8.78).[482] It is clear that global warming and land-use changes are already impacting animal and plant species on a global scale, and in most cases, negatively, with decreasing diversity.[483–485] In addition, there is a steadily increasing problem with illegal international wildlife trade.[486] Since animals are the source of most epidemic and pandemic organisms, the

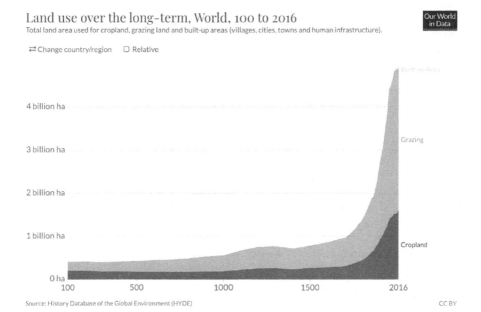

Land use over the long-term, World, 100 to 2016
Total land area used for cropland, grazing land and built-up areas (villages, cities, towns and human infrastructure).

⇄ Change country/region   ○ Relative

Source: History Database of the Global Environment (HYDE)   CC BY

Figure 8.78. Estimated increases in land use for cropland and grazing. 100AD to 2016.[482] With permission.

above trends and their effects on animals could be very important related to the future risk of global infectious diseases.[486,487,507,508] As an example, bats, one animal species with clear importance related to global infectious diseases, have actually experienced increasing diversity during the last century (Figure 8.79).[488] Could this be a factor in the recent appearance of SARS, MERS and SARS-CoV-2? Further work is needed to understand these global trends and their impact on pandemic diseases.

One last consideration that could be one of the most important reasons for the increasingly rapid appearance of new infectious diseases is the asymptotic global population growth. As described in Chapter 7, in the last 10,000 years, there has been an increased frequency of emerging infectious diseases (EIDs). It was also noted that this was associated with increased city size and a steadily increasing global population. Chapter 7 did not discuss whether pandemics are increasing in frequency. In Figure 8.80, the time course of EIDs can be seen in comparison to the increasing global population since humanity first appeared roughly 3 million years ago.[489–503] The estimated time of the first appearance of pandemics caused

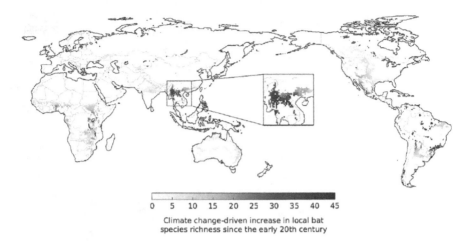

Climate change-driven increase in local bat
species richness since the early 20th century

Figure 8.79. Estimated increase in the local number of bat species due to shifts in their geographical ranges driven by climate change between the 1901–1930 and 1990–2019 periods. The zoomed-in area represents the likely spatial origin of the bat-borne ancestors of SARS-CoV-1 and 2.[488] With permission.

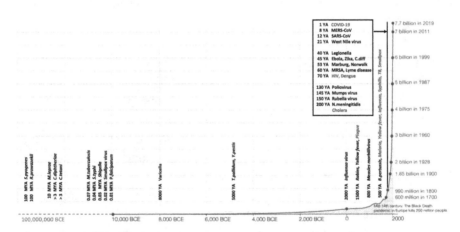

Figure 8.80. The appearance of historically important emerging infectious diseases in relationship to the global population.[484–497] Dates were taken from Tables 19 and 20 in Chapter 7 (see molecular clock discussion) and Table 23 in Chapter 8. The first known appearance of pandemics is shown in red for the 11 organisms thought to cause pandemics.

TB = *M. tuberculosis*, Plague = *Y. pestis*, Malaria = *P. falciparum*, Syphilis = *T. pallidum*, COVID-19 = *SARS-CoV-2*, HIV = *human immunodeficiency virus*, Dengue = *Dengue virus*, Cholera = *V. cholerae*, Yellow Fever = *yellow fever virus*, Influenza = *influenza virus*, Smallpox = *smallpox virus*. The global population curve is taken from the ourworldindata.org website with permission. Graph created by Sherertz.

by the 11 different organisms discussed in this chapter is shown in red. The earliest known pandemic was thought to be the first plague pandemic, approximately 1,500 years ago, which likely spread along known trade routes in Europe. However, by utilizing new technologies, such as probing for the DNA-encoding virus-interactive proteins in large human genome databases, it has recently been possible to show that a large-scale coronavirus epidemic occurred in Asia approximately 25,000 years ago, suggesting we may not yet know when the first pandemic occurred.[504]

Most known pandemics have occurred much more recently in human history. Six of the pandemics first occurred globally associated with exploration and colonization beginning about 500 years ago (malaria, yellow fever, influenza, syphilis, tuberculosis, smallpox), although prior regional pandemics in Africa and Asia are likely to have occurred with malaria, yellow fever, and smallpox. Four of the pandemics have appeared in the last 200 years (cholera, HIV, dengue, and COVID-19). Figure 8.80 suggests that pandemics are likely to keep happening at an even faster pace and that we have to better figure out how to deal with them on a global scale.

7. Summary of Factors Leading to Pandemics

To conclude, we will directly compare the 11 pandemic-causing organisms discussed above (Table 8.25). For all organisms, there is minimal pre-existing immunity, and international travel is necessary for global spread. For all organisms except syphilis, there is a high rate of transmission. Seven of the organisms had their greatest mortality pre-Germ Theory, likely related to the lack of knowledge about how to prevent and control the infection, and the lack of availability of vaccines and treatments (excluding smallpox with a vaccine since 1800). Public health measures can have significant impacts on all 11 of these infections and are especially important related to vector-borne agents (controlling vectors), sexually transmitted agents (syphilis, HIV — contact tracing), and infections where vaccines are available (vaccine programs). Comparing SARS-CoV-2 with the other pandemic organisms, the only organism similar in most aspects is influenza A (Table 8.25).

Table 8.25. Summary of factors predisposing to pandemics.

Pandemic	Pandemic(s) Worse Pre-Germ Theory (1870)	International Travel Augments	High Transmission (R_0)	Transmission Route	Pre-existing Herd Immunity	Effective Vaccine	Effective Treatment	Public Health Measures Reduce Risk
Plague	Yes	Yes	Yes	A, V	No	No	Yes	Yes
Syphilis	Yes	Yes	No	B	No	No	Yes	Yes
Tuberculosis	Yes	Yes	Yes	A	No	Yes	Yes	Yes
Smallpox	Yes	Yes	Yes	A	No	Yes	No	Yes
Yellow Fever	Yes	Yes	Yes	V	No	Yes	No	Yes
Malaria	Yes	Yes	Yes	V	No	No	Yes	Yes
Cholera	Yes	Yes	Yes	F	No	No	Yes	Yes
Dengue	No	Yes	Yes	V	No	No	No	Yes
HIV	No	Yes	Yes	B	No	No	Yes	Yes
Influenza A	No	Yes	Yes	A	No	No	Yes	Yes
COVID-19	No	Yes	Yes	A	No	No	Yes	Yes

A = airborne and/or droplet, B = body fluid, F = fecal/oral, V = vector (flea, mosquito, louse).

Influenza vaccine — no long-lasting immunity, no immunity that protects against a pandemic strain.

To gain a better understanding of SARS-CoV-2, we did a more detailed comparison of it with 1918 influenza A (Table 8.26). They are both RNA viruses with a high frequency of mutation, which makes developing a long-lasting vaccine difficult. They both have complex life cycles that involve animal hosts in nature, including flying animals (bats, birds). They both cause respiratory tract illnesses with similar frequencies of symptomatic infection, similar R_0s, and similar abilities to airborne transmit.

They have some striking differences with disease pathogenesis, including different respiratory tract infection binding sites, different lung pathologies (Chapter 4), different mortalities in different age ranges, and a different primary cause of death. The latter was influenced by the lack of

Table 8.26. Pandemic SARS-CoV-2 versus pandemic 1918 Influenza A.

Organism	SARS-CoV-2	Influenza A (1918 pandemic)
Similarities		
Virus type	RNA (positive strand)	RNA (negative strand)
Mutation frequency	~10^{-3} subs/site/yr	~10^{-3} subs/site/yr
Reservoirs in nature	Bats, pangolins?	Birds, swine, bats, others
Type of infection	Respiratory tract	Respiratory tract
Frequency of symptomatic infection	60–80%	40–80+%
Frequency of asymptomatic infection	18–40%	6–59%
R_0 average	1.2–6.5	1.8
R_0 highest	>30	>30
Airborne transmission distance	>6 feet	>6 feet
Mortality	0.5–2%	1–2%
Differences		
Respiratory viral receptor	ACE-2 receptor	Sialic acid
Duration of viral spreading	>10 days	~5 days
Duration of symptomatic illness	30% >9 months	~7 days
Risk of mortality by age	>age 60	> age 60, also <1, 20–40
Cause of mortality	90% viral LRTI	90% bacterial LRTI
Pulmonary pathology	Capillary thrombi	Interstitial edema

availability of antibiotics in 1918. Perhaps most remarkable, COVID-19 has more prolonged symptoms associated with more prolonged viral shedding.

Questions to be addressed:

1. In the last 200 years, greater than 80% of emerging infectious diseases have come either directly from animals or indirectly from animals via vectors (Chapter 7 and 8).[508] During this same time frame, the global human population has increased asymptotically (Chapter 8, Figure 8.80), associated with a near asymptotic increase in land use (Chapter 8, Figure 8.78). Are these findings related?

2. The 1918 influenza A flu strain and SARS-CoV-2 are very similar in how they are transmitted. Can this be leveraged to obtain a better understanding of viral airborne transmission in general?

3. Since 1950, the amount of global shipping has gone up greater than 6-fold, and the amount of air travel has gone up more than 1,000-fold (Chapter 8, Figure 8.76).[478,479] How important are these findings in facilitating pandemics, and what can be done to decrease the risk?

4. Global warming is increasing steadily, with the likely result being the ultimate thawing of the arctic permafrost and the exposure of humans to microorganisms that have been frozen for many thousands of years (Chapter 8, Figure 8.77).[509–513] Some of these organisms are well-known pathogens (1918 pandemic influenza, anthrax, smallpox); many will be organisms that modern-day humanity has never experienced before and for which we may not have treatments or vaccines.[509,510] Will this be a source of future pandemics? If yes, what can be done to mitigate the risk?

Key Points: Factors Leading to Pandemics
1. Minimal pre-existing immunity.
2. High rate of transmission (except syphilis, offset by silent transmission).
3. Pre-Germ Theory ignorance facilitated 7 of the 11 pandemics.
4. Public Health Measures since the Germ Theory have allowed more rapid control.
5. Vector control is very important for certain organisms.
6. Vaccines and therapies can dramatically reduce mortality.
7. Increased shipping and air travel likely play a very important role.
8. Disruption of animal habitat may turn out to be very important, especially for bats.
9. Increasing global population is likely the most important factor.

References

1. CDC. (nd) Lesson 1: Introduction to epidemiology. Section 11: Epidemic disease occurrence. Centers for Disease Control and Prevention. https://www.cdc.gov/csels/dsepd/ss1978/lesson1/section11.html

2. CDC. (nd) Lesson 6: Investigating an outbreak. Section 2: Steps of an outbreak investigation. Centers for Disease Control and Prevention. https://www.cdc.gov/csels/dsepd/ss1978/lesson6/section2.html#step2

3. Tsang TK, Wu P, Lin Y, *et al.* (2020) Effect of changing case definitions for COVID-19 on the epidemic curve and transmission parameters in mainland China: A modelling study. *Lancet Public Health* **5**:e289–e296.

4. Anonymous, CDC. (nd) Interpretation of Epidemic (Epi) curves during ongoing outbreak investigations. Centers for Disease Control and Prevention. https://www.cdc.gov/foodsafety/outbreaks/investigating-outbreaks/epi-curves.html

5. WHO. (2020) Report of the WHO-China Joint Mission on Coronavirus Disease 2019 (COVID-19). World Health Organization, February 28. https://www.who.int/publications-detail/report-of-the-who-china-joint-mission-on-coronavirus-disease-2019-(covid-19)

6. CDC. (nd) Lesson 1: Introduction to Epidemiology. Section 11: Epidemic Disease Occurrence. Epidemic Patterns. Centers for Disease Control and Prevention. https://www.cdc.gov/csels/dsepd/ss1978/lesson1/section11.html

7. Delamater PL, Street EJ, Leslie TF, *et al.* (2019) Complexity of the basic reproduction number (R_0). *Emerging Infectious Diseases* **25**:1–4.

8. Farrington CP, Whitaker HJ. (2003) Estimation of effective reproduction numbers for infectious diseases using serological survey data. *Biostatistics* **4**:621–632.

9. Aronson JK, Brassey J, Mahtani KR. (2020) "When will it be over?" An introduction to viral reproduction numbers, R_0 and R_e. The Centre for Evidence-Based Medicine. https://www.cebm.net/covid-19/when-will-it-be-over-an-introduction-to-viral-reproduction-numbers-r0-and-re/

10. Pascapurnama DN, Murakami A, Chagan-Yasutan H, *et al.* (2016) Prevention of tetanus outbreak following natural disaster in Indonesia: lessons learned from previous disasters. *Tohoku Journal of Experimental Medicine* **238**:219–227.

11. Pennington H. (2019) The impact of infectious disease in war time: A look back at WWI. *Future Microbiology* **14**:165–168.

12. Rochlin I, Ninivaggi DV, Benach JL. (2019) Malaria and Lyme disease — the largest vector-borne US epidemics in the last 100 years: Success and failure of public health. *BMC Public Health* **19**:804.

13. Mercante JW, Morrison SS, Desai HP, *et al.* (2016) Genomic analysis reveals novel diversity among the 1976 Philadelphia Legionnaire's Disease outbreak isolates and additional ST36 strains. *PLOS One*, September 28. DOI:10.1371/journal.pone.0164074

14. Herwaldt L, Marra AR. (2018) Legionella: A reemerging pathogen. *Current Opinion in Infectious Diseases* **31**:325–333.

15.   Shaheen M, Scott C, Ashbolt NJ. (2019) Long-term persistence of infectious Legionella with free-living amoebae in drinking water biofilms. *International Journal of Hygiene and Environmental Health* **222**(4):678–686. https://doi.org/10.1016/j.ijheh.2019.04.007

16.   Chancey C, Grinev A, Volkova E, Rios M. (2015) The global ecology and epidemiology of West Nile virus. *Biomed Res Int.* **2015**:376230. doi: 10.1155/2015/376230.

17.   Velasco-Villa A, Escobar LE, Sanchez A, *et al.* (2017) Successful strategies implemented towards the elimination of canine rabies in the Western Hemisphere. *Antiviral Research* **143**:1–12.

18.   Gunn JS, Marshall JM, Baker S, *et al.* (2014) Salmonella chronic carriage: Epidemiology, diagnosis and gallbladder persistence. *Trends in Microbiology* **22**:648–655.

19.   Pitzer VE, Meiring J, Martineau FP, *et al.* (2019) The invisible burden: Diagnosing and combating typhoid fever in Asia and Africa. *Clinical Infectious Diseases* **69**(S5):S395–S401.

20.   Antillon M, Warren JL, Crawford FW, *et al.* (2017) The burden of typhoid fever in low- and middle-income countries: A meta-regression approach. *PLOS Neglected Tropical Diseases* **11**:e0005376. DOI:10.1371/journal.pntd.0005376

21.   Marineli F, Tsoucalas G, Karamanou M, Androutsos G. (2013) Mary Mallon (1869–1938) and the history of typhoid fever. *Annals of Gastroenterology* **26**:132–134.

22.   Hsiao A, Toy T, Seo HJ, Marks F. (2016) Interaction between Salmonella and schistosomiasis: A review. *PLOS Pathogens* **12**:e1005928.

23.   Kramer HD. (1942) History of the public health movement in the United States, 1850 to 1900. PhD Thesis, University of Iowa. https://ir.uiowa.edu/etd/5070

24.   Cutler D, Miller G. (2005) The role of public health improvements in health advances: The 20th century United States. *Demography* **42**:1–22.

25.   Wray A. (2015) Water quality, morbidity, and mortality in London, 1906–1926. Doctoral thesis, Northwestern University Economics Department. https://scholar.google.com/scholar?q=Water+quality,+morbidity,+and+mortality+in+London,+1906%E2%80%931926.++Doctoral+thesis,+Northwestern+University+Economics+Department.&hl=en&as_sdt=0&as_vis=1&oi=scholart

26.   CDC. Antibiotic use in the United States, 2017: progress and opportunities. Centers for Disease Control and Prevention. https://www.cdc.gov/antibiotic-use/stewardship-report/hospital.html

27. Gupta A, Khanna S. (2014) Community-acquired Clostridium difficile infection: An increasing public health threat. *Infection and Drug Resistance* **14**:63–72.

28. Das M, Diana D, Wedderburn A, *et al.* (2020) Molecular epidemiology and transmission dynamics of leprosy among multicase families and case-contact pairs. *International Journal of Infectious Diseases* **96**:172–179. https://doi.org/10.1016/j.ijid.2020.04.064

29. WHO. (2021) Global leprosy (Hansen disease) update, 2020: impact of COVID-19 on global leprosy control. **96**:421–444. https://www.who.int/publications/i/item/who-wer9636-421-444.

30. Eichenwald HF, Kotsevalov O, Fasso LA. (1960) The "Cloud Baby": An example of bacterial-viral interaction. *American Journal of Diseases of Children* **100**:161–173.

31. Sherertz RJ, Reagan DR, Hampton KD, *et al.* (1996) A cloud adult: the Staphylococcus aureus — virus interaction revisited. *Annals of Internal Medicine* **124**:539–547.

32. Friedman ND, Kaye KS, Stout JE, *et al.* (2002) Health care-associated bloodstream infection in adults: A reason to change the accepted definition of community-acquired infections. *Annals of Internal Medicine* **137**:791–797.

33. Huang SS, Septimus E, Kleinman K, *et al.* (2013) Targeted versus universal decolonization to prevent ICU infection. *New England Journal of Medicine* **368**:2255–2265.

34. Jain R, Kralovic SM, Evans ME, *et al.* (2011) Veterans Affairs Initiative to prevent methicillin-resistant Staphylococcus aureus infections. *New England Journal of Medicine* **364**:1419–1430.

35. Hampson K, Dushoff J, Cleaveland S, *et al.* (2009) Transmission dynamics and prospects for the elimination of canine rabies. *PLOS Biology* **7**:e1000053.

36. Otete EH, Ahankari AS, Jones H, *et al.* (2013) Parameters for the mathematical modelling of Clostridium difficile acquisition and transmission: A systematic review. *PLOS One* **8**:e84224.

37. Pitzer VE, Feasey NA, Msefula C, *et al.* (2015) Mathematical modeling to assess the drivers of the recent emergence of typhoid fever in Blantyre, Malawi. *Clinical Infectious Diseases* **61**(Suppl):S251–8.

38. Malheiro L, Pinto SC, Sarmento A, Santos L. (2016) Comparison and contrast of the elimination campaigns for poliomyelitis and leprosy: Which is more feasible? *Acta Médica Portuguesa* **29**:279–283.

39. Cooper BS, Kypraios T, Batra R, *et al.* (2012) Quantifying type-specific reproduction numbers for nosocomial pathogens: evidence for heightened

transmission of an Asian sequence type 239 MRSA clone. *PLOS Computational Biology* **8**:e1002454.

40. Kugeler KJ, Griffith KS, Gould LH, *et al.* (2011) A review of death certificates listing Lyme Disease as a cause of death in the United States. *Clinical Infectious Diseases* **52**:364–367.

41. Philpott DCE, Nolan M, Evert N, *et al.* (2019) Acute and delayed deaths after West Nile Virus infection, Texas, USA, 2002–2012. *Emerging Infectious Diseases* **25**:263–271.

42. Roush SW, Murphy TV; Vaccine-Preventable Disease Table Working Group. (2007) Historical comparisons for vaccine-preventable diseases in the United States. *JAMA* **298**:2155–2163.

43. Phin N, Parry-Ford F, Harrison T, *et al.* (2014) Epidemiology and clinical management of Legionnaire's disease. *Lancet Infectious Diseases* **14**:1011–1021.

44. Lessa F, Mu Y, Bamberg WM, *et al.* (2015) Burden of Clostridium difficile infection in the United States. *New England Journal of Medicine* **372**:825–834.

45. Pieters Z, Saad NJ, Antillon M, *et al.* (2017) Case fatality rate of enteric fever in endemic countries: A systematic review and meta-analysis. *Clinical Infectious Diseases* **67**:628–638.

46. Gay F. (1918) *Typhoid Fever Considered as a Problem of Scientific Medicine.* New York, The Macmillan Company.

47. Friedman ND, Kaye KS, Stout JE, *et al.* (2002) Health Care–associated bloodstream infections in adults: A reason to change the accepted definition of community-acquired infections. *Annals of Internal Medicine* **137**: 791–797.

48. Steere AC, Sikand VK, Schoen RT, Nowakowski J. (2003) Asymptomatic infection with Borrelia burgdorferi. *Clinical Infectious Diseases* **37**:528–532.

49. Sejvar JJ. (2016) West Nile virus infection. *Microbiology Spectrum* **4**(3):EI10-0021-2016. DOI:10.1128/microbiolspec.EI10-0021-2016

50. Boshuizen HC, Neppelenbroek SE, van Vliet H, *et al.* (2001) Subclinical Legionella infection in workers near the source of a large outbreak of Legionnaires Disease. *Journal of Infectious Diseases* **184**:515–518.

51. Furuya-Kanamori L, Marquess J, Yakob L, *et al.* (2015) Asymptomatic Clostridium difficile colonization: Epidemiology and clinical implications. *BMC Infectious Diseases* **15**:516 DOI:10.1186/s12879-015-1258-4

52. Gunn JS, Marshall JM, Baker S, *et al.* (2014) Salmonella chronic carriage: Epidemiology, iagnosis and gallbladder persistence. *Trends in Microbiology* **22**:648–655.

53. Talty S. (2009) *The Illustrious Dead. The Terrifying Story of How Typhus Killed Napoleon's Greatest Army.* Crown Publishing Group, New York City.

54. Strong RP. (1920) *Typhus Fever with Particular Reference to the Serbian Epidemic.* Harvard University Press, Cambridge.

55. Stone L, He D, Lehnstaedt S, Artzy-Randrup Y. (2020) Extraordinary curtailment of massive typhus epidemic in the Warsaw Ghetto. *Science* **6**(30). DOI:10.1126/sciadv.abc0927

56. Schellekens J. (1996) Irish famines and English mortality in the eighteenth century. *Journal of Interdisciplinary History* **27**:29–42.

57. Raoult D, Ndihokubwayo JB, Tissot-Dupont H, *et al.* (1998) Outbreak of epidemic typhus associated with trench fever in Burundi. *Lancet* **352**:353–358. https://doi.org/10.1016/S0140-6736(97)12433-3

58. Umulisa I, Omolo J, Muldoon KA, *et al.* (2012) A mixed outbreak of epidemic typhus fever and trench fever in a youth rehabilitation center: Risk factors for illness from a case-control study, Rwanda. *American Journal of Tropical Medicine and Hygiene* **95**:452–456.

59. Faucher J-F, Socolovschi C, Aubry C. (2012) Brill-Zinsser Disease in Moroccan man, France 2011. *Emerging Infectious Diseases* **18**:171–172.

60. Ai J-W, Zhang Y, Zhang W. (2016) Zika virus outbreak: "A perfect storm". *Emerging Microbes & Infections* **5**(3):e21.

61. Lessler J, Chaisson LH, Kucirka LM, *et al.* (2016) Assessing the global threat from Zika virus. *Science* 353. DOI:10.1126/science.aaf8160

62. De Oliveira WK, de Franca VA, Carmo EH, *et al.* (2017) Infection-related microcephaly after the 2015 and 2016 Zika virus outbreaks in Brazil: A surveillance-based analysis. *Lancet* **390**:861–870.

63. CDC. (2011) Updated Norovirus outbreak management and disease prevention guidelines. *Morbidity and Mortality Weekly Report* **60**(RR03):1–15.

64. Ohfuji S, Kondo K, Ito K, *et al.* (2019) Nationwide epidemiologic study of norovirus-related hospitalization among Japanese older adults. *BMC Infectious Diseases* **19**:400.

65. Kerneis S, Guerin PJ, von Seidlein L, *et al.* (2009) A look back at an ongoing problem: Shigella dysenteriae type 1 epidemics in refugee settings in central Africa (1993–1995). *PLOS One* **4**:e4494.

66. Birmingham ME, Lee LA, Ntakibirora M, *et al.* (1997) A household survey of dysentery in Burundi: Implications for the current pandemic in sub-Saharan Africa. *Bulletin of the World Health Organization* **75**:45–53.

67. Kotloff KL, Winickoff JP, Ivanoff B, *et al.* (1999) Global burden of Shigella infections: Implications for vaccine development and implementation of control strategies. *Bulletin of the World Health Organization* **77**:651–666.

68. Chen T, Leung RK-k, Zhou Z, *et al.* (2014) Investigation of key interventions for shigellosis outbreak control in China. *PLOS One* **9**:e95006.

69. Kothary MH, Babu US. (2007) Infective dose of foodborne pathogens in volunteers: A review. *Journal of Food Safety* **21**:49–68. https://doi.org/10.1111/j.1745-4565.2001.tb00307.x

70. Nathanson N, Kew OM. (2010) From emergence to eradication: The epidemiology of poliomyelitis deconstructed. *American Journal of Epidemiology* **172**:1213–1219.

71. Alleman MM, Jorba J, Henderson E, *et al.* (2021) Update on vaccine-derived poliovirus outbreaks — worldwide, January 2020-June 2021. *MMWR* **70**(49):1691–9. https://www.cdc.gov/mmwr/volumes/70/wr/mm7049a1.htm

72. Szreter S. (2014) The prevalence of syphilis in England and Wales on the eve of the Great War: Re-visiting the estimates of the Royal Commission on Venereal Diseases 1913–1916. *Social History of Medicine* 27:508–529.

73. Armstrong GL, Conn LA, Pinner RW. (1999) Trends in infectious disease mortality in the United States during the 20th century. *JAMA* **281**:61–66.

74. WHO. Marburg virus disease. August 7, 2021. https://www.who.int/newsroom/fact-sheets/detail/marburg-virus-disease

75. CDC. (nd) 2014–2016 Ebola Outbreak in West Africa. Centers for Disease Control and Prevention. https://www.cdc.gov/vhf/ebola/history/2014-2016-outbreak/index.html

76. Munster VJ, Bausch DG, de Wit E, *et al.* (2018) Outbreaks in a rapidly changing central Africa — Lessons from Ebola. *New England Journal of Medicine* **379**:1198–1201.

77. Malvy D, McElroy AK, de Clerck H, *et al.* (2019) Ebola virus disease. *Lancet* **393**:936–948.

78. Plowright RK, Peel AJ, Streicker DG, *et al.* (2016) Transmission of within-host dynamics driving pulses of zoonotic viruses in reservoir-host populations. *PLOS Neglected Tropical Diseases* **10**(8):e0004796. DOI:10.1371/journal.pntd.0004796

79. Amman BR, Carroll SA, Reed ZD, *et al.* (2012) Seasonal pulses of Marburg virus circulation in juvenile Rousettus aegyptiacus bats coincide with periods of increased risk of human infection. *PLOS Pathogens* **8**:e1002877.

80. Mulangu S, Dodd LE, Davey RT Jr, *et al.* (2019) A randomized, controlled trial of ebola virus disease therapeutics. *New England Journal of Medicine* **381**:2293–2303.

81. Branswell H. (2020) "Against all odds": The inside story of how scientists across three continents produced an Ebola vaccine. STAT, January 7. https://www.statnews.com/2020/01/07/inside-story-scientists-produced-world-first-ebola-vaccine/

82. Park M, Thwaites RS, Openshaw PJM. (2020) COVID-19 Lessons from SARS and MERS. *European Journal of Immunology* **50**:308–316.

83. Weisse AB. (1995) Tuberculosis: Why "The White Plague". *Perspectives in Biology and Medicine* **39**:132–138.

84. Barberis I, Bragazzi NL, Galluzzo L, Martini M. (2017) The history of tuberculosis: From the first historical records to the isolation of Koch's bacillus. *Journal of Preventive Medicine and Hygiene* **58**:E9–12.

85. WHO. (nd) Tuberculosis. Key facts. World Health Organization, 2021. https://www.who.int/news-room/fact-sheets/detail/tuberculosis

86. Mindra G, Wortham JM, Haddad MB, Powell KM. (2017) Tuberculosis outbreaks in the United States. *Public Health Reports* **132**:157–163.

87. Dye C, Harries AD, Maher D, *et al.* (2006) Tuberculosis. In: *Disease and Mortality in Sub-Saharan Africa*, 2nd edition, eds. Jamison DT, Fechem RG, Makgoba MW, *et al.* The World Bank, Washington DC, pp. 179–193.

88. Brown TS, Challagundla L, Baugh EH, *et al.* (2019) Pre-detection history of extensively drug-resistant tuberculosis in KwaZulu-Natal, South Africa. *Proceedings of the National Academy of Sciences* **116**:23284-91.

89. Roy A, Eisenhut M, Harris RJ, *et al.* (2014) Effect of BCG vaccination against Mycobacterium tuberculosis infection in children: Systematic review and meta-analysis. *BMJ* **349**:g4643.

90. Glaziou P, Sismanidis C, Floyd K, Raviglione M. (2015) Global epidemiology of Tuberculosis. *Cold Spring Harbor Perspectives in Medicine* **5**:a017798.

91. CDC. (2010) Estimates of deaths associated with seasonal influenza — United States, 1976–2007. *Morbidity and Mortality Weekly Report* **59**:1057–1062.

92. CDC. (nd) Disease burden of influenza, 2010–2020. Centers for Disease Control and Prevention. https://www.cdc.gov/flu/about/burden/index.html

93. CDC. (nd) FastStats, influenza. Centers for Disease Control and Prevention. https://www.cdc.gov/nchs/fastats/flu.htm

94. Paget J, Spreeuwenberg P, Charu V, *et al.* (2019) Global mortality associated with seasonal influenza epidemics: New burden estimates and predictors from the GLaMOR Project. *Journal of Global Health* **9**:020421. DOI:10.7189/jogh.09.020421

95. Taubenberger JK, Morens DM. (2006) 1918 Influenza: The mother of all pandemics. *Emerging Infectious Diseases* **12**:15–22.

96. Simonsen L, Reichert TA, Viboud C, *et al.* (2005) Impact of influenza vaccination on seasonal mortality in the US elderly population. *Archives of Internal Medicine* **165**:265–272.

97. Foppa IM, Cheng P-Y, Reynolds SB, *et al.* (2015) Deaths averted by influenza vaccination in the US during the seasons 2005/06 through 2013/14. *Vaccine* **33**:3003–3009.

98. Wang C-B, Chiu M-L, Lin P-C, *et al.* (2015) Prompt oseltamivir therapy reduces medical care and mortality for patients with influenza infection. *Medicine* **94**:1–6.

99. Lytras T, Mouratidou E, Andreopoulou A, *et al.* (2019) Effect of early oseltamivir treatment on mortality in critically ill patients with different types of Influenza: A multiseason cohort study. *Clinical Infectious Diseases* **69**:1896–1902.

100. Karki BR, Sedhai YR, Bokhari SRA. (2019) *Water-Friderichsen Syndrome.* StatPearls, NCBI Bookshelf. https://www.ncbi.nlm.nih.gov/books/NBK551510/

101. Van de Beek D, de Gans J, Spanjaard L, *et al.* (2004) Clinical features and prognostic factors in adults with bacterial meningitis. *New England Journal of Medicine* **351**:1849–1859.

102. Theodoridou MN, Vasilopoulou, Atsali EE, *et al.* (2007) Meningitis registry of hospitalized cases in children: Epidemiological patterns of acute bacterial meningitis throughout a 32-year period. *BMC Infectious Diseases* **7**:101. DOI:10.1186/1471-2334-7-101

103. GBD 2016 Meningitis Collaborators. (2018) Global, regional, and national burden of meningitis, 1990–2016: A systematic analysis for the Global Burden of Disease Study 2016. *Lancet Neurology* **17**:1061–1782.

104. Nadel S, Ninis N. (2018) Invasive meningococcal disease in the vaccine era. *Frontiers in Pediatrics* **6**:1. https://www.frontiersin.org/articles/10.3389/fped.2018.00321/full

105. WHO. (nd) Meningococcal meningitis. World Health Organization. https://www.who.int/news-room/fact-sheets/detail/meningococcal-meningitis

106. Zimmerman LA, Knapp JK, Antoni S, Grant GB, Reef SE. (2022) Progress toward Rubella and congenital Rubella syndrome control and elimination. *MMWR* **71**:196–201. DOI: 10.15585/mmwr.mm7106a2

107. Gershon AA, Breuer J, Cohen JI, *et al.* (2015) Varicella zoster virus infection. *Nature Reviews* **1**:1.

108. Rubin S, Eckhaus M, Rennick LJ, *et al.* (2015) Molecular biology, pathogenesis and pathology of Mumps virus. *Journal of Pathology* 235–252.

109. Masarani M, Wazalt H, Dinneen M. (2006) Mumps orchitis. *Journal of the Royal Society of Medicine* **99**:573–575.

110. Metcalf CJE, Bjornstad ON, Grenfell BT, Andreasen V. (2009) Seasonality and comparative dynamics of six childhood infections in pre-vaccination Copenhagen. *Proceedings of the Royal Society* **B 276**:4111–4118.

111. Becker AD, Wesolowski A, Bjornstad ON, Grenfell BT. (2019) Long-term dynamics of measles in London: Titrating the impact of wars, the 1918 pandemic, and vaccination. *PLOS Computational Biology* **15**:e1007305.

112. Choisy M, Rohani P. (2012) Changing spatial epidemiology of pertussis in continental USA. *Proceedings of the Royal Society B* **279**:4574–4581.

113. Grenfell BT, Bjornstad ON, Kappey J. (2001) Travelling waves and spatial hierarchies in measles epidemics. *Nature* **414**:716–723.

114. Logan WPD. (1949) Scarlet fever, diphtheria, measles, and whooping cough in Glasgow from 1916 to 1945. *Glasgow Medical Journal* **30**:131–139.

115. Besa NC, Coldiron ME, Bakri A, *et al.* (2014) Diphtheria outbreak with high mortality in northeastern Nigeria. *Epidemiology and Infection* **142**:797–802.

116. Spencer RC. (1995) Invasive streptococci. *European Journal of Clinical Microbiology & Infectious Diseases* **14**(Suppl):S26–S32.

117. Brady DB, Kaiser AD. (1950) *Fifty Years of Health in Rochester New York.* Health Bureau, Rochester NY.

118. Harries HER, Gale AH. (1943) Variations in the mortality and incidence of the common infectious diseases of childhood over a century. *Journal of the Royal Society of Medicine.* https://doi.org/10.1177/003591574303600301

119. Tulchinsky TH. (2018) *Case Studies in Public Health.* Academic Press, Elsevier, San Diego CA.

120. Plotkin S. (2014) History of vaccination. *Proceedings of the National Academy of Sciences* 111:1283–1287.

121. Plotkin S, Orenstein W, Offit P. (2008) *Vaccines*, 5th edition. Elsevier Inc., Philadelphia.

122. Gould K. (2016) Antibiotics from prehistory to the present day. *Journal of Antimicrobial Chemotherapy* **71**:572–575.

123. Aminov RI. (2010) Brief history of the antibiotic area, lessons learned and challenges for the future. *Frontiers in Microbiology* **134**:1–7.

124. Liu Y, Lillepold K, Semenza JC, *et al.* (2020) Reviewing estimates of the basic reproduction number for dengue, Zika and chikungunya across global climate zones. *Environmental Research* **182**:109114.

125. Joh RI, Hoekstra RM, Barzilay EJ, *et al.* (2013) Dynamics of shigellosis epidemics: Estimating individual-level transmission and reporting rates from national epidemiologic data sets. *American Journal of Epidemiology* **178**:1319–1326.

126. Matsuyama R, Miura F, Nishiura H. (2017) The transmissibility of noroviruses: Statistical modeling of outbreak events with known route of transmission in Japan. *PLOS One* **12**:e0173996.

127. Tsuzuki S, Yamaguchi T, Nishiura H. (2018) Time series transition of basic reproduction number of syphilis in Japan. *International Journal of Infectious Disease* **7(Suppl)**:337.

128. Chowell G, Hengartner NW, Castillo-Chavez C, *et al.* (2004) The basic reproductive number of Ebola and the effects of public health measures: The cases of Congo and Uganda. *Journal of Theoretical Biology* **229**:119–126.

129. Ajelli M, Merler S. (2012) Transmission potential and design of adequate control measures for Marburg hemorrhagic fever. *PLOS One* **7**:e50948.

130. Ma Y, Horsburgh CR Jr, White LF, Jenkins HE. (2018) Quantifying TB transmission: A systematic review of reproduction number and serial interval estimates for tuberculosis. *Epidemiology and Infection* **146**:1478–1494.

131. Chowell G, Castillo-Chavez C, Fenimore PW, *et al.* (2004) Model parameters and outbreak control for SARS. *Emerging Infectious Diseases* **10**:1258–1263.

132. Killerby ME, Biggs HM, Midgley CM, *et al.* (2020) Middle East Respiratory Syndrome coronavirus transmission. *Emerging Infectious Diseases* **26**:191–198.

133. Biggerstaff M, Cauchemez S, Reed C, *et al.* (2014) Estimates of the reproduction number for seasonal, pandemic, and zoonotic influenza: A systematic review of the literature. *BMC Infectious Diseases* **14**:480. http://www.biomedcentral.com/1471-2334/14/480

134. Trotter CL, Gay NJ, Edmunds WJ. (2005) Dynamic models of meningococcal carriage, disease, and the impact of serogroup C conjugate vaccination. *American Journal of Epidemiology* **162**:89–100.

135. Marangi L, Mirinaviciute G, Flem E, *et al.* (2016) The natural history of varicella zoster virus infection in Norway: Further insights on exogenous boosting and progressive immunity to herpes zoster. *PLOS One* **12**(5):e0176845.

136. McGirr AA, Tuite AR, Fisman DN. (2013) Estimation of the underlying burden of Pertussis in adolescents and adults in southern Ontario, Canada. *PLOS One* **8**(12):e83850.

137. Bechah Y, Capo C, Mege J-L, Raoult D. (2008) Epidemic typhus. **8**:417–426.

138. Da Cunha AJLA, de Magalhaes-Barbosa MC, Medronho R de A, Prata-Barbosa A. (2017) Microcephaly case fatality rate associated with Zika virus infection in Brazil. *Pediatric Infectious Disease Journal* **36**:528–530.

139. Bardhan P, Faruque ASG, Naheed A, Sack DA. (2010) Decrease in shigellosis-related deaths without Shigella spp.-specific interventions, Asia. *Emerging Infectious Diseases* **16**:1718–1723.

140. GBD 2016 Diarrhoeal Disease Collaborators. (2018) Estimates of the global, regional, and national morbidity, mortality, aetiologies of diarrhea

in 195 countries: A systematic analysis for the Global Burden of Disease Study 2016. *Lancet Infectious Diseases* **18**:1211–1228.

141. Robilotti E, Deresinski S, Pinsky BA. (2015) Norovirus. *Clinical Microbiology Reviews* **28**:134–163.

142. Nathanson N, Kew OM. (2010) From emergence to eradication: The epidemiology of poliomyelitis deconstructed. *American Journal of Epidemiology* **172**:1213–1229.

143. Armstrong GL, Conn LA, Pinner RW. (1999) Trends in infectious disease mortality in the United States during the 20ᵗʰ century. *JAMA* **281**:61–66.

144. Mulangu S, Dodd LE, Davey RT Jr, *et al.* (2019) A randomized controlled trial of Ebola virus disease therapeutics. *New England Journal of Medicine* **381**:2293–2303.

145. CDC. (nd) Chronology of Marburg hemorrhagic fever outbreaks. Centers for Disease Control and Prevention. https://www.cdc.gov/vhf/marburg/outbreaks/chronology.html

146. Abdullahi OA, Ngari MM, Sanga D, *et al.* (2019) Mortality during treatment for tuberculosis; a review of surveillance data in a rural county in Kenya. *PLOS One*, July 11. https://doi.org/10.1371/journal.pone.0219191

147. Tiemersma EW, van der Werf MJ, Borgdorff MW, *et al.* (2011) Natural history of tuberculosis: Duration and fatality of untreated pulmonary tuberculosis in HIV negative patients: A systematic review. *PLOS One* **6**:e17601. DOI:10.1371/journal.pone.0017601

148. Park M, Thwaites RS, Openshaw PJM. (2020) COVID-19 Lessons from SARS and MERS. *European Journal of Immunology* **50**:308–316.

149. Paget J, Spreeuwenberg P, Charu V, *et al.* (2019) Global mortality associated with seasonal influenza epidemics: New burden estimates and predictors from the GLaMOR Project. *Journal of Global Health* **9**:020421. DOI:10.7189/jogh.09.020421

150. Mathuri SG, Venkatesan S, Myles PR, *et al.* (2014) Effectiveness of neuraminidase inhibitors in reducing mortality in patients admitted to hospital with influenza A H1Npdm09 virus infection: A meta-analysis of individual participant data. *Lancet Respiratory Medicine* **2**:395–404.

151. Branger J, van der Meer JTM, van Ketel RJ, *et al.* (2009) High incidence of asymptomatic syphilis in HIV-infected MSM justifies routine screening. *Sexually Transmitted Diseases* **36**:84–85.

152. Swartz MN. (2004) Bacterial meningitis — a view of the past 90 years. *New England Journal of Medicine* **351**:1826.

153. Chow MYK, Khandaker G, McIntyre P. (2016) Global childhood deaths from Pertussis: A historical review. *Clinical Infectious Diseases* **63**:S134–S141.

154. Faucher J-F, Socolovschi C, Aubry C, *et al.* (2012) Brill-Zinsser disease in Moroccan man, France, 2011. *Emerging Infectious Diseases* **18**:171–172.

155. Haby MM, Pinart M, Elias V, Reveiz L. (2018) Prevalence of asymptomatic Zika virus infection: A systematic review. *Bulletin of the World Health Organization* **96**:402–413.

156. Bliss J, Bouhenia M, Hale P, *et al.* (2018) High prevalence of Shigella or enterinvasive Escherichia coli carriage among residents of an internally displaced persons camp in South Sudan. *American Journal of Tropical Medicine and Hygiene* **98**:595–597.

157. Robilotti E, Deresinski S, Pinsky. (2015) Norovirus. *Clinical Microbiology Reviews* **28**:134–164.

158. Martinez-Bakker M, King AA, Rohani P. (2015) Unraveling the transmission ecology of Polio. *PLOS Biology* **13**:e102172.

159. Kenyon C, Osbak KK, Apers L. (2018) Repeat syphilis is more likely to be asymptomatic in HIV-infected individuals: A retrospective cohort analysis with important implications for screening. *Open Forum Infectious Diseases* DOI:10.1093/ofid/ofy096

160. Glynn JR, Bower H, Johnson S, *et al.* (2017) Asymptomatic infection and unrecognized Ebola virus disease in Ebola-affected households in Sierra Leone: A cross-sectional study using a new non-invasive assay for antibodies to Ebola virus. *Lancet Infectious Diseases* **17**:645–653.

161. Borchert M, Mulangu S, Swanepoel R, *et al.* (2006) Serosurvey on household contacts of Marburg hemorrhagic fever patients. *Emerging Infectious Diseases* **12**:433–439.

162. Drain PK, Bajema KL, Dowdy D, *et al.* (2018) Incipient and subclinical tuberculosis: A clinical review of early stages and progression of infection. *Clinical Microbiology Reviews* **3**:e00021-18.

163. Che X-Y, Di B, Zhao G-P, *et al.* (2006) A patient with asymptomatic Severe Acute Respiratory Syndrome (SARS) and antigenemia from the 2003–2004 community outbreak of SARS in Guangzhou, China. *Clinical Infectious Diseases* **43**:e1–5.

164. Wilder-Smith A, Teleman MD, Heng BH, *et al.* (2005) Asymptomatic SARS coronavirus infection among healthcare workers, Singapore. *Emerging Infectious Diseases* **11**:1142–1145.

165. Song Y-J, Yang J-S, Yoon HJ, *et al.* (201) Asymptomatic Middle East Respiratory Syndrome coronavirus infection using a serologic survey in Korea. *Epidemiology Health* **40**:e2018014.

166. Leung NHL, Xu C, Ip DKM, Cowling BJ. (2015) The fraction of influenza virus infections that are asymptomatic: A systematic review and meta-analysis. *Epidemiology* **26**:862–872.

167. Cooper LV, Kristiansen PA, Christensen H, *et al.* (2019) Meningococcal carriage by age in the African meningitis belt: A systematic review and meta-analysis. *Epidemiology and Infection* **147**:e228.

168. Fogel A, Gerichter CB, Rannon L, *et al.* (1976) Serologic studies in 11,460 pregnant women during the 19721 rubella epidemic in Israel. *American Journal of Epidemiology* **103**:51–59.

169. Plotkin SA, Reef SE, Cooper LZ, *et al.* (2011) Rubella. In: *Infectious Diseases of the Fetus and Newborn Infant*, 7th edition, eds. Remington JS, Klein JO, Wilson CB, *et al.* Elsevier, Philadelphia, pp. 861–898.

170. Gershon AA, Gershon MD. (2013) Pathogenesis and current approaches to control of Varicella-Zoster virus infections. *Clinical Microbiology Reviews* **26**:728–743.

171. Wagenvoort JHT, Harmsen M, Boutahar-Trouw BJK, *et al.* (1980) Epidemiology of mumps in the Netherlands. *Journal of Hygiene* **85**:313–326.

172. Bonwitt J, Kawakami V, Wharton A, *et al.* (2017) Absence of asymptomatic mumps virus shedding among vaccinated college students during a mumps outbreak-Washington, February–June 2017. *Morbidity and Mortality Weekly Report* **47**:1307–1308.

173. Udgaonkar US, Dharmadhikari CA, Kulkarni RD, *et al.* (1989) Study of diphtheria carriers in Miraj. *Indian Pediatrics* **26**:435–439.

174. Grosse-Kock S, Kolodkina V, Schwalbe E, *et al.* (2017) Genomic analysis of endemic clones of toxigenic and non-toxigenic Corynebacterium diphtheriae in Belarus during and after the major epidemic in 1990s. *BMC Genomics* **18**:873.

175. DeMuri GP, Wald ER. (2014) The group A streptococcal carrier state reviewed: Still an enigma. *Pediatric Infectious Disease Journal* **3**:336–342.

176. Edmonson MB, Addiss DG, McPherson JT, *et al.* (1990) Mild measles and secondary vaccine failure during a sustained outbreak in a highly vaccinated population. *JAMA* **263**:2467–2471.

177. Aoyama T, Takeuchi Y, Goto A, *et al.* (1992) Pertussis in adults. *American Journal of Diseases of Children* **146**:163–166.

178. Cherry JD. (2016) Pertussis in young infants throughout the world. *Clinical Infectious Diseases* **63**:S119–S122.

179. Mattern S. (2011) The art of medicine. Galen and his patients. *Lancet* **378**:478–479.

180. Eli SR. (1984) Immunity as a factor in the epidemiology of medieval plague. *Reviews of Infectious Diseases* **6**:866.

181. Dennis DT, Mead PS. (2006) Plague. In: *Tropical Infectious Diseases*, 2nd edition. ScienceDirect, Elsevier, pp. 471–481. 10.1016/B978-0-443-06668-9.50047-8

182. Rascovan N, Sjogren K-G, Kristiansen K, *et al.* (2019) Emergence and spread of basal lineages of Yersinia pestis during the Neolithic Decline. *Cell* **176**:295–306.

183. Fornaciari A. (2017) Environmental microbial forensics and archeology of past pandemics. *Microbiology Spectrum* **5**:EMF-0011-2016.

184. Procopius. (1914) *History of the Wars*, 7 Vols, trans. Dewing HB. Harvard University Press. **1**:451–473.

185. Cohn SK. (2002) *The Black Death transformed: Disease and Culture In Early Renaissance Europe.* Arnold, London.

186. Dean KR, Krauer F, Walloe L, *et al.* (2018) Human ectoparasites and the spread of plague in Europe during the second pandemic. *Proceedings of the National Academy of Sciences* **115**:1304–1309.

187. Gomez JM, Verdu M. (2017) Network theory may explain the vulnerability of medieval human settlements to the Black Death Pandemic. *Scientific Reports* **7**:43467.

188. Yu RPH, Lee HF, Wu CYH. (2017) Trade routes and plague transmission in pre-industrial Europe. *Scientific Reports* **7**:12973.

189. Xu L, Stige LC, Kausrud KL, *et al.* (2014) Wet climate and transportation routes accelerate spread of human plague. *Proceedings of the Royal Society B* **281**:20133159.

190. Simpson F. (1920) Methods of Plague control. *American Journal of Public Health* **10**:845–850.

191. Verma SK, Tuteja U. (2016) Plague vaccine development: Current research and future trends. *Frontiers in Immunology* **7**:1–8.

192. Behbehani AM. (1983) The Smallpox story: Life and death of an old disease. *Microbiological Reviews* **47**:455–509.

193. Acuna-Soto R, Stahle DW, Cleaveland MK, Therrell MD. (2002) Megadrought and megadeath in 16th century Mexico. *Emerging Infectious Diseases* **8**:360–362.

194. Breman JG, Henderson DA. (2002) Diagnosis and management of Smallpox. *New England Journal of Medicine.* **346**:1300–1308.

195. Duncan SR, Scott S, Duncan CJ. (1994) Modelling the different Smallpox epidemics in England. *Philosophical Transactions of the Royal Society B* **346**:407–419.

196. Rusnock A. (2009) Catching cowpox: The early spread of smallpox vaccination, 1798–1810. *Bulletin History Medicine* **83**:17–36.

197. Davenport RJ, Boulton J, Schwarz L. (2016) Urban inoculation and the decline of smallpox mortality in eighteenth century cities — a reply to Razzell. *Economic History Review* **69**:188–214.

198. Belongia EA, Naleway AL. (2003) Smallpox vaccine: The good, the bad, and the ugly. *Clinical Medicine & Research* **1**:87–92.

199. Stewart L. (1985) The edge of utility: Slaves and Smallpox in the early eighteenth century. *Medical History* **29**:54–70.

200. Tandy EC. (1923) Local quarantine and inoculation for Smallpox in the American Colonies (1620–1775). *American Journal of Public Health* **13**:203–207.

201. Aragon TJ, Ulrich S, Fernyak S, Rutherford GW. (2003) Risks of serious complications and death from Smallpox vaccination: A systematic review of the United States experience, 1963–1968. *BMC Public Health* **3**:26.

202. Ferguson NM, Keeling MJ, Edmunds WJ, *et al.* (2003) Planning for Smallpox outbreaks. *Nature* **425**:681–685.

203. Nishiura H, Kashiwagi T. (2009) Smallpox and season: Reanalysis of historical data. *Interdisciplinary Perspectives on Infectious Diseases* DOI:10.1155/2009/591935

204. Galvani AP, Slatkin M. (2003) Evaluating plague and smallpox as historical selective pressures for the CCR5-delta32 HIV-resistance allele. *Proceedings of the National Academy of Sciences* **100**:15276–15279.

205. Rogers DJ, Wilson AJ, Hay SI, Graham AJ. (2006) The global distribution of yellow fever and dengue. *Advances in Parasitology* **62**:181–220.

206. Garske T, Van Kerkhove MD, Yactayo S, *et al.* (2014) Yellow Fever in Africa: Estimating the burden of disease and impact of mass vaccination from outbreak and serological data. *PLOS Medicine* **11**:e1001638.

207. Chippaux J-P, Chippaux A. (2018) Yellow fever in Africa and the Americas: A historical and epidemiological perspective. *Journal of Venomous Animals and Toxins including Tropical Diseases* **24**:20. https://doi.org/10.1186/s40409-018-0162-y

208. Boyce R. (1911) The history of yellow fever in West Africa. *BMJ* **1**(2613):181–185.

209. Ndeffo-Mbah ML, Pandey A. (2019) Global risk and elimination of Yellow Fever epidemics. *Journal of Infectious Diseases* **221**(12):2026–2034. DOI:10.1093/infdis/jiz375

210. Smith BG. (2013) *Ship of Death: The Voyage that Changed the Atlantic World.* Yale University Press, New Haven, CT.

211. Patterson KD. (1992) Yellow Fever epidemics and mortality in the United States, 1693–1905. *Social Science & Medicine* **34**:855–865.

212. Duffy J. (1968) Yellow fever in the continental United States during the nineteenth century. *Bulletin of the New York Academy of Medicine* **44**:687–701.

213. Bryant JE, Holmes EC, Barrett ADT. (2007) Out of Africa: A molecular perspective on the introduction of yellow fever virus into the Americas. *PLOS Pathogens* **3**:e75.

214. McCullough D. (1977) *The Path Between the Seas. The Creation of the Panama Canal. 1870–1914.* Simon & Schuster, New York.

215. Gardner CL, Ryman KD. (2010) Yellow Fever: A reemerging threat. *Clinics in Laboratory Medicine* **30**:237–260.

216. WHO. (nd) Yellow fever, key facts. World Health Organization. https://www.who.int/news-room/fact-sheets/detail/yellow-fever

217. Thomas SJ, Endy TP, Rothman AL, Barrett AD. (2015) Flaviviruses (dengue, yellow fever, Japanese encephalitis, West Nile encephalitis, St. Louis encephalitis, tick-borne encephalitis, Kyasanur Forest disease, Alkhurma hemorrhagic fever, Zika). In: *Mandell, Douglas and Bennett's Principles and Practice of Infectious Diseases*, 8th edition, eds. Bennett JE, Dolin R, Blaser MJ. ScienceDirect, Elsevier, pp. 1881–1903.

218. Blake LE, Garcia-Blanco MA. (2014) Human genetic variation and Yellow Fever mortality during 19th century US epidemics. *mBio* **5**:e01253-14.

219. Norrby E. (2007) Yellow fever and Max Theiler: The only Nobel Prize for a virus vaccine. *Journal of Experimental Medicine* **204**:2779–2784.

220. WHO. (nd) Yellow fever vaccination booster not needed. World Health Organization. https://www.who.int/mediacentre/news/releases/2013/yellow_fever_20130517/en/#:~:text=The%20vast%20majority%20of%20reported,at%20highest%20risk%20of%20infection

221. Gotuzzo E, Yactayo S, Cordova E. (2013) Review article: Efficacy and duration of immunity after yellow fever vaccination: Systematic review on the need for a booster every 10 years. *American Journal of Tropical Medicine and Hygiene* **89**:434–444.

222. Emeribe AU, Abdullahi IN, Ajagbe OOR, *et al.* Incidence, drivers and global health implications of the 2019/2020 yellow fever sporadic outbreaks in Sub-Saharan Africa, Pathogens and Disease, Volume 79, Issue 4, June 2021, ftab017, https://doi.org/10.1093/femspd/ftab017

223. Domingo C, Fraissinet J, Ansah PO, *et al.* (2019) Long-term immunity against yellow fever in children vaccinated during infancy: A longitudinal cohort study. *Lancet* **19**:1363–1370.

224. Shearer FM, Mayes CL, Pigott DM, *et al.* (2017) Global yellow fever vaccination coverage from 1970 to 2016: An adjusted retrospective analysis. *Lancet Infectious Diseases* **17**:1109–1117.

225. Gubler DJ. (2004) The changing epidemiology of yellow fever and Dengue, 1900 to 2003: Full circle? *Comparative Immunology, Microbiology & Infectious Diseases* **27**:319–330.

226. Ferede G, Tiruneh M, Abate E. (2018) Distribution and larval breeding habitats of Aedes mosquito species in residential areas of northwest Ethiopia. *Epidemiology and Health* **40**:e2018015.

227. Faria NR, Kraemer MUG, Hill SC. (2018) Genomic and epidemiological monitoring of yellow fever virus transmission potential. *Science* **361**:894–899.

228. Sutherst RW. (2004) Global change and human vulnerability to vector-borne diseases. *Clinical Microbiology Reviews* **17**:136–173.

229. Ooi EE. (2015) The re-emergence of dengue in China. *BMC Medicine* **13**:99.

230. Dick OB, San Martin JL, Montoya RH, *et al.* (2012) Review: The history of Dengue outbreaks in the Americas. *American Journal of Tropical Medicine and Hygiene* **87**:584–593.

231. Amarasinghe A, Kuritsky JN Letson GW, Margolis HS. (2011) Dengue virus infection in Africa. *Emerging Infectious Diseases* **17**:1349–1354

232. Messina JP, Brady OJ, Scott TW, *et al.* (2014) Global spread of Dengue virus types: Mapping the 70-year history. *Trends in Microbiology* **22**:138–146.

233. Powell JR. (2018) Mosquito-borne human viral diseases: Why Aedes aegypti? *American Journal of Tropical Medicine and Hygiene* **98**:1563–1565.

234. Simmons CP, Farrar JJ, Van Vinh Chau N, Wills B. (2012) Dengue. *New England Journal of Medicine* **366**:1423–1432.

235. Katzelnick LC, Gresh L, Halloran ME, *et al.* (2017) Antibody-dependent enhancement of severe dengue disease in humans. *Science* **358**:929–932.

236. Laul A, Laul P, Merugumala V, *et al.* (2016) Clinical profiles of Dengue infection during an outbreak in northern India. *Journal of Tropical Medicine.* http://dx.doi.org/10.1155/2016/5917934

237. Wang W-H, Urbina AN, Chang MR, *et al.* (2020) Dengue hemorrhagic fever — a systemic literature review of current perspectives on pathogenesis, prevention and control. *Journal of Microbiology, Immunology and Infection* **53**(6):963–978. https://doi.org/10.1016/j.jmii.2020.03.007

238. WHO. Dengue and severe dengue. https://www.who.int/news-room/fact-sheets/detail/dengue-and-severe-dengue

239. Neff JM, Morris L, Gonzalez-Alcover R, *et al.* (1967) Dengue fever in a Puerto Rican community. *American Journal of Epidemiology* **86**:162–184.

240. Zhao ZG. (1986) Epidemiological study on dengue fever in Hainan Island. *Chinese Journal of Epidemiology* **7**:29–32.

241. Murray NE-A, Quam MB, Wilder-Smith A. (2013) Epidemiology of dengue: Past, present and future prospects. *Clinical Epidemiology* **5**:299–309.

242. Gubler DJ. (2011) Dengue, urbanization and globalization: The unholy trinity of the 21st century. *Tropical Medicine and Health* **39**(Suppl 4):3–11.

243. Kyle JL, Harris E. (2008) Global spread and persistence of Dengue. *Annual Review of Microbiology* **62**:71–92.

244. Messina JP, Brady OJ, Golding N, *et al.* (2019) The current and future global distribution and population at risk of dengue. *Nature Microbiology* **4**:1508–1515.

245. Ryan SJ, Carlson CJ, Mordecai EA, Johnson LR. (2019) Global expansion and redistribution of Aedes-borne virus transmission risk with climate change. *PLOS Neglected Tropical Diseases* **13**:e0007213.

246. Campbell LP, Luther C, Moo-Llanes D, *et al.* (2015) Climate change influences on global distributions of dengue and chikungunya virus vectors. *Philosophical Transactions of the Royal Society B* **370**:20140135.

247. Souza-Neto JA, Powell JR, Bonizzoni M. (2019) Aedes aegypti vector competence studies: A review. *Infection Genetics Evolution* **67**:191–209.

248. Muturi EJ, Buckner E, Bara J. (2017) Superinfection interference between dengue-2 and dengue-4 viruses in *Aedes aegypti* mosquitoes. *Tropical Medicine & International Health* **22**:399–406.

249. Snow GE, Haaland B, Ooi EE, Gubler DJ. (2014) Review article: Research on dengue during World War II revisited. *American Journal of Tropical Medicine and Hygiene* **91**:1203–1217.

249A. Utarini A, Indriani C, Ahmad RA, et al. Efficacy of Wolbachia-infected mosquito deployments of the control of Dengue. NEJM, June 10, 2021; 384:2177-86. DOI: 10.1056/NEJMoa2030243

249B. van den Hurk AF, Hall-Mendelin S, Pyke AT, Frentiu FD, McElroy K, Day A, Higgs S, O'Neill SL. Impact of Wolbachia on infection with chikungunya and yellow fever viruses in the mosquito vector Aedes aegypti. PLoS Negl Trop Dis. 2012;6(11):e1892. doi: 10.1371/journal.pntd.0001892.

249C. Caragata EP, Rocha MN, Pereira TN, Mansur SB, Dutra HLC, Moreira LA. Pathogen blocking in Wolbachia-infected Aedes aegypti is not affected by Zika and dengue virus coinfection. PLoS Negl Trop Dis 2019;13(5): e0007443. https://doi.org/10.1371/journal.pntd.0007443

249D. Amuzu HE, Tsyganov K, Koh C, Herbert RI, Powell DR, McGraw EA. Wolbachia enhances insect-specific flavivirus infection in Aedes aegypti mosquitoes. Ecol Evol. 2018 May 8;8(11):5441–5454. doi: 10.1002/ece3.4066.

250. Arrow KJ, Panosian C, Gelband H, eds. (2004) *A Brief History of Malaria, in Saving Lives, Buying Time. Economics of Malaria Drugs in an Age of Resistance*. National Academies Press. http://www.nap.edu/catalog/11017.html

251. Carter R, Mendis KN. (2002) Evoluntionary and historical aspects of the burden of Malaria. *Clinical Microbiology Reviews* **15**:564–594.

252. Tanabe K, Mita T, Jombart T, *et al.* (2010) *Plasmodium falciparum* accompanied the human expansion out of Africa. *Current Biology* **20**:1283–1289.

253. Yalcindag E, Elguero E, Arnathau C, *et al.* (2012) Multiple independent introductions of *Plasmodium falciparum* in South America. *Proceedings of the National Academy of Sciences* **109**:511–516.

254. Rodrigues PT, Valdivia HO, De Oliveira TC, *et al.* (2018) Human migration and the spread of malaria parasites to the New World. *Scientific Reports* 8(1):1993. DOI:10.1038/s41598-018-19554-0

255. Cowman AF, Healer J, Marapana D, Marsh K. (2016) Malaria: Biology and diseases. *Cell* **167**:610–624.

256. White NJ. (2003) The management of severe falciparum malaria. *American Journal of Respiratory and Critical Care Medicine* **167**:673–677.

257. Gething PW, Casey DC, Weiss DJ, *et al.* (2016) Mapping Plasmodium falciparum mortality in Africa between 1990 and 2015. *New England Journal of Medicine* **375**:2435–2445.

258. Kwiatkowski DP. (2005) How Malaria has affected the human genome and what human genetics can teach us about malaria. *American Journal of Human Genetics* **77**:171–192.

259. Kevin Esoh, Ambroise Wonkam, Evolutionary history of sickle-cell mutation: implications for global genetic medicine, Human Molecular Genetics, Volume 30, Issue R1, 1 March 2021, Pages R119–R128, https://doi.org/10.1093/hmg/ddab004

260. Selemani M, Msengwa AS, Mrema S, *et al.* (2016) Assessing the effects of mosquito nets on malaria mortality using a space time model: A case study of Rufiji and Ifakara Health and Demographic Surveillance System sites in rural Tanzania. *Malaria Journal* **15**:257.

261. The Nobel Prize. (nd) The Nobel Prize in Physiology or Medicine 1948. https://www.nobelprize.org/prizes/medicine/1948/summary/

262. Carson R. (1962) *Silent Spring*. Houghton Mifflin, Boston.

263. Berry-Caban CS. (2011) DDT and Silent Spring: Fifty years after. *Journal of Military and Veterans' Health* **19**:19–24.

264. Van den Berg H, Manuweera G, Konradsen F. (2017) Global trends in the production and use of DDT for control of malaria and other vector-borne diseasses. *BioMed Central* **16**:401.

265. Roberts DR, Laughlin LL, Hsheih P, Legters LJ. (1997) DDT, global strategies, and a malaria control crisis in South America. *Emerging Infectious Diseases* **3**:295–302.

266. WHO. (nd) WHO gives indoor use of DDT a clean bill of health for controlling malaria. World Health Organization. https://www.who.int/media-centre/news/releases/2006/pr50/en/

267. Pedercini M, Blanco SM, Kopainsky B. (2011) Application of the malaria management model to the analysis of costs and benefits of DDT versus non-DDT malaria control. *PLOS One* **6**:e27771.

268. Enayati A, Hemingway J. (2010) Malaria management: Past, present, and future. *Annual Review of Entomology* **55**:569–591.

269. Tognotti E. (2009) The rise and fall of syphilis in Renaissance Europe. *Journal of Medical Humanities* **30**:1–30.

270. Rothschild BM. (2005) History of syphilis. *Clinical Infectious Diseases* **40**:1454–1463.

271. Baughn RE, Musher DM. (2005) Secondary syphilitic lesions. *Clinical Microbiology Reviews* **18**:205–216.

272. Gall GEC, Lautenschlager S, Bagheri HC. (2016) Quarantine as a public health measure against an emerging infectious disease: Syphilis in Zurich at the dawn of the modern era (1496–1585). *GMS Hygiene and Infection Control* **11**:1–10.

273. Dobay A, Gall GEC, Rankin DJ, Bagheri HC. (2013) Renaissance model of an epidemic with quarantine. *Journal of Theoretical Biology* **317**:348–358.

274. Benedek TG, Erlen J. (1999) The scientific environment of the Tuskegee Study of Syphilis, 1920–1960. *Perspectives in Biology and Medicine* **43**:1–30.

275. Szreter S. (2014) The prevalence of Syphilis in England and Wales on the eve of the Great War: Re-visiting the estimates of the Royal Commission on Venereal Diseases 1913–1916. *Social History of Medicine* **27**:508–529.

276. WHO. New study highlights unacceptably high global prevalence of syphilis among men who have sex with men. July 9, 2021. https://www.who.int/news/item/09-07-2021-new-study-highlights-unacceptably-high-global-prevalence-of-syphilis-among-men-who-have-sex-with-men

277. Gottlieb MS, Schanker HM, Fam PT, *et al.* (1981) Pneumocystis pneumonia --- Los Angeles. *Morbidity and Mortality Weekly Report* **30**:1–3.

278. Deeks SG, Overbaugh J, Phillips A, Buchbinder S. (2015) HIV infection. *Nature Reviews* **1**:1–22.

279. GBD 2015 HIV Collaborators. (2016) Estimates of global, regional and national incidence, prevalence, and mortality of HIV, 1980–2015: The Global Burden of Disease Study 2015. *Lancet HIV* **3**:e361.

280. Dwyer-Lindgren L, Cork MA, Sligar A, *et al.* (2019) Mapping HIV prevalence in sub-Saharan Africa between 2000 and 2017. *Nature* **570**:189–209.

281. Bulstra CA, Hontelez JAC, Giardina F, et al. (2020) Mapping and characterizing areas with high levels of HIV transmission in sub-Saharan Africa: A geospatial analysis of national survey data. PLOS Medicine **17**:e1003042.

282. Committee on a National Strategy for AIDS. (1986) Confronting AIDS: Directions for public health, health care, and research. Institute of Medicine. http://www.nap.edu/catalog/938.html, pp. 1–374.

283. Moylett EH, Shearer WT. (2002) HIV: Clinical manifestations. *Journal of Allergy and Clinical Immunology* **110**:3–116.

284. Coovadia HM, Hadingham J. (2005) HIV/AIDS: Global trends, global trends and delivery bottlenecks. *Gobalization and Health.* DOI:10.1186/1744-8603-1-13.

285. Palella FJ, Delaney KM, Moorman AC, et al. (1998) Declining morbidity and mortality among patients with advanced human immunodeficiency virus infection. *New England Journal of Medicine* **338**:853–860.

286. Pollitzer R. (1954) Cholera studies. History of the disease. *Bulletin of the World Health Organization* **10**:421–461.

287. Stewart-Tull DES. (2001) Vaba, Haiza, Kholera, Foklune or Cholera: In any language still the disease of seven pandemics. *Journal of Applied Microbiology* **91**:580–591.

288. Ali M, Nelson AR, Lopez AL, Sack DA. (2015) Updated global burden of cholera in endemic countries. *PLOS Neglected Tropical Diseases* **9**:e0003832.

289. WHO. Cholera, Key facts. March 30, 2022. https://www.who.int/newsroom/fact-sheets/detail/cholera?gclid=Cj0KCQjw--2aBhD5ARIsALiRlwA8ySwkcb2jgAoXyfAqW-taDm9lX51NFuNcu6WDI6l7qIrS_ykK8IwaArr1EALw_wcB

290. Harris JB, LaRocque RC, Qadri F, et al. (2012) Cholera. *Lancet* **379**:2466–2476.

291. Azman AS, Rudolph KE, Cummings DAT, Lessler J. (2013) The incubation period of Cholera: A systematic review. *Journal of Infection* **66**:432–438.

292. Hartley DM, Morris JG, Smith DL. (2006) Hyperinfectivity: A critical element in the ability of *V. cholerae* to cause epidemics? *PLOS Medicine* **3**:e7.

293. Pascual M, Koelle K, Dobson AP. (2006) Hyperinfectivity in Cholera: A new mechanism for an old epidemiological model. *PLOS Medicine* **3**:e280.

294. Chowdhury FR, Nur Z, Hassan N, et al. (2017) Pandemics, pathogenicity and changing molecular epidemiology of cholera in the era of global warming. *Annals of Clinical Microbiology and Antimicrobials* **16**:10.

295. Almagro S, Taylor RK. (2013) Cholera: Environmental reservoirs and impact on disease transmission. *Microbiology Spectrum* **1**(2):OH-0003-2012. DOI:10.1128/microbiolspec.OH-0003-2012

296. Laviad-Shitrit S, Izhaki I, Halpern M. (2019) Accumulating evidence suggests that some waterbird species are potential vectors of Vibrio cholerae. *PLOS Pathogens* **15**:e1007814.

297. Senderovich Y, Izhaki I, Halpern M. (2010) Fish as reservoirs and vectors of Vibrio cholerae. *PLOS One* **5**:e8607.

298. Cohen NJ, Slaten DD, Marano N, *et al.* (2012) Preventing maritime transfer of toxigenic Vibrio cholerae. *Emerging Infectious Diseases* **18**:1680–1682.

299. Ojaveer H, Galil BS, Carlton JT, *et al.* (2018) Historical baselines in marine bio-invasions: Implications for policy and management. *PLOS One* **13**:e0202383.

300. Moore SM, Azman AS, Zaitchik BF, *et al.* (2017) El Nino and the shifting geography of cholera in Africa. *Proceedings of the National Academy of Sciences* **114**:4436–4441.

301. Orata FD, Keim PS, Boucher Y. (2014) The 2010 cholera outbreak in Haiti: How science solved a controversy. *PLOS Pathogens* **10**:e1003967.

302. Lewnard JA, Antillon M, Gonsalves G, *et al.* (2016) Strategies to prevent cholera introduction during international personnel deployments: A computational modeling analysis based on the 2010 Haiti outbreak. *PLOS Medicine* **13**:e1001947.

303. Frith J. (2014) History of Tuberculosis. Part 1 — Phthisis, consumption and the White Plague. *Journal of Military and Veterans' Health* **22**:29–35.

304. Bunyan J. (1860) The life and death of Mr. Badman. In: *The Entire Works of John Bunyan by Henry Stebbing*. Google Books, p. 61.

305. Hermans S, Horsburgh CR, Wood R. (2015) A century of Tuberculosis epidemiology in the northern and southern hemisphere: The differential impact of control interventions. *PLOS One* **10**:1–13.

306. Glaziou P, Floyd K, Raviglione MC. (2018) Global epidemiology of tuberculosis. *Seminars in Respiratory and Critical Care Medicine* **39**:271–285.

307. Dawson K. (2017) "The captain of all these men of death". Aspects of the medical history of tuberculosis. Masters of Public Health Thesis, Massey University, Manawatu, New Zealand. https://www.semanticscholar.org/paper/'The-captain-of-all-these-men-of-death'-%3A-aspects-%3A-Dawson/f851b688f08b9c248b156c393e2fcda0e9e831a6

308. Sepkowitz KA. (1996) How contagious is tuberculosis. *Clinical Infectious Diseases* **23**:954–962.

309. Haddad MB, Mitruka K, Oeltmann JE, *et al.* (2015) Characteristics of tuberculosis cases that started outbreaks in the United States, 2002–2011. *Emerging Infectious Diseases* **21**:508–510.

310. Mah MW, Fanning EA. (1991) An epidemic of primary tuberculosis in a Canadian aboriginal community. *Canadian Journal of Infectious Diseases* **2**:133–141.

311. Valway SE, Sanchez MPC, Shinnick TF, *et al.* (1998) An outbreak involving extensive transmission of a virulent strain of *Mycobacterium tuberculosis*. *New England Journal of Medicine* **338**:633–639.

312. Houk VN. (1980) Spread of Tuberculosis via recirculated air in a naval vessel: The Byrd study. *Annals of the New York Academy of Sciences* **353**:10–24.

313. Suzuki S, Nakabayashi K, Ohkouchi H, *et al.* (1997) Tuberculosis in the crew of a submarine. *Nihon Kyobu Shikkan Gakkai Zasshi (Japanese Journal of Thoracic Diseases)* **35**:61–66.

314. CDC. (1995) Exposure of passengers and flight crew to *Mycobacterium tuberculosis* on commercial aircraft, 1992–1995. *Morbidity and Mortality Weekly Report* **44**:137–140.

315. Kenyon TA, Valway SE, Ihle WW, *et al.* (1996) Transmission of multidrug-resistant *Mycobacterium tuberculosis* during a long airplane flight. *New England Journal of Medicine* **334**:933–938.

316. Escombe AR, Moore DAJ, Gilman RH, *et al.* (2008) The infectiousness of tuberculosis patients co-infected with HIV. *PLOS Medicine* **5**:e188.

317. Riley RL, Mills C, O'Grady F, *et al.* (1962) Infectiousness of air from a tuberculosis ward. Ultraviolet irradiation of infected air: Comparative infectiousness of different patients. *American Review of Respiratory Disease* **85**:511–525.

318. Riley RL, Mills CC, Nyka W. (1959) Aerial dissemination of pulmonary TB — a two year study of contagion on a tuberculosis ward. *American Journal of Epidemiology* **70**:185–196.

319. Churchyard G, Kim P, Shah S, *et al.* (2017) What we know about tuberculosis transmission: An overview. *Journal of Infectious Diseases* **216**(Suppl):S629–S635.

320. Vynnycky E, Fine PEM. (1999) Interpreting the decline in tuberculosis: The role of secular trends in effective contact. *International Journal of Epidemiology* **28**:327–334.

321. Kramer HD. (1942) History of the public health movement in the United States, 1850 to 1900. PhD Thesis, University of Iowa, 1942. https://ir.uiowa.edu/etd/5070

322. Howard-Jones N. (1975) The scientific background of the international sanitary conferences, 1851–1938. World Health Organization, Geneva. http://whqlibdoc.who.int/publications/1975/14549_eng.pdf.

323. Cutler D, Miller G. (1942) The role of public health improvements in health advances, the 20th century United States. *Demography* **42**:1–22.

324. Ramakrishnan CV, Andrews RH, Devadatta S, *et al.* (1961) Influence of segregation of tuberculosis patients for one year on the attack rate of tuberculosis in a 5-year period in close family contacts in South India. *Bulletin of the World Health Organization* **24**:129–148.

325. Kamat SR Dawson JJY, Devadatta S, *et al.* (1966) A controlled study of the influence of segregation of tuberculosis patients for one year on the attack rate of tuberculosis in a 5-year period in close family contacts in South India. *Bulletin of the World Health Organization* **34**:517–532.

326. Wright CM, Westerkamp L, Korver S, Dobler CC. (2015) Community-based directly observed therapy (DOT) versus clinic DOT for Tuberculosis: A systematic review and meta-analysis of comparative effectiveness. *BMC Infectious Diseases* **15**:210.

327. Colditz GA, Brewer TF, Berkey CS, *et al.* (1994) Efficacy of BCG vaccine in the prevention of Tuberculosis. *JAMA* **271**:698–702.

328. Begun M, Newall AT, Marks GB, Wood JG. (2013) Contact tracing of Tuberculosis: A systematic review of transmission modeling studies. *PLOS One* **8**:e72470.

329. CDC. (2005) Guidelines for preventing the transmission of *Mycobacterium tuberculosis* in healthcare settings. *Morbidity and Mortality Weekly Report* **54**:1–144.

330. Dharmadhikari AS, Mphahlele M, Stoltz A, *et al.* (2012) Surgical face masks worn by patients with multidrug-resistant tuberculosis. Impact on infectivity of air on a hospital ward. *American Journal of Respiratory and Critical Care Medicine* **185**:1104–1109.

331. WHO. (nd) Tuberculosis. World Health Organization. https://www.who.int/news-room/fact-sheets/detail/tuberculosis

332. Janssens J-P, Rieder HL. (2008) An ecological analysis of incidence of tuberculosis and per capita gross domestic product. *European Respiratory Journal* **32**:1415–1416.

333. Dye C, Lonnroth K, Jaramillo E, *et al.* (2009) Trends in tuberculosis incidence and their determinants in 134 countries. *Bulletin of the World Health Organization* **87**:683–691.

334. Taubenberger JK, Morens DM. (2009) Pandemic influenza — including a risk assessment of H5N1. *Revue Scientifique et Technique* **28**:187–202.

335. Taubenberger JK, Kash JC. (2010) Influenza virus evolution, host adaptation and pandemic formation. *Cell Host & Microbe* **7**:440–451.

336. Taubenberger JK, Morens DM. (2006) 1918 Influenza: The mother of all pandemics. *Emerging Infectious Diseases* **12**:15–22.

337. Barry J. (2004) *The Great Influenza: The Story of the Deadliest Pandemic in History*. Penguin Books, New York.

338. Zhao P, Sun L, Xiong J, *et al.* (2019) Semiaquatic mammals might be intermediate hosts to spread avian influenza viruses from avian to humans. *Scientific Reports* **9**:11641.

339. Parrish CR, Murcia PR, Holmes EC. (2015) Influenza virus reservoirs and intermediate hosts: Dogs, horses, and new possibilities for Influenza exposure of humans. *Journal of Virology* **89**:2990–2994.

340. Kuchipudi SV, Nissly RH. (2018) Novel flu viruses in bats and cattle: "Pushing the envelope of influenza infection". *Veterinary Sciences* **5**:71.

341. Wallensten A. (2007) Influenza virus in wild birds and mammals other than man. *Microbial Ecology in Health and Disease* **19**:122–139.

342. Tong S, Zhu X, Li Y, *et al.* (2013) New World bats harbor diverse influenza A viruses. *PLOS Pathogens* **9**:e1003657.

343. Luis AD, Hayman DTS, O'Shea TJ, *et al.* (2013) A comparison of bats and rodents as reservoirs of zoonotic viruses: Are bats special? *Proceedings of the Royal Society B* **280**:20122753. http://doi.org/10.1098/rspb.2012.2753

344. Ma EJ, Hill NJ, Zabilansky J, *et al.* (2016) Reticulate evolution is favored in influenza niche switching. *Proceedings of the National Academy of Sciences* **113**:5535–5539.

345. Bui CM, Chughtai AA, Adam DC, MacIntyre CR. (2017) An overview of the epidemiology and emergence of influenza A infection in humans over time. *Archives of Public Health* **75**:1–7.

346. Kramer F, Smith GJD, Fouchier RAM, *et al.* (2018) Influenza. *Nature Reviews Disease Primers* **4**:1–21.

347. Carrat F, Vergu E, Ferguson, *et al.* (2008) Time-lines and disease in human Influenza: A review of volunteer challenge studies. *American Journal of Epidemiology* **167**:775–785.

348. Chen SC, Liao CM. (2008) Modelling control measures to reduce the impact of pandemic influenza among schoolchildren. *Epidemiology and Infection* **136**:1035–1045.

349. Hsieh Y-H, Tsai C-A, Lin C-Y, *et al.* (2014) Asymptomatic ratio for seasonal H1N1 influenza infection among schoolchildren in Taiwan. *BMC Infectious Diseases* **14**:80.

350. Ip DKM, Lau LLH, Leung NHL, *et al.* (2017) Viral shedding and transmission potential of asymptomatic and paucisymptomatic influenza virus infections in the community. *Clinical Infectious Diseases* **64**:736–742.

351. Mills CE, Robins JM, Lipsitch M. (2004) Transmissibility of 1918 pandemic influenza. *Nature* **432**:904–906.

352. White LF, Pagano M. (2008) Transmissibility of the Influenza virus in the 1918 pandemic. *PLOS One* **3**:e1498.

353. Moser MR, Bender TR, Margolis HS, *et al.* (1979) An outbreak of Influenza aboard a commercial airliner. *American Journal of Epidemiology* **110**:1–6.

354. Bischoff WE, Swett K, Leng I, Peters TR. (2013) Exposure to Influenza virus aerosols during routine patient care. *Journal of Infectious Diseases* **207**: 1037–1046.

355. Morens DM, Taubenberger JK, Fauci AS. (2008) Predominant role of bacterial pneumonia as a cause of death in pandemic Influenza: Implications for pandemic Influenza preparedness. *Journal of Infectious Diseases* **198**: 962–970.

356. Roser M. (nd) International arrivals by world region. University of Oxford. https://ourworldindata.org/tourism

357. MacIntyre CR, Chughtai AA, Rahman B. (2017) The efficacy of medical masks and respirators against infection in healthcare workers. *Influenza and Other Respiratory Viruses* **11**:511–517.

358. Smith JD, MacDougall CC, Johnstone J, *et al.* (2016) Effectiveness of N95 respirators versus surgical masks in protecting health care workers from acute respiratory infection: A systematic review and meta–analysis. *Canadian Medical Association Journal* **188**:567–574.

359. Radonovich LJ, Simberkoff MS, Bessesen MT, *et al.* (2019) N95 respirators vs medical masks for preventing Influenza among health care personnel. A randomized clinical trial. *JAMA* **322**:824–833.

360. Ahmed F, Zviedrite N, Uzicanin A. (2018) Effectiveness of workplace social distancing measures in reducing Influenza transmission: A systematic review. *BMC Public Health* **18**:518.

361. The Council of Economic Advisers. (2019) Mitigating the impact of pandemic influenza through vaccine innovation. https://www.hsdl.org/?view&did=831583

362. Muthuri SG, Venkatesan S, Myles PR, *et al.* (2014) Effectiveness of neuraminidase inhibitors in reducing mortality in patients admitted to hospital with Influenza A H1N1pdm09 virus infection: A meta-analysis of individual participant data. *Lancet Respiratory Medicine* **2**:395–404.

363. Heneghan CJ, Onakpoya I, Jones MA, *et al.* (2016) Neuraminidase inhibitors for Influenza: A systematic review and meta-analysis of regulatory and mortality data. *Health Technology Assessment* **20**:1–274.

364. Ferguson NM, Cummings DAT, Fraser C, *et al.* (2006) Strategies for mitigating an Influenza pandemic. *Nature* **442**:448–452.

365. Polgreen PM, Chen Y, Pennock DM, *et al.* (2008) Using Internet searches for influenza surveillance. *Clinical Infectious Diseases* **47**:1443–1448.

366. Zhang Y, Yakob L, Bonsall MB, Hu W. (2019) Predicting seasonal Influenza epidemics using cross-hemisphere Influenza surveillance data and local internet query data. *Scientific Reports* **9**:3262.

367. Hatchett RJ, Mecher CE, Lipsitch M. (2007) Public health interventions and epidemic intensity during the 1918 Influenza pandemic. *Proceedings of the National Academy of Sciences* **104**:7582–7587.

368. Markel H, Lipman HB, Navarro JA, *et al.* (2007) Nonpharmaceutical interventions implemented by US cities during the 1918–1919 Influenza pandemic. *JAMA* **298**:644–655.

369. SCMP. (2020) Coronavirus: China's first confirmed Covid-19 case traced back. *South China Morning Post*, March 13. https://www.scmp.com/news/ china/society/article/3074991/coronavirus-chinas-first-confirmed-covid-19- case-traced-back

370. Wu Z, McGoogan J. (2020) Characteristics of and important lessons from the coronavirus disease 2019 (COVID-19) outbreak in China. Summary of a report of 72 314 cases from the Chinese Center for Disease Control and Prevention. *JAMA* **323**(13):1239–1242. DOI:10.1001/jama.2020.2648

371. WHO. (nd) WHO receives first report. World Health Organization. https:// www.who.int/emergencies/diseases/novel-coronavirus-2019/events-as-they-happen

372. JHU. (nd) Coronavirus Resource Center, Johns Hopkins University. https:// coronavirus.jhu.edu/us-map

373. Morawska L, Milton DK. (2020) It is time to address airborne transmission of COVID-19. *Clinical Infectious Diseases*, July. https://doi.org/10.1093/cid/ciaa939

374. Yu ITS, Li Y, Wong TW, *et al.* (2004) Evidence of airborne transmission of the severe acute respiratory syndrome virus. *New England Journal of Medicine* **350**:1731–1739.

375. Miller S, Nazaroff WW, Jimenezet JL, *et al.* (2020) Transmission of SARS-CoV-2 by inhalation of respiratory aerosol in the Skagit Valley Chorale superspreading event. *medRxiv*. https://doi.org/10.1101/2020.06.15.2013 2027

376. Buonanno G, Morawska L, Stabile L, *et al.* (2020) Quantitative assessment of the risk of airborne transmission of SARS-CoV-2 infection: Prospective and retrospective applications. Environmental International https://doi.org/10.1016/j.envint.2020.106112

377. Li Y, Qian H, Hang Jian, *et al.* (2020) Evidence for probable aerosol transmission of SARS -CoV -2 in a poorly ventilated restaurant .Building and Environment. https://doi.org/10.1016/j.buildenv.2021.107788

378. Santarpia JL, Rivera DN, Herra V, *et al.* (2020) Transmission potential of SARS-CoV-2 in viral shedding observed at the University of Nebraska Medical Center. *medRxiv*, March 26. DOI:10.1101/2020.03.23.20039446

379.   Van Doremalen N, Morris DH, Holbrook MG, *et al.* (2020) Aerosol and surface stability of SARS-CoV-2 as compared with SARS-CoV-1. *New England Journal of Medicine* **382**:1564–1567.

380.   Lauer SA, Grantz KH, Qifang B, *et al.* (2020) The incubation period of coronavirus disease (COVID-19) from publicly reported confirmed cases: Estimation and application. *Annals of Internal Medicine.* https://doi.org/10.7326/M20-0504

381.   Mizumoto K, Kagaya K, Zarebski A, Chowell G. (2020) Estimating the asymptomatic proportion of coronavirus disease 2019 (COVID-19) cases on board the Diamond Princess cruise ship, Yokohama, Japan, 2020. **25**:e200180.

382.   Workman J. (2020) The proportion of COVID-19 cases that are asymptomatic in South Korea: Comment on Nishiura *et al. International Journal of Infectious Disease* **96**:398.

383.   Oran DP, Topol EJ. (2020) Prevalence of asymptomatic SARS-CoV-2 infection. A narrative review. *Annals of Internal Medicine.* https://doi.org/10.7326/M20-3012

384.   Lavezzo E, Franchin E, Ciavarella C, *et al.* (2020) Suppression of a SARS-CoV-2 outbreak in the Italian municipality of Vo. *Nature.* https://doi.org/10.1038/s41586-020-2488-1

385.   Byambasuren O, Cardona M, Bell K, *et al.* (2020) Estimating the extent of true asymptomatic COVID-19 and its potential for community transmission: Systematic review and meta-analysis. Official Journal of the Association of Medical Microbiology and Infectious Disease Canada. DOI:10.3138/jammi-2020-0030

386.   Furukawa NW, Brooks JT, Sobel J. (2020) Evidence supporting transmission of Severe Acute Respiratory Syndrome Coronavirus 2 while presymptomatic or asymptomatic. *Emerging Infectious Diseases* **26**:e1.

387.   Arons MM, Hatfield KM, Reddy SC, *et al.* (2020) Presymptomatic SARS-CoV-2 infections and transmission in a skilled nursing facility. *New England Journal of Medicine* **382**:2081–2090.

388.   Anonymous . Ending Isolation and Precautions for People with COVID-19: Interim Guidance https://www.cdc.gov/coronavirus/2019-ncov/hcp/duration-isolation.html#:~:text=In%20certain%20high%2Drisk%20congregate,day%20isolation%20period%20for%20residents.

389.   Folgueira MD, Luczkowiak J, Lasala F, *et al.* (2020) Persistent SARS-CoV-2 replication in severe COVID-19. *medRxiv*, June 12. https://doi.org/10.1101/2020.06.10.20127837

390. Li J, Zhang L, Liu B, Song D. (2020) Case report: Viral shedding for 60 days in a woman with COVID-19. *American Journal of Tropical Medicine and Hygiene* **102**:1210–1213.

391. Carfi A, Bernabei R; Gemelli Against COVID-19 Post-Acute Care Study Group. (2020) Persistent symptoms in patients after acute COVID-19. *JAMA*, July 9. https://jamanetwork.com/journals/jama/fullarticle/2768351

392. Lu J, Gu J, Li K, *et al*. (2020) COVID-19 outbreak associated with air conditioning in restaurant, Guangzhou, China, 2020. *Emerging Infectious Diseases* **26**:1628–1631.

393. Hamner L, Dubbel P, Capron I, *et al*. (2020) High SARS-CoV-2 attack rate following exposure at a choir practice — Skagit County, Washington, March 2020. *Morbidity and Mortality Weekly Report* **69**:606–610.

394. Ioannidis JPA. (2020) The infection fatality rate of COVID-19 inferred from seroprevalence data. *Bulletin of the World Health Organization*. DOI: 10.2471/BLT.20.265892

395. The WHO Rapid Evidence Appraisal for COVID-19 Therapies (REACT) Working Group. (2020) Association between administration of systemic corticosteroids and mortality among critically ill patients with COVID-19. A meta-analysis. *JAMA* **324**(13):1330–1341. https://jamanetwork.com/journals/jama/fullarticle/2770279

396. Tritschler T, Mathieu M-E, Skeith L, *et al*. (2020) Anticoagulant interventions in hospitalized patients with COVID-19: A scoping review of randomized controlled trials and call for international collaboration. *Journal of Thrombosis and Haemostasis* **18**(11):2958–2967. https://doi.org/10.1111/jth.15094

397. Libster R, Marc GP, Wappner D, *et al*. (2021) Early high-titer plasma therapy to prevent severe COVID-19 in older adults. *New England Journal of Medicine* **384**:610–618. DOI:10.1056/NEJMoa2033700

398. NIH. (nd) Potential antiviral drugs under evaluation for the treatment of COVID-19. Remdesivir. National Institutes of Health. https://www.covid19treatmentguidelines.nih.gov/antiviral-therapy/. Updated: August 27, 2020.

399. NIH. (nd) COVID treatment guidelines. Anti-SARS-CoV-2 monoclonal antibodies. National Institutes of Health. https://www.covid19treatmentguidelines.nih.gov/anti-sars-cov-2-antibody-products/anti-sars-cov-2-monoclonal-antibodies/

400. NIH. (nd) COVID treatment guidelines. The COVID-19 Treatment Guidelines Panel's statement on the use of tocilizumab for the treatment of

COVID-19. National Institutes of Health. https://www.covid19treatment-guidelines.nih.gov/statement-on-tocilizumab/

401. Holmdahl I, Buckee C. (2020) Wrong but useful — what COVID-19 epidemiologic models can and cannot tell us. *New England Journal of Medicine* **383**:303–305.

402. Jewell NP, Lewnard JA, Jewell BL. (2020) Caution warranted: Using the Institute for Health Metrics and Evaluation model for predicting the course of the COVID-19 pandemic. *Annals of Internal Medicine*, April 14. DOI:10.7326/M20-1565

403. Shen Z, Ning F, Zhou W, *et al*. (2004) Superspreading SARS events Beijing, 2003. *Emerging Infectious Diseases* **10**:256–260.

404. Galvani AP, May RM. (2005) Dimensions of superspreading. *Nature* **438**: 293–295.

405. Lloyd-Smith JO, Schreiber SJ, Kopp PE, Getz WM. (2005) Superspreading and the effect of individual variation on disease emergence. *Nature* **438**:355–359.

406. Bassetti S, Bischoff WE, Sherertz RJ. (2005) Are SARS superspreaders cloud adults? *Emerging Infectious Diseases* **11**:637–638.

407. Bischoff WE, Wallis ML, Tucker BK, *et al*. (2006) "Gesundheit!" Sneezing, common colds, allergies, and *Staphylococcus aureus* dispersion. *Journal of Infectious Diseases* **194**:1119–1126.

408. Stein RA. (2011) Super-spreaders in infectious diseases. *International Journal of Infectious Disease* **15**:e510.

409. Bischoff WE, Swett K, Leng I, Peters TR. (2013) Exposure to Influenza virus aerosols during routine patient care. *Journal of Infectious Diseases* **207**:1037–1046.

410. Wong G, Liu W, Liu Y, *et al*. (2015) MERS, SARS, and Ebola: The role of super-spreaders in infectious disease. *Cell Host & Microbe* **18**:398–401.

411. Lau MSY, Dalziel BD, Funk S, *et al*. (2017) Spatial and temporal dynamics of superspreading events in the 2014–2015 West Africa Ebola epidemic. *Proceedings of the National Academy of Sciences* **114**:2337–2342.

412. Nandi A, Allen LJS. (2019) Stochastic two-group models with transmission dependent on host infectivity or susceptibility. *Journal of Biological Dynamics* **13**:201–224.

413. Al-Tawfiq JA, Rodriguez-Morales AJ. (2020) Super-spreading events and contribution to transmission of MERS, SARS, and SARS-CoV-2 (COVID-19). *Journal of Hospital Infection* **105**(2):111–112. https://doi.org/10.1016/j.jhin.2020.04.002

414. Liu Y, Eggo RM, Kucharski AJ. (2020) Secondary attack rate and super-spreading events for SARS-CoV-2. *Lancet* **395**:347.

415. Roy M, Zinck RD, Bouma MJ, Pascual M. (2014) Epidemic cholera spreads like wildfire. *Scientific Reports* **4**:3710.

416. Pinto OA, Munoz MA. (2011) Quasi-neutral theory of epidemic outbreaks. *PLOS One* **6**:e21946.

417. Finkenstadt BF, Bjornstad ON, Grenfell BT. (2002) A stochastic model for extinction and recurrence of epidemics: Estimation and inference for measles outbreaks. *Biostatistics* **3**:493–510.

418. Eichenwald HF, Kotsevalov O, Fasso LA. (1960) The "cloud baby": An example of bacterial-viral interaction. *American Journal of Diseases of Children* **100**:161–173.

419. Bassetti S, Dunagan DP, D'Agostino RB, Sherertz RJ. (2001) Nasal carriage of Staphylococcus aureus among patients receiving allergen-injection immunotherapy: Associated factors and quantitative nasal cultures. *Infection Control & Hospital Epidemiology* **22**:741–745.

420. Bourouiba L. (2020) Turbulent gas clouds and respiratory pathogen emissions. Potential implications for reducing transmission of COVID-19. *JAMA* **323**(18):1837–1838.

421. Wheatley LM, Togias A. (2015) Allergic rhinitis. *New England Journal of Medicine* **372**:456–463.

422. De Magalhaes JP, Curado J, Church GM. (2009) Meta-analysis of age-related expression profiles identifying common signatures of aging. *Bioinformatics* **25**:875–881.

423. Saltiel AR, Olefsky JM. (2017) Inflammatory mechanisms linking obesity and metabolic disease. *Journal of Clinical Investigation* **127**:1–4.

424. McMichael TM, Currie DW, Clark S, *et al.* (2020) Epidemiology of COVID-19 in a long-term care facility in King County, Washington. *New England Journal of Medicine* **382**:2005–2011. https://doi.org/10.1056/NEJMoa2005412

425. Ghinai I, Woods S, Ritger KA, *et al.* (2020) Community transmission of SARS-CoV-2 at two family gatherings — Chicago, Illinois, February– March 2020. *Morbidity and Mortality Weekly Report* **69**:446–450. https://doi.org/10.15585/mmwr.mm6915e1

426. The Guardian. (2020) South Korean city on high alert as coronavirus cases soar at "cult" church. *The Guardian*, February 20. https://www.theguardian.com/world/2020/feb/20/south-korean-city-daegu-lockdown-coronavirus-outbreak-cases-soar-at-church-cult-cluster

427. James A, Eagle L, Phillips C, *et al*. (2020) High COVID-19 attack rate among attendees at events at a church — Arkansas, March 2020. *Morbidity and Mortality Weekly Report* **69**:632–635.

428. Althouse BM, Wenger AE, Miller JC, *et al*. (2020) Stochasticity and heterogeneity in the transmission dynamics of SARS-CoV-2. *arXiv*, May 27. arXiv:2005.13689v1

429. Asadi S, Wexler AS, Cappa CD, *et al*. (2019) Aerosol emission and super-emission during human speech increase with voice loudness. *Scientific Reports* **9**:2348. https://doi.org/10.1038/s41598-019-38808-z

430. Sneppen K, Taylor RJ, Simonsen L. (2020) Impact of superspreaders of dissemination and mitigation of COVID-19. Proceedings of the National Academy of Sciences. 10.1073/pnas.2016623118

431. Zhao S, Musa S, Hebert JT, *et al*. (2020) Modelling the effective reproduction number of vector-borne diseases: The yellow fever outbreak in Luanda, Angola 2015–2016 as an example. *PeerJ* **8**:e8601. DOI:10.7717/peerj.8601.

432. Sanches RP, Massad E. (2016) A comparative analysis of three different methods for the estimation of the basic reproduction number of dengue. *Infectious Disease Modelling* **1**:88–100. http://dx.doi.org/10.1016/j.idm.2016.08.002

433. Smith DL, McKenzie FE, Snow RW, Hay SI. (2007) Revisiting the basic reproductive number for malaria and its implications for malaria control. *PLOS Biology* **5**:e42.

434. Nguyen VK, Parra-Rojas C, Hernandez-Vargas EA. (2018) The 2017 plague outbreak in Madagascar: Data descriptions and epidemic modelling. *Epidemics* **25**:20–25.

435. Mukandavire Z, Morris JG Jr. (2015) Modeling the epidemiology of cholera to prevent disease transmission in developing countries. *Microbiology Spectrum* **3**:1–10.

436. Tsuzuki S, Yamaguchi T, Nishiura H. (2018) Time series transition of basic reproduction number of Syphilis in Japan. *International Journal of Infectious Disease* **73**:337. https://doi.org/10.1016/j.ijid.2018.04.4180

437. Nsubuga RN, White RG, Mayanja BN, Shafer LA. (2014) Estimation of the HIV basic reproduction number in rural south west Uganda: 1991–2008. *PLOS One* **9**:e83778.

438. Liu Y, Gayle AA, Wilder-Smith A, Rocklov J. (2020) The reproductive number of COVID-19 is higher compared to SARS coronavirus. *International Society of Travel Medicine* **27**(2):taaa021. DOI:10.1093/jtm/taaa021

439. Mills CE, Robins JM, Lipsitch M. (2004) Transmissibility of 1918 pandemic influenza. *Nature* **432**:904–906.

440. Gani R, Leach S. (2001) Transmission potential of smallpox in contemporary populations. *Nature* **414**:748–751.

441. Blake LE, Garcia-Blanco MA. (2014) Human genetic variation and Yellow Fever mortality during the 19th century U.S. epidemics. *mBio* **5**:e01253-14.

442. Romano APM, Costa ZGA, Ramos DG, *et al.* (2014) Yellow fever outbreaks in unvaccinated populations, Brazil, 2008–2009. *PLOS Neglected Tropical Diseases* **8**:e2740.

443. Kuno G. (2009) Emergence of the severe syndrome and mortality associated with Dengue and Dengue-like illness: Historical records (1890 to 1950) and their compatibility with current hypotheses on the shift of disease manifestation. *Clinical Microbiology Reviews* **22**:186–201.

444. White NJ. (2003) The management of severe falciparum malaria. *American Journal of Respiratory and Critical Care Medicine* **167**:673–677.

445. DeWitte SH. (2014) Mortality risk and survival in the aftermath of the medieval Black Death. *PLOS One* **9**:e96513.

446. Forrester JD, Apangu T, Griffith K, *et al.* (2017) Patterns of human Plague in Uganda, 2008–2016. *Emerging Infectious Diseases* **23**:1517–1521.

447. Phelps M, Perner ML, Pitzer VE, *et al.* (2018) Cholera epidemics of the past offer new insight into an old enemy. *Journal of Infectious Diseases* **217**: 641–649.

448. Barzilay EJ, Schaad N, Magloire R, *et al.* (2013) Cholera surveillance during the Haiti epidemic — the first 2 years. *New England Journal of Medicine* **368**:599–609.

449. Baughn RE, Musher DM. (2005) Secondary syphilitic lesions. *Clinical Microbiology Reviews* **18**:205–216.

450. Boulle A, Schomaker M, May MT, *et al.* (2014) Mortality win patients with HIV-1 infection starting antiretroviral therapy in South Africa, Europe, or North America: A collaborative analysis of prospective studies. *PLOS Medicine* **11**:e1001718.

451. JHU. (nd) Mortality analyses. Johns Hopkins Coronavirus Resource Center. https://coronavirus.jhu.edu/data/mortality

452. Taubenberger JK, Morens DM. (2006) 1918 Influenza: The mother of all pandemics. *Emerging Infectious Diseases* **12**:15–22.

453. Viboud C, Simonsen L, Fuentes R, *et al.* (2016) Global mortality impact of the 1957–1959 influenza pandemic. *Journal of Infectious Diseases* **213**:738–745.

454. Glezen WP. (1996) Emerging infections: Pandemic influenza. *Epidemiologic Reviews* **18**:64–76.

455. CDC. (nd) 2009 H1N1 pandemic (H1Npdm09 virus). Centers for Disease Control and Prevention. https://www.cdc.gov/flu/pandemic-resources/2009-h1n1-pandemic.html

456. Simonsen L, Spreeuwenberg P; the GLaMOR Collaborating Teams, *et al.* (2013) Global mortality estimates for the 2009 Influenza pandemic from the GLaMOR Project: A modeling study. *PLOS Medicine* **10**(11):e1001558.

457. Medical Research Council. (1948) Streptomycin treatment of pulmonary tuberculosis. *BMJ* **2**:769–782.

458. da Silva Escada RO, Velasque L, Ribeiro SR, *et al.* (2017) Mortality in patients with HIV-1 and tuberculosis co-infection in Rio de Janeiro, Brazil — associated factors and causes of death. *BMC Infectious Diseases* **17**:373.

459. Lin C-H, Lin C-J, Kuo Y-W, *et al.* (2014) Tuberculosis mortality: Patient characteristics and causes. *BMC Infectious Diseases* **14**:5.

460. Tiemersma EW, van der Werf MJ, Borgdorff MW, *et al.* (2011) Natural history of tuberculosis: Duration and fatality of untreated pulmonary tuberculosis in HIV negative patients: A systematic review. *PLOS One* **6**:e17601.

461. Ellner PD. (1998) Smallpox: Gone but not forgotten. *Infection* **26**:263–269.

462. Johansson MA, Vasconcelos PFC, Staples JE. (2014) The whole iceberg: Estimating the incidence of yellow fever virus infection from the number of severe cases. *Transactions of the Royal Society of Tropical Medicine & Hygiene* **108**:482–487.

463. Ly S, Fortas C, Duong V, *et al.* (2019) Asymptomatic dengue virus infections, Cambodia, 2012–2013. *Emerging Infectious Diseases* **25**:1354–1362.

464. Ten Bosch QA, Clapham HE, Lambrechts L, *et al.* (2018) Contributions from the silent majority dominate dengue virus transmission. *PLOS Pathogens* **14**:e1006965.

465. Buchwald AG, Sixpence A, Chimenya M, *et al.* (2019) Clinical implications of asymptomatic Plasmodium falciparum infections in Malawi. *Clinical Infectious Diseases* **68**:106–114.

466. Marshall JD, Quy DV, Gibson FL. (1967) Asymptomatic pharyngeal plague infection in Vietnam. *American Journal of Tropical Medicine and Hygiene* **16**:175–177.

467. Legters LJ, Cottingham AJ, Hunter DG. (1969) Comparison of serological and bacteriological methods in the confirmation of plague infections. *Bulletin of the World Health Organization* **41**:859–863.

468. Harris JB, LaRocque RC, Qadri F, *et al.* (2012) Cholera. *Lancet* **379**:2466–2476.

469. Mammone A, Pezzotti P, Regine V, *et al.* (2016) How many people are living with undiagnosed HIV infection? An estimate for Italy, based on surveillance data. *AIDS* **30**:1131–1136.

470. CDC. (2019) Estimated HIV incidence and prevalence in the United States 2010–2016. HIV Surveillance Supplemental Report 24, No. 1, Centers for Disease Control and Prevention. http://www.cdc.gov/hiv/library/reports/hiv-surveillance.html

471. Oran DP, Topol EJ. (2020) Getting a handle on asymptomatic SARS-CoV-2 infection. Scripps Research, September 22. https://www.scripps.edu/science-and-medicine/translational-institute/about/news/sarc-cov-2-infection/

472. Mizumoto K, Kagaya K, Zarebski A, Chowell G. (2020) Estimating the asymptomatic proportion of coronavirus 2019 (COVID-19) cases on board the Diamond Princess cruise ship, Yokohama, Japan 2020. *Eurosurveillance* **25**:2000180.

473. Fraser C, Cummings DAT, Klinkenberg D, *et al.* (2011) Influenza transmission in households during the 1918 pandemic. *American Journal of Epidemiology* **174**:505–514.

474. Hsieh Y-H, Tsai C-A, Lin C-Y, *et al.* (2014) Asymptomatic ratio for seasonal H1N1 influenza infection among schoolchildren in Taiwan. *BMC Infectious Diseases* **14**:80.

475. Ip DKM, Lau LLH, Leung NH, *et al.* (2017) Viral shedding and transmission potential of asymptomatic and paucisymptomatic influenza virus infections in the community. *Clinical Infectious Diseases* **64**:736–742.

476. Achkar JM, Jenny-Avital ER. (2011) Incipient and subclinical tuberculosis: Defining early disease states in the context of host immune response. *Journal of Infectious Diseases* **204**(Suppl):S1179–S1186.

477. Milton DK. (2012) What was the primary mode of smallpox transmission? Implications for biodefense. *Frontiers in Cellular and Infection Microbiology* **2**:1–7.

478. Corbett JJ, Winebrake J, Energy and Environmental Research Associates (US). (2008) Global Shipping 1948–2008. Global Forum on Transport and Environment in a Globalizing World, November 10–12, Guddalajara, Mexico.

479. Qualman D. (2017) Too much tourism: Global air travel and climate change. Darrin Qualman, February 7. https://www.darrinqualman.com/global-air-travel-climate-change/

480. Berkeley Earth. (2019) Global temperature report. 1850–2019. http://berkeleyearth.org/2019-temperatures/

481. Gonchar M. (2019) Teach about climate change with these 24 New York Times graphs. *NY Times*, February 18. https://www.nytimes.com/2019/02/28/learning/teach-about-climate-change-with-these-24-new-york-times-graphs.html

482. Our World in Data. (nd) Our world in data. https://ourworldindata.org/land-use

483. Kyle JL, Harris E. (2008) Global spread and persistence of dengue. *Annual Review of Microbiology* **62**:71–92. DOI:10.1146/annurev.micro.62.081307.163005.

484. Root, TL, Price JT, Hall KR, *et al*. (2003) Fingerprints of global warming on wild animals and plants. *Letters to Nature* **421**:57–60.

485. Horton KG, La Sorte FA, Sheldon D, *et al*. (2020) Phenology of nocturnal avian migration has shifted at the continental scale. *Nature Climate Change* **10**:63–68.

486. Borsky S, Hennighausen H, Leiter A, *et al*. (2020) CITES and the zoonotic disease content in international wildlife trade. *Environmental & Resource Economics* **76**:1001–1017. https://doi.org/10.1007/s10640-020-00456-7

487. Altizer S, Bartel R, Han BA. (2011) Animal migration and infectious disease risk. *Science* **331**:296–302.

488. Beyer RM, Manica A, Mora C. (2021) Shifts in global bat diversity suggest a possible role of climate change in the emergence of SARS-CoV-1 and SARS-CoV-2. *Science of the Total Environment* **767**:145413. https://doi.org/10.1016/j.scitotenv.2021.145413

489. Our World in Data. (nd) Smallpox mortality in London, 1629–1902. Redrawn from https://ourworldindata.org/grapher/deaths-from-smallpox-in-london

490. Our World in Data. (nd) Smallpox mortality in Sweden, 1774–1899. Redrawn from https://ourworldindata.org/grapher/deaths-from-smallpox-per-1000-population?time=1774..1899&country=SWE

491. Carter R, Mendis KN. (2002) Evolutionary and historical aspects of the burden of malaria. *Clinical Microbiology Reviews* **15**:564–594. Redrawn.

492. Office of National Statistics. (nd) Tuberculosis mortality, England and Wales 1836–1960. Redrawn from data from the Office of National Statistics.

493. CDC. (nd) Influenza/Pneumonia Mortality Rates 1900–1960s. Redrawn from data from the Vital Statistics of the United States, Historical Statistics of the United States — Colonial Times to 1970 Part 1, US Department of Health and Human Services. https://books.google.com/books?id=qgX5SvRPCKUC&pg=RA1-PA76&lpg=RA1-PA76&dq=Influenza/Pneumonia+mortality+rates+historical+statistics+of+the+united+states+colonial+times+to+1970&source=bl&ots=UKiX8nilIA&sig=ACfU3U3yvat6Y57KNLnan3CpoPQ-IgHaKQ&hl=en&sa=X&ved=2ahUKEwjY7Pbbrc74AhVCJEQIHZR1Df8Q6AF6BAgbEAM#v=onepage&q=Influenza%2FPneumonia%20mortality%20rates%20historical%20statistics%20of%20the%20united%20states%20colonial%20times%20to%201970&f=false

494. Office of National Statistics. (nd) Scarlet fever mortality, England and Wales 1860–1960. Redrawn from data from the Office of National Statistics.

495. Office of National Statistics. (nd) Cholera mortality, England and Wales 1975–1820. Redrawn from data from the Office of National Statistics.

496. Louisiana Division New Orleans Public Library. (nd) Yellow fever deaths, New Orleans, 1817–1905. https://www.google.com/url?sa=t&rct=-j&q=&esrc=s&source=web&cd=2&ved=2ahUKEwjbuPLXg9rhAh-WHIlQKHZW6A7AQFjABegQICxAE&url=http%3A%2F%2Fnutrias.org%2Ffacts%2Ffeverdeaths.htm&usg=AOvVaw23nLyyRB8Nd2N0u6FrI-wIH

497. World Population Review. (nd) New Orleans population statistics. http://worldpopulationreview.com/us-cities/new-orleans-population/

498. Office of National Statistics. (nd) Pertussis mortality, England and Wales 1838–1966. Redrawn from data from the Office of National Statistics.

499. Office of National Statistics. (nd) Measles mortality, England and Wales 1838–1966. Redrawn from data from the Office of National Statistics.

500. Office of National Statistics. (nd) Diphtheria mortality, England and Wales 1838–1966. Redrawn from data from the Office of National Statistics.

501. World Bank. (nd) HIV mortality, Subsaharan Africa, 1990–2010. Drawn from data posted on two Worldbank websites. https://data.worldbank.org/region/sub-saharan-africa. http://blogs.worldbank.org/opendata/global-state-aids-4-charts

502. New York Health Department. (nd) Epidemic meningitis mortality, 1965–1935. Redrawn from New York City, New York Health Department data.

503. Krylova O, Earn DJD. (2020) Patterns of smallpox mortality in London, England, over three centuries. *PLOS Biology*, December 21. https://doi.org/10.1371/journal.pbio.3000506

504. Souilmi Y, Lauterbur ME, Tobler R, *et al.* (2021) An ancient viral epidemic involving host coronavirus interacting genes more than 20,000 years ago in East Asia. *Current Biology* **31**(16):3504–3514. https://doi.org/10.1016/j.cub.2021.05.067

505. Rogers DJ, Wilson AJ, Hay SI, Graham AJ. (2006) The global distribution of yellow fever and dengue. *Advances in Parasitology* **62**:181–220. DOI:10.1016/S0065-308X(05)62006-4

506. Messina JP, Brady OJ, Scott TW, *et al.* (2014) Global spread of dengue virus types: Mapping the 70 year history. *Trends in Microbiology* **22**(3):138–146. DOI:10.1016/j.tim.2013.12.011

507. Symes WS, Edwards DP, Miettinen J, *et al.* (2018) Combined impacts of deforestation and wildlife trade on tropical biodiversity are severely

underestimated. *Nature Communications* **9**:4052. https://doi.org/10.1038/s41467-018-06579-2

508. Jones KE, Patel NG, Levy MA, *et al.* (2008) Global trends in emerging infectious diseases. *Nature* **451**:990–994.

509. Miner KR, Edwards A, Miller C. (2020) Deep frozen arctic microbes are waking up. *Scientific American*, November 20. https://www.scientificamerican.com/article/deep-frozen-arctic-microbes-are-waking-up/

510. Fox-Skelly J. (2017) There are diseases hidden in ice, and they are waking up. *BBC News*, May 4. http://www.bbc.com/earth/story/20170504-there-are-diseases-hidden-in-ice-and-they-are-waking-up

511. Revich BA, Podolnaya MA. (2011) Thawing of permafrost may disturb historic cattle burial grounds in East Siberia. *Global Health Action*, November 21. https://doi.org/10.3402/gha.v4i0.8482

512. BBC. (2016) Russia anthrax outbreak affects dozens in north Siberia. *BBC News*, August 2. https://www.bbc.com/news/world-europe-36951542

513. Taubenberger JK, Hultin JV, Morens DM. (2007) Discovery and characterization of the 1918 pandemic influenza virus in historical context. *Antiviral Therapy* **12**:581–591. https://pubmed.ncbi.nlm.nih.gov/17944266/

514. Biagini P, Theves C, Geraut A, *et al.* (2012) Variola virus in a 300-year-old Siberian mummy. *New England Journal of Medicine* **367**:2057–2059. DOI:10.1056/NEJMc1208124

9 Are There Geopolitical Solutions?

"Our message for change is clear: no more pandemics. If we fail to take this goal seriously, we will condemn the world to successive catastrophes."

The Independent Panel
COVID-19: Make it the Last Pandemic
May 2021

"Insanity is doing the same thing over and over and expecting different results."

Rita Mae Brown,
Author of, Sudden Death

Contents

1. Improve WHO and member countries pandemic capabilities
2. Determine the impact of mitigation strategies on global economies
3. Study the relationship between longCOVID and persistent SARS-CoV-2 infection
4. Evaluate the relationship between the immune system and 2nd SARS-CoV-2 infections
5. Find ways to decrease global vaccine inequity
6. Improve education for all ages during a pandemic
7. Understand the importance of bat reservoirs related to SARS-CoV-2 evolution and human adaptation
8. Investigate the reasons for the asymptotic increase in global epidemic/pandemic infectious diseases
9. Learn from all countries how best to handle future pandemics (investigation, early mitigation, global treatment trials, vaccine development and deployment)

Introduction

In this chapter, we note some of the topics and questions that could prove helpful for dealing with the ongoing and future pandemics. Chapter 9 is written so that the topics and questions are listed under the specific chapters where more detailed information can be found related to the questions being asked.

1. Improve WHO and member countries pandemic capabilities

Chapters 2 and 3

Topic 1. Improving the capabilities of the WHO and member countries so they are better prepared to prevent pandemics and more effectively deal with pandemics when they occur.

Question to be addressed:

How can the major issues that negatively affected the WHO's ability to prevent and/or lessen the impact of COVID-19 be overcome for this and future pandemics?

Issue and possible solutions:

The WHO was criticized by various countries and outside groups for its initial response to the COVID-19 pandemic. In response to this criticism, the WHO Director-General requested that the Independent Oversight and Advisory Committee (IOAC) for the WHO Health Emergencies Program review the WHO's response during the time period January through April 2020.[1] The IOAC was established in 2017 to provide oversight and monitoring of the development and performance of the WHO Emergency Program. The IOAC had issued reports on various outbreaks in the past, including those due to Zika and Ebola viruses. The IOAC issued a preliminary report in May 2020 on the WHO's COVID-19 pandemic response, which noted the extent of the various problems that the WHO and countries encountered during the first four months of the pandemic and highlighted areas that needed to be strengthened, including (1) the limitations of the International Health Regulations (IHR), the legally binding agreement created in 2005 for how the WHO and its member countries would work to ensure global health security, (2) the issuance and timing of the Public Health Emergency of International Concern (PHEIC), (3) the role of the WHO in providing travel advice, (4) the WHO Emergency Program's capacity and funding, and (5) the development of a multilateral governance mechanism to ensure equitable access to therapeutics and vaccines (see Chapter 2 for details on each of these areas). No specific recommendations on how to fix these problems were issued in the preliminary report.

The report was discussed at the May 2020 World Health Assembly (WHA) meeting, and the members issued a resolution requesting the Director-General appoint a second independent group to provide an impartial and comprehensive evaluation of the international health response to COVID-19. In July 2020, the Director-General established the Independent Panel for Pandemic Preparedness and Response. In January 2021, the Panel reported its preliminary findings that included[2]:

1. The world was not prepared for the COVID-19 pandemic, and must do better.
2. The pandemic response has deepened inequalities.
3. The global pandemic alert system is not fit for purpose.
4. There has been a failure to take seriously the already known existential risks posed by pandemic threats.
5. The WHO has been underpowered to do the job expected of it.
6. The COVID-19 pandemic must be a catalyst for fundamental and systemic change in preparedness for future such events, from the local community all the way to the highest international levels.
7. The full potential of vaccines cannot be realized if narrow national interests and economic power determine who gets access, instead of basic principles of fairness and ensuring that allocation will optimize their public health impact.

The Panel also noted that these issues have been known for years and examined by various commissions and panels during the past decade (Table 9.27). Recommendations have been made in the past, and some have advanced the world's ability to deal with various aspects of pandemics. However, the COVID-19 pandemic provided definitive proof that much more remains to be done. The WHO has repeatedly been asked to take on more responsibility to lessen the impact of outbreaks, epidemics and pandemics but has not been provided the necessary resources and authority to implement a coherent strategy. Furthermore, to solve the various problems, countries will need to move away from a nationalistic to a global approach.

Table 9.27. Twelve different commissions and panels have examined outbreaks, epidemics, and pandemics, and the International Health Regulations (2005) during the past decade.[2]*

Disease	Year	Committee
COVID-19	2020	Review Committee on the Functioning of the International Health Regulations (2005) during the COVID-19 Response
COVID-19	2020	Independent Oversight Advisory Committee for the WHO Health Emergencies Programme
COVID-19	2020	Global Preparedness Monitoring Board, Annual Report, A World in Disorder
COVID-19	2019	2019 Global Preparedness Monitoring Board, Annual Report, A World At Risk
COVID-19	2019	Independent Oversight Advisory Committee for the WHO Health Emergencies Programme
COVID-19	2017	UN Global Health Crises Task Force
COVID-19	2017	Independent Oversight Advisory Committee for the WHO Health Emergencies Programme
COVID-19	2016	UN High-Level Panel on the Global Response to Health Crises
Ebola	2016	Director General's Advisory Group on Reform of WHO's Work in Outbreaks and Emergencies
Ebola	2016	Commission on a Global Health Risk Framework for the Future: A Framework to Counter Infectious Disease Crises
Ebola	2015	Ebola Interim Assessment Panel
Ebola	2015	Review Committee on Second Extensions for Establishing National Public Health Capacities and on IHR Implementation
Influenza HiN1	2011	Review Committee on the Functioning of the International Health Regulations (2005) in relation to Pandemic (H1N1) 2009

* Modified from reference 2.

In May 2021, the Panel issued a final report that included definitive recommendations.[3] The Panel noted their deep concern that the failure to enact fundamental change despite the warnings issued has left the world dangerously exposed, as the COVID-19 pandemic proves. They highlight that the ongoing inequity in distribution of COVID19 vaccines between high-income and most other countries provides a poignant example to examine what might be possible since it is in each country's self-interest to equitably share the vaccine and thereby shorten the duration of the pandemic.

The Panel made seven overarching recommendations for transforming the international system for pandemic preparedness and response.[3]

1. Elevate leadership to prepare for and respond to global health threats to the highest levels to ensure just, accountable and multi-sectoral action.

2. Focus and strengthen the independence, authority and financing of the WHO.

3. Invest in preparedness now to create fully functional capacities at the national, regional and global levels.

4. Establish a new international system for surveillance, validation and alert.

5. Establish a pre-negotiated platform for tools and supplies.

6. Raise new international financing for the global public goods of pandemic preparedness and response.

7. Countries should establish the highest level of national coordination for pandemic preparedness and response.

Each of these overarching recommendations is accompanied by specific recommendations that are included in the Independent Panel's report and notes what entities should do what and when (Table 9.28). The Panel noted that it conducted its work independently and impartially with

Table 9.28. A timetable for immediate action. Who needs to do what, and when created by the Independent Panel for Pandemic Preparedness and Response for the WHO Executive Board.[3]

Action	Main Actor	When
Apply non-pharmaceutical public health measures systematically and rigorously in every country at the scale the epidemiological situation requires. All countries to have an explicit strategy agreed to at the highest level of government to curb COVID-19 transmission.	National governments	Immediately
High income countries with a vaccine pipeline for adequate coverage should, alongside their scale up, commit to provide to the 92 low and middle-income countries of the Gavi COVAX Advance Market Commitment, at least one billion vaccine doses no later than 1 September 2021 and more than two billion doses by mid-2022, to be made available through COVAX and other coordinated mechanisms.	National governments	Immediately

(Continued)

Table 9.28. *(Continued)*

Action	Main Actor	When
G7 countries to commit to providing 60% of the US$19 billion required for ACT-A in 2021 for vaccines, diagnostics, therapeutics and strengthening health systems with the remainder being mobilized from others in the G20 and other higher income countries. A formula based on ability to pay should be adopted for predictable sustainable, and equitable financing of such global public goods on an ongoing basis.	G7, G20 and national governments of high-income countries, foundations	Immediately
WTO and WHO to convene major vaccine producing countries and manufacturers to get agreement on voluntary licensing and technology transfer arrangements for COVID-19 vaccines (including through the Medicines Patent Pool [MPP]). If actions do not occur within 3 months, a waiver of TRIPS intellectual property rights should come into force immediately.	WTO, WHO and vaccine- producing countries and manufacturers	Immediately
Production of and access to COVID-19 tests and therapeutics, including oxygen, scaled up urgently in low and middle-income countries with full funding of US$1.7 billion for needs in 2021 and the full utilization of the US$3.7 billion in the Global Fund's COVID-19 Response Mechanism Phase 2 for procuring tests, strengthening laboratories, and running surveillance and tests.	Test- and therapeutics producing countries and manufacturers/ Global Fund to Fight AIDS, tuberculosis and malaria	Immediately
WHO to develop immediately a road map for the short term and within a 3-month scenario for the medium and long-term response to COVID-19, with clear goals, targets and milestones to guide and monitor the implementation of country and global efforts towards ending the COVID-19 pandemic.	WHO	Immediately

a focus on data, facts and science as the basis for the recommendations. The title of this report, "COVID-19: Make it the Last Pandemic", speaks to the boldness of the recommendations, all well thought out, pragmatic and achievable if global leadership commits to them.

Each of the high-level and specific recommendations deserves consideration and to be improved upon, where possible. However, if these recommendations are ignored or postponed, as has happened too often in the past, the world will continue to experience increasing numbers of outbreaks and pandemics, especially if countries continue to take a national versus global approach to finding and implementing solutions.

2. Determine the impact of mitigation strategies on global economies

Topic 2. The impact of the COVID-19 pandemic on mortality differed substantially between various countries.

Question to be addressed:

What is the relationship between the intensity of containment and mitigation policies and the economic impact of these policies on countries?

Issue and possible solutions:

The data suggest that widespread testing in combination with geographically focused lockdowns over limited periods of time in conjunction with social distancing and masks are the most effective ways to decrease the health impact of the pandemic. Even in countries that do not have the capacity to do widespread testing, implementing these other measures will substantially decrease the incidence of disease. Furthermore, taking these steps would likely cause less disruption of the economy over a several-year period. The January 2021 report by the Independent Panel for Pandemic Preparedness and Response concluded that implementing strict public health control measures will help the economies of countries recover faster than in countries that do not implement and/or enforce stringent measures while averting significantly more death and illness.[2] This is a powerful conclusion that should help inform the approach that countries take in dealing with ongoing or new COVID-19 waves and in future pandemics.

Question to be addressed:

What are the best ways to separate political influences from science-based public health recommendations?

Issue and possible solutions:

In various countries most impacted by the pandemic, there was substantial political interference with public health recommendations from the WHO and national public health agencies. The WHO is continuously dealing with political issues as it is governed by over 190 countries and a substantial amount of its funding comes from these countries, particularly the high-income countries. A poignant example of political interference with the functioning of the WHO occurred in May 2020 when President Trump threatened to permanently withdraw from the WHO and stop paying its annual dues payment because he was unhappy with various issues related to the WHO, including how the Director-General was dealing with China.[4] Soon thereafter, the Director-General did reach an agreement with China to send an independent team into China to investigate how the pandemic started, but it would be many months before China let them visit. Even after the team went to China, this important question has not been resolved because of the government's unwillingness to provide all of the information requested. This is just one of many examples where the WHO is encumbered by competing political interests of various countries. At this point in time, the Director-General's best tool is to create independent groups, such as the Independent Panel for Pandemic Preparedness and Response,[2,3] which can help call out political interference when it is present. However, the WHO will not be able to fully meet its mission until this problem is fully resolved.

The WHO was not alone in public health outcomes being endangered by political interference. This occurred in various countries. The US was one of the main culprits, as noted by the Trump administration's interference on numerous occasions with moving CDC recommendations forward.[5] Various solutions have been proposed to help avoid political interference with public health recommendations, and one we find particularly appealing is to have the US Congress create an independent board that oversees the CDC.[6]

There is precedent for this type of independent governance of Federal Agencies in the US, including the Federal Trade Commission, the National Labor Relations Board, the Securities and Exchange Commission, and the Federal Reserve Board. The independence of these boards has proven to be important on multiple occasions. For example, in the first few years of his presidency, Trump criticized Jerome Powell, the Chairman of the Federal Reserve Board, on multiple occasions for interest rates being too high. However, Trump was unable to replace Powell due to the protection created by Congress.[7] During the current pandemic, this type of independent oversight group would also have been helpful for the FDA commissioner, Stephan Hahn, when the Trump administration threatened to fire him because he would not speed up the process for evaluating the Pfizer and Moderna COVID-19 vaccines so that they would be approved for use prior to the end of his presidential term.[8]

An independent group overseeing the public health response should also be considered by other countries since the US was not the only country where politics substantially impaired the public health response. For example, the public health responses in England, Brazil and India were also negatively impacted by political interference.[9–11] An additional potential solution that could help overcome political interference is to reinstitute the PREDICT initiative, which is discussed later on this chapter.

3. Study the relationship between longCOVID and persistent SARS-CoV-2 infection

Chapter 4

1. Topic 3. Persistent SARS-CoV-2 infections occur in a subgroup of patients with normal immune systems (Chapter 4, Case #9 – long haulers), particularly in the gastrointestinal tract, and persisting even longer in humans with compromised immune systems (Chapter 4, Case #7),[12–20] with the associated finding in both cases of ongoing viral evolution (mutation) with resultant new viral variants.[17–20] An important mechanism in this regard is the continuous formation of new viral quasispecies and what factors influence the development of new SARS-CoV-2 variants (Figure 9.81).[21]

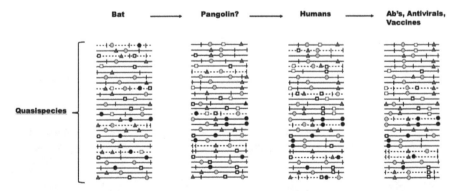

Figure 9.81. Viral quasi-species are an important mechanism for the evolution of new coronavirus species. Once a virus is exposed to a new host, the most-fit quasispecies will become the consensus species for the new host. Further, modifications can occur within the host through the evolutionary pressure provided by the use of viral therapeutics (antibodies, antivirals, vaccines) or by the lack of an immune response, as seen in immunocompromised hosts. This figure was modified from reference 21.

Questions to be addressed:

1. What human genetic and viral factors allow persistent SARS-CoV-2 infection in patients with normal immune systems (long haulers, Chapter 4, Case #9),[12-16] persisting especially in the gastrointestinal tract,[15] and what is the SARS-CoV-2 mutational rate in these patients?

2. In immunocompromised hosts, there seems to be a more rapid rate of SARS-CoV-2 mutation. Could this mean that immunocompromised hosts are the likely source of the new SARS-CoV-2 variants described in Chapter 5?

3. Does the subset of patients with persistent symptoms and an increased risk of blood clots (arterial or venous thrombosis) with resultant increased risk of acute coronary disease, deep venous thrombosis/pulmonary embolus, and/or stroke have identifiable viral genome or human genome characteristics?[14]

Issues and possible solutions:

The US National Institute of Health has set aside $1.15 billion in funding to examine the Post-Acute Sequelae of SARS-CoV-2 infection.[22] It is hoped that the answers to the above questions and others will occur as part of this initiative, and similar initiatives in other countries.

4. Evaluate the relationship between the immune system and 2nd SARS-CoV-2 infections

Topic 4. SARS-CoV-2 reinfection occurs and can be fatal (Chapter 4, Case #4).

Pre-existing antibodies to SARS-CoV-2 do not guarantee protection against a second infection (up to 1/3 can have a second infection).[23] There are increasing numbers of genomically well documented second SARS-CoV-2 infections with a strain of SARS-CoV-2 virus that is distinct from the one causing the first infection.[24-27]

Questions to be addressed:

1. What role does immunity (both antibody and cell-mediated) play in reinfection (Chapter 4, SARS-CoV-2 Mutation/Pathogenesis discussion; Chapter 10, Immunocompetent Adults)?[28,29]
2. What role does viral evolution play in reinfection (Chapter 4, SARS-CoV-2 Mutation/Pathogenesis discussion; Chapter 10, Long-COVID = Persistent Infection, Immunocompromised Patients, SARS-CoV-2 Mutations)?[30–37]
3. What role do human genetic factors play in reinfection (Chapter 4, Case #2 discussion)?[38,39]

Issues and possible solutions:

The Human COVID Genetic Effort is a global consortium that will attempt to determine the human genetic and immunologic basis for the diversity of SARS-CoV-2's clinical course.[22] It is likely that questions related to SARS-CoV-2 reinfection and the importance of the immune system, viral evolution, and human genetics will be looked at by this group.

5. Find ways to decrease global vaccine inequity

Chapter 5

Topic 5. As of mid-2021, there continues to be a severe inequity between vaccine availability in high-income countries and most other countries.

Question to be addressed:

Is there a way to address the vaccine inequity problem going forward?

Issue and possible solutions:

The COVAX facility and program was created to equitably distribute COVID-19 vaccines across the world based on the population size of each country. While almost all countries agreed to participate, when the first wave caused a substantial amount of disease in high-income countries, the governments of many of these countries hoarded vaccine doses. High-income countries that vaccinated most of those who wanted the vaccine are now beginning to send vaccine to countries in need, but this approach is likely to prolong the pandemic, and result in more deaths and economic problems than had vaccine distribution been done equitably initially.[2,3] Despite the creation of COVAX, inequitable distribution is likely to persist for several more years during this and future pandemics, unless additional steps are taken to address this problem.

A patent waiver approach has been proposed as a potential solution to help create an equitable distribution of vaccines and other needed medical products to combat the COVID-19 pandemic. The World Trade Organization (WTO) members have been discussing this proposal since October 2020 when India and South Africa requested the WTO suspend certain intellectual property protections for COVID-19 vaccines, diagnostics and therapeutics.[40,41] Both countries claimed the international patent protections, which were part of the Agreement on Trade-Related Aspects of Intellectual Property Rights (TRIPS), had slowed production of and access to COVID-19 vaccines. As of May 2021, over 100 countries, mostly low and middle-income, and a number of organizations have joined India and South Africa in calling for a waiver of TRIPS for COVID-19 vaccines and related products. Many of the high-income countries and pharmaceutical companies have indicated their opposition to this waiver,[42,43] but US President Biden has indicated his support for the waiver.[44]

Figure 9.82 shows the countries who are either in favor or against waiving patent protections as of May 28, 2021.[45] Those countries and organizations favoring the waiver argue that existing vaccine manufacturing capacities in the developing world remain underutilized because of intellectual property barriers, and hence insufficient amounts of vaccines were being produced to end the pandemic. In their view, the waiver proposal represents an open and expedited global solution to allow uninterrupted collaboration in the production and supply of health products and technologies required for an effective COVID-19 response.[3,45,46] Those arguing against the waiver believe the major barrier to producing greater quantities of vaccine is the manufacturing capacity rather than the patent protection.[42,43] The WTO needs to wrap up the analysis of the pros and cons of waiving TRIPS by determining to what degree the inequitable supply of vaccines is occurring due to patent protections versus inadequate manufacturing capacity. The most likely answer is that solutions to fix both issues are needed, and time is of the essence.

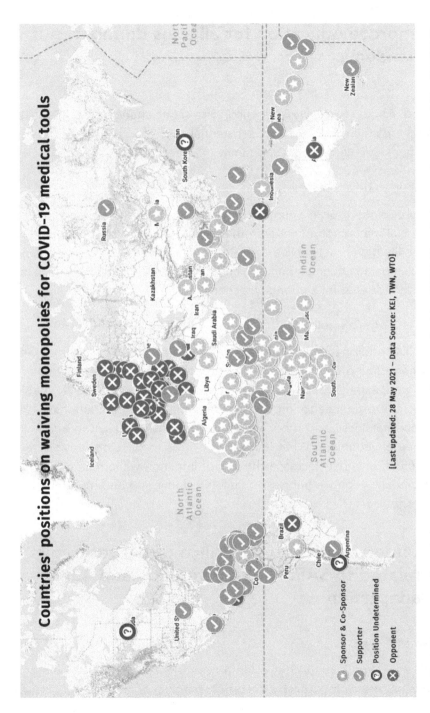

Figure 9.82. A map outlines which countries support or oppose the move of waiving COVID-19 medical patents. Last updated: May 28, 2021.[45]

6. Improve education for all ages during a pandemic

Chapter 6

Topic 6. Finding better ways for children to safely attend school in person during a pandemic that do not substantially increase the risk of disease for other students, teachers and family members.

Question to be addressed:

School closings result in a number of serious limitations to learning and the emotional maturation of children that cannot be fixed by increasing the availability of Internet services. Are there ways children can safely attend school in person during a pandemic that would not substantially increase the risk of disease for students, teachers, and family members?

Issue and possible solutions:

The CDC published a plan in March 2021 to safely send children back to school during the COVID-19 pandemic, but the required mitigation steps were expensive, and only a small percentage of schools were able to find the resources to implement all of the recommendations.[47] It is unlikely that these and other recommendations will result in a COVID risk-free environment. What is needed now is to develop feasible recommendations that decrease the risk of infection while minimizing the substantially negative impact on childhood learning and maturation as well as their families.

7. Understand the importance of bat reservoirs related to SARS-CoV-2 evolution and human adaptation

Chapter 7.

Topic 7. In late 2019, SARS-CoV-2, a novel, RNA coronavirus, emerged from a bat reservoir to quickly become a pandemic.

Bats are increasingly recognized as a unique source of historical and recent EIDs, as shown by the partial listing of RNA viral human pathogens displayed in Table 9.29. Unique features of bats pertinent to the pandemic

Table 9.29. Well known RNA human pathogens with bat reservoirs.

Human Pathogen (*Genus species*)	Human Disease	Virus Type	Molecular Clock Appearance Date	Bat Species Host
SARS-CoV-2 (*Betacoronavirus sarbecovirus*)	Pneumonia	Positive sense, single stranded RNA	~1948 (Chapter 7)	Horseshoe bats (*Rhinolophus pearsoni* and *macrotis*)
SARS-CoV (*Betacoronavirus SARS-CoV*)	Pneumonia	Positive sense, single stranded RNA	~1952 (Chapter 7)	Horseshoe bats (*Rhinolophus sinicus*)
MERS-CoV (*Betacoronavirus MERS-CoV*)	Pneumonia	Positive sense, single stranded RNA	~2010	*Taphozous perforatus, Rhinopoma hardwickii, Pipistrellus kuhlii*
Ebola (*Ebolavirus zaire* and 5 other species)	Hemorrhagic fever	Negative sense, Single-stranded RNA	~1945–1975	Fruit bats: *Hypsignathus monstrosus, Epomops franqueti, Myonycteris torquata*
Marburg (*Marburgvirus*, 1 species, 2 variants: Victoria, Ravn	Hemorrhagic fever	Negative sense, Single-stranded RNA	~1967	Egyptian fruit bat: *Rousettus aegyptiacus*
Nipah (*Henipavirus nipah, Henipavirus hendra*, 3 other species)	Nipah and Hendra: lower respiratory infection, encephalitis	Negative sense, Single-stranded RNA	Nipah ~1998 Hendra ~1994	Fruit bats: Nipah (*Pteropodidae medius*), Hendra (*Pteropodidae alecto*)
Rabies (*Lyssavirus rabies*)	Encephalitis	Negative sense, Single-stranded RNA	888–1459 YA (transitioned from bats to carnivores as primary reservoir)	Many species (insectivorous >> hematophagous > frugivorous)

and other emerging infectious diseases include the following. They are the second most common animal species globally, after rodents. As part of global warming, the number of bat and rodent species has increased, whereas many other animal species have declined.[48–50] The number of viral species per bat species is greater than that seen per rodent species, and the likelihood of viral transmission between bat species was 3.9 times greater than between rodent species.[51,52] Different bat species have different coronavirus species, demonstrating evolutionary adaptation to the bat host.[53] In spite of these many unique bat characteristics relevant to EIDs, it has been suggested by one large study looking at virus-reservoir relationships that bats are not uniquely related to emerging infectious diseases and simply transmit a lot of viruses because there are so many bat species.[54] However, and perhaps most remarkably, in the last 20 years, there have been two global coronavirus epidemics originating from bats (SARS, MERS) and one coronavirus pandemic originating from bats (COVID-19), and no similar global events attributable to rodents or other animals.

A recent study by the PREDICT Consortium, a USAID Emerging Pandemic Threat initiative, investigated in 20 countries perceived to be EID hotspots the likelihood that bats, rodents and shrews, and nonhuman primates would have identifiable coronavirus RNA.[53] Strikingly, 8.6% of bats were positive for coronavirus versus 0.2% of rodents or nonhuman primates. Among the 1,065 bats found positive for coronavirus, they found 91 distinct coronavirus species and that global diversity and the distribution of coronaviruses were nonrandom. They mathematically predicted that there would be at least 3,204 coronavirus species in the world's bat population. The dominant evolutionary mechanisms driving this diversity were host switching (evolutionary adaptation of a microorganism to a new host) and co-speciation (microorganism causes the host to evolve to a new species). These findings strongly suggest bats are unique in their ability to start zoonotic epidemics and/or pandemics, and we need to understand why.

Question to be addressed:

Is co-evolution of SARS-CoV, MERS-CoV and SARS-CoV-2 with their bat hosts (Table 9.29) the likely explanation for the ability of these coronaviruses to cause human disease?[52,54,55] Does this involve viral quasispecies shifting toward a new consensus species (Figure 9.83)?[21]

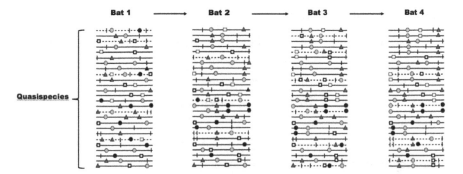

Figure 9.83. Viral quasi-species are an important mechanism for the evolution of new coronavirus species. Once a virus is exposed to a new host, the most-fit quasispecies will become the consensus species for the new host. Thus, when a coronavirus is exposed to a new bat species, there is the ability for a new coronavirus consensus species to develop. This figure was modified from reference 21.

Issue and possible solutions:

It seems promising that a comparison of genomes from bats where the above viruses reside versus control bat genomes (not infected by these three organisms) should lead to a better understanding of how these three important coronaviruses are successful pathogens in humans.[56–63]

Question to be addressed:

Are the human tissue tropisms and disease pathogenesis of other bat-derived human RNA virus pathogens, such as Ebola, Marburg, Nipah and Hendra (Table 9.29), also a product of virus/bat co-evolution?

Issue and possible solutions:

Comparing bat genomic data (from bats colonized with these pathogens versus a control group) with viral genomic data (pathogens versus non pathogens) should help provide a much better understanding of the different human tissue tropisms exhibited by these viruses and how this relates to viral persistence in bats.[64–70]

Question to be addressed:

Can developing a bat model of coronavirus infection help answer some of the virus human pathogenesis questions?

Issues and possible solutions:

1. Bat models of virus infection should allow a better understanding of the natural history of coronavirus infection, the duration of viral persistence, and the likelihood of *in vivo* evolution.

2. Bat models should facilitate studying how co-evolution affects viral human tissue tropisms.

3. By adding a second species of coronavirus to each bat model, it should be possible to explore whether *in vivo* evolution is more likely to occur in the presence of a second virus and how likely are the two coronavirus strains to exchange RNA.

Question to be addressed:

Why does the bat ecological research community not interact significantly with the human infectious disease-focused community?[72]

Issue and possible solutions:

Given the recent importance of bats in SARS, MERS and COVID-19, it should be quite possible to organize scientific meetings to bring these two communities together to facilitate collaboration to better approach some of the questions noted above and a myriad of other important questions that were not mentioned.

8. Investigate the reasons for the asymptotic increase in global epidemic/pandemic infectious diseases

Chapter 8

Topic 8. The frequency of historically important emerging infectious diseases is increasing at a near logarithmic rate and the SARS-CoV-2 pandemic is just a piece of this much larger puzzle (Chapter 7, Figure 7.70; Chapter 8, Figure 8.80).

With each passing year of the 21st century, our understanding of what causes epidemics and pandemics has exploded. Related to the COVID pandemic, there were over 200,000 scientific publications in 2020.[73] This represented a greater than 90% increase over the previous year, with 6% of all health and medicine titles indexed in PubMed being COVID-19-related.[73] This unprecedented increase in scientific knowledge bodes well for the future, but unfortunately, as noted previously, politics frequently gets in the way of science. China tried to suppress all early information related to its Wuhan investigation, but some leaked out, including warnings from various individuals, particularly the physician Li Wenliang.[74,75] Russia cut corners in their efforts to develop a COVID-19 vaccine, delayed the release of data on their vaccine, and when the vaccine data was finally released, the Russian population did not participate well in getting the vaccine, and Brazil refused to accept the Russian vaccine they had ordered until further testing was done.[76] In the US, President Trump subjected his scientific advisors to gag orders preventing them from speaking freely about COVID-19.[77] Globally, it has become clear that we presently lack the political will to be transparent and rise above nationalism.[78]

Question to be addressed:

Can we decrease the rate of emerging infectious diseases occurring globally, and how might that be accomplished?

Issues and possible solutions:

1. A global pandemic treaty has been proposed by the European Council and the WHO Director-General.[79] In this publication, they argue that, "with the proposal for a global pandemic treaty by the European Council, endorsed by more than 25 heads of state and the WHO Director-General, the question has arisen as to what such a treaty should do. We argue that it should focus on reducing the risk of pathogens jumping from animals to humans".

2. The scientific approach that might form the core of such a global pandemic treaty has already been proposed as a multi-country,

multi-continent, global collaboration, such as the PREDICT Initiative discussed in Topic 7 above, which could be expanded to look for all conceivable EIDs, utilizing target surveillance, new mathematical modeling, diagnostics, communications, and informatics technologies to identify and report EIDs in real-time, as well as assist with the identification of what strategies might be effective at controlling them.[80] The PREDICT Initiative started in 2009 and continued until March 2020 when the program was ended by the Trump administration, again demonstrating political interference with the science that is needed to help protect humanity. We must come together globally to understand and manage the increasing threat of emerging infectious diseases before it is too late.

9. Learn from all countries how best to handle future pandemics (investigation, early mitigation, global treatment trials, vaccine development and deployment)

Topic 9. Some Potential Future Pandemic Management Steps to Consider

Phase 1:   The Investigation

1. Determine that you have an outbreak.
2. Determine that it has spread regionally, internationally (i.e., become a pandemic), and notify the world as soon as possible. This should be done using the WHO and other international resources.
3. Determine the causative organism's epidemiologic characteristics:
    a. Determine its route of transmission: airborne, vector or other
    b. Calculate the organisms R_0
4. Isolate the organism.
5. Identify and sequence the organism's genome.

Phase 2:   Early Interventions (Assuming Airborne)
1. Early interventions attempt to slow the pandemic (flatten the curve) until more definitive interventions become available (see R&D below).

2. Initiate containment interventions:
   a. Educate the public without political overtones
   b. A pre-pandemic essential services plan needs to be in place before stay-at-home orders are issued.
   c. Cancellation of nonessential meetings
   d. Travel restrictions, especially air travel
3. Initiate transmission interventions based on the known route of transmission:
   a. Restrict nonessential person-to-person interactions
   b. A large stockpile of masks needs to exist prior to making mask wearing mandatory for essential person-to-person interactions, so that supply is adequate until mask production is ramped up.
   c. Eye protection, if transmission data supports
   d. If mortality is very high, martial law may become necessary

Phase 3:   R&D
1. Arrange multinational collaborations to accelerate disease understandings.
2. Determine disease pathogenesis.
3. Based on disease pathogenesis, initiate treatment trials and new drug development.
4. Based on disease pathogenesis, initiate vaccine development efforts.
5. Make all findings available globally and instantaneously.

Phase 4:   Global Vaccination
1. Focus vaccination efforts globally in areas of highest disease mortality and ensure equitable distribution.
2. Prioritize further based on identified epidemiologic risk factors.
3. If one dose of vaccine gives adequate protection against severe disease, then give one dose to all before a second dose is given. Otherwise give two doses to each person, before trying to vaccinate everyone.

References

1. Independent Oversight and Advisory Committee for the WHO Health Emergencies Programme. (2020) Interim report on WHO's response to COVID-19 January–April 2020. World Health Organization, May 12. https://www.who.int/publications/m/item/interim-report-on-who-s-response-to-covid---january---april-2020

2. Independent Panel for Pandemic Preparedness & Response. (2021) Second report on progress. https://theindependentpanel.org/wp-content/uploads/2021/01/Independent-Panel_Second-Report-on-Progress_Final-15-Jan-2021.pdf

3. Independent Panel for Pandemic Preparedness & Response. (2021) COVID-19: Make it the last pandemic. May. https://theindependentpanel.org/wp-content/uploads/2021/05/COVID-19-Make-it-the-Last-Pandemic_final.pdf

4. Wang C. (2020) Trump threatens to permanently cut off WHO funding, withdraw U.S. membership. CNBC, May 18. https://www.cnbc.com/2020/05/19/trump-threatens-to-permanently-cut-off-who-funding-withdraw-us-membership.html

5. The New York Times. (2020) A letter from more than 1,000 current and former "disease detectives" decries the politicization of the CDC. NY Times Coronavirus Briefing, October 16.

6. Salwa J, Roberston C. (2021) Designing an Independent public health agency. *New England Journal of Medicine* **384**:1684–1687. DOI:10.1056/NEJMp2033970

7. Conti-Brown P. (2019) What happens if Trump tries to fire Fed chair Jerome Powell? The Brookings Institution, September 9. https://www.brookings.edu/blog/up-front/2019/09/09/what-happens-if-trump-tries-to-fire-fed-chair-jerome-powell/

8. Levin B. (2020) The White House threatens to fire FDA Chief if he doesn't approve the Pfizer vaccine today. *Vanity Fair*, December 11. https://www.vanityfair.com/news/2020/12/white-house-stephen-hahn-vaccine-threat

9. Savarese M. (2020) Brazil's Bolsonaro rejects COVID-19 shot, calls masks taboo. *ABC News*, November 27. https://abcnews.go.com/International/wireStory/brazils-bolsonaro-rejects-covid-19-shot-calls-masks-74428885

10. VOA. (2020) British Prime Minister takes responsibility for COVID-19 response. *VOA News*, July 8. https://www.voanews.com/covid-19-pandemic/british-prime-minister-takes-responsibility-covid-19-response

11. Gettleman J, Scjmall E, Mashal M. (2021) India cuts back on vaccine exports as infections surge at home. *NY Times*, April 22. https://www.nytimes.com/2021/03/25/world/asia/india-covid-vaccine-astrazeneca.html

12. Huang C, Huang L, Wang Y, *et al.* (2021) 6-month consequences of COVID-19 in patients discharged from hospital: A cohort study. *Lancet* **397**(10270):220–232. DOI:10.1016/S0140-6736(20)32656-8

13. Logue JK, Franko NM, McCulloch DJ, *et al.* (2021) Sequelae in adults at 6 months after COVID-19 infection. *JAMA* 4(2):e210830. DOI:10.1001/jamanetworkopen.2021.0830

14. Al-Aly Z, Xie Y, Bowe B. (2021) High-dimensional characterization of post-acute sequalae of COVID-19. *Nature* **594**:259–264. https://doi.org/10.1038/s41586-021-03553-9

15. Hu F, Chen F, Ou Z, *et al.* (2020) A compromised specific humoral immune response against the SARS-CoV-2 receptor-binding domain is related to viral persistence and periodic shedding in the gastrointestinal tract. *Cellular & Molecular Immunology* **17**:1119–1125. https://doi.org/10.1038/s41423-020-00550-2

16. Rodriguez-Grande C, Adan-Jimenez J, Catalan P, *et al.* (2021) Inference of active viral replication in cases with sustained positive reverse transcription-PCR results for SARS-CoV-2. *Journal of Clinical Microbiology* **59**(2):e02277-20. DOI:10.1128/JCM.02277-20

17. Kemp SA, Collier DA, Datir RP, *et al.* (2021) SARS-CoV-2 evolution during treatment of chronic infection. *Nature* **592**:277–282. https://doi.org/10.1038/s41586-021-03291-y

18. Choi B, Choudhary MC, Regan J, *et al.* (2020) Persistence and evolution of SARS-CoV-2 in an immunocompromised host. *New England Journal of Medicine* **383**:2291–2293.

19. Avanzato VA, Matson MJ, Seifert SN, *et al.* (2020) Case study: Prolonged infectious SARS-CoV-2 shedding from an asymptomatic immunocompromised cancer patient. *Cell* **183**:1901–1912.

20. Karim F, Moosa MYS, Gosnell BI, *et al.* (2021) Persistent SARS-CoV2 infection and intra-host evolution in association with advanced HIV infection. *medRxiv.* https://doi.org/10.1101/2021.06.03.21258228

21. Domingo E, Perales C (2019) Viral quasispecies. *PLOS Genetics* **15**(10):e1008271. https://doi.org/10.1371/journal.pgen.1008271

22. Marx V. (2021) Scientists set out to connect the dots on long COVID. *Nature Methods* **18**:449–453.

23. Hall V, Foulkes S, Charlett A, *et al.* (2020) Do antibody positive healthcare workers have lower SARS-CoV-2 infection rates than antibody negative healthcare workers? Large multi-centre prospective cohort study (the SIREN study), England: June to November. *medRxiv.* https://doi.org/10.1101/2021.01.13.21249642

24. To KKW, Hung IF-N, Ip JD, *et al.* (2020) COVID-19 re-infection by a phylogenetically distinct SARS-coronavirus-2 strain confirmed by whole genome sequencing. *Clinical Infectious Diseases* **73**(9):e2946–e2951. https://doi.org/10.1093/cid/ciaa1275

25. Prado-Vivar B, Becerra-Wong M, Guadalupe JJ, *et al.* (2020) COVID-19 re-infection by a phylogenetically distinct SARS-CoV-2 variant, first confirmed event in South America. https://papers.ssrn.com/sol3/papers.cfm?abstract_id=3686174

26. Tillett R, Sevinsky J, Hartleyet P, *et al.* (2020) Genomic evidence for a case of reinfection with SARS-CoV-2. *SSRN.* https://doi.org/10.2139/ssrn.3680955

27. Gupta V, Bhoyar RC, Jain A, *et al.* (2020) Asymptomatic reinfection in two healthcare workers from India with genetically distinct SARS-CoV-2. *Clinical Infectious Diseases* 73(9):e2823–e2825. DOI:10.1093/cid/ciaa1451

28. Ibarrondo FJ, Fulcher JA, Goodman-Meza D, *et al.* (2020) Rapid decay of anti-SARS-CoV-2 antibodies in persons with mild COVID-19. *New England Journal of Medicine* **383**(11):1085–1087. https://www.nejm.org/doi/full/10.1056/nejmc2025179

29. Huang AT, Garcia-Carreras B, Hitchings MDT, *et al.* (2020) A systematic review of antibody mediated immunity to coronaviruses: Antibody kinetics, correlates of protection, and association of antibody responses with severity of disease. *Nature Communications* **11**,4. https://doi.org/10.1101/2020.04.14.20065771

30. CDC. (2021) Science brief: Emerging SARS-CoV-2 variants. Centers for Disease Control and Prevention, January 28. https://www.cdc.gov/coronavirus/2019-ncov/more/science-and-research/scientific-brief-emerging-variants.html

31. Tseng A, Seiler J, Issema R, *et al.* (2021) Summary of SARS-CoV-2 novel variants. Washington State Department of Health, Alliance for Pandemic Preparedness: University of Washington, Start Center. February 5.

32. Davies NG, Abbott S, Barnard RC, *et al.* (2021) Estimated transmissibility and impact of SARS-CoV-2 lineage B.1.1.7 in England. *Science* **372**(6538):eabg3055. DOI:10.1126/science.abg3055

33. Tegally H, Wilkinson E, Giovanetti M, *et al.* (2020) Emergence and rapid spread of a new severe acute respiratory syndrome-related coronavirus 2 (SARS-CoV-2) lineage with multiple spike mutations in South Africa. *medRxiv.* https://www.medrxiv.org/content/10.1101/2020.12.21.20248640v1

34. Faria NR, Mellan TA, Whittaker C, *et al.* (2021) Genomics and epidemiology of a novel SARS-CoV-2 lineage in Manaus, Brazil. Science. https://www.science.org/doi/10.1126/science.abh2644

35. Wang P, Nair MS, Liu L, *et al.* (2021) Antibody Resistance of SARS-CoV-2 Variants B.1.351 and B.1.1.7. *Nature* **593**:130–135. https://doi.org/10.1038/s41586-021-03398-2

36. Cele S, Gazy I, Jackson L, *et al*. (2021) Escape of SARS-CoV-2 401 Y.V2 variants from neutralization by convalescent plasma. *medRxiv*. https://www.medrxiv.org/content/10.1101/2021.01.26.21250224v1

37. Chen RE, Zhang X, Case JB, *et al*. (2021) Resistance of SARS-CoV-2 variants to neutralization by monoclonal and serum-derived polyclonal antibodies. *Nature Medicine* **27**(4):717–726. https://doi.org/10.1038/s41591-021-01294-w

38. The Severe Covid-19 GWAS Group. (2020) Genomewide association study of severe Covid-19 with respiratory failure. *New England Journal of Medicine* **383**:1522–1534. DOI:10.1056/NEJMoa2020283

39. Pairo-Castineira E, Clohisey S, Klaric L, *et al*. (2020) Genetic mechanisms of critical illness in Covid-19. *Nature* **591**:92–98. https://doi.org/10.1038/s41586-020-03065-y

40. WTO. (2021) Members discuss TRIPS waiver, LDC transition period and green tech role for small business. World Trade Organization, March 11. https://www.wto.org/english/news_e/news21_e/trip_11mar21_e.htm

41. Ravelo JL. (2021) Winnie Byanyima asks World Bank to "align with us" and support the TRIPS waiver. Devex, March 30. https://www.devex.com/news/winnie-byanyima-asks-world-bank-to-align-with-us-and-support-the-tripswaiver-99523

42. Lee T, Holt C. (2021) Intellectual Property, COVID-19 Vaccines, and the Proposed TRIPS Waiver. American Action Forum, May 10. https://www.americanactionforum.org/insight/intellectual-property-covid-19-vaccines-and-the-proposed-trips-waiver/

43. PhRMA. (2021) PhRMA statement on WTO TRIPS intellectual property waiver. Press Release, Pharmaceutical Research and Manufacturers of America, May 5. https://www.phrma.org/en/Press-Release/PhRMA-Statement-on-WTO-TRIPS-Intellectual-Property-Waiver

44. Widakuswara P. (2021) Biden agrees to waive COVID-19 vaccine patents, but it's still complicated. *VOA News*, May 5. https://www.voanews.com/covid-19-pandemic/biden-agrees-waive-covid-19-vaccine-patents-its-still-complicated

45. MSF. (2021) Countries obstructing COVID-19 patent waiver must allow negotiations to start. Press Release, Medecins Sans Frontières, March 9. https://www.msf.org/countries-obstructing-covid-19-patent-waiver-must-allow-negotiations

46. MSF. (nd) WTO COVID-19 TRIPS waiver proposal Myths, realities and an opportunity for governments to protect access to lifesaving medical tools in a pandemic. Medecins Sans Frontières. https://msfaccess.org/wto-covid-19-trips-waiver-proposal-myths-realities-and-opportunity-governmentsprotect-access

47. Rice KL, Miller GF, Coronado F, Meltzer MI. (2020) Estimated resource costs for implementation of CDC's Recommended COVID-19 mitigation strategies in pre-kindergarten through grade 12 public schools — United States, 2020–21 school year. *Morbidity and Mortality Weekly Report*. https://www.cdc.gov/mmwr/volumes/69/wr/pdfs/mm6950e1-H.pdf

48. Beyer RM, Manica A, Mora C. (2021) Shifts in global bat diversity suggest a possible role of climate change in the emergence of SARS-CoV-1 and SARS-CoV- 2. *Science of the Total Environment* **767**:145413. https://doi.org/10.1016/j.scitotenv.2021.145413

49. Jiang G, Liu J, Xu L, *et al.* (2013) Climate warming increases biodiversity of small rodents by favoring rare or less abundant species in a grassland ecosystem. *Integrative Zoology* **8**(2):162–174. DOI:10.1111/1749-4877.12027

50. Root, TL, Price JT, Hall KR, *et al.* (2003) Fingerprints of global warming on wild animals and plants. *Nature* **421**:57–60.

51. Luis AD, Hayman DTS, O'Shea TJ, *et al.* (2013) A comparison of bats and rodents as reservoirs of zoonotic viruses: are bats special? *Proceedings of the Royal Society B* **280**:20122753. http://dx.doi.org/10.1098/rspb.2012.2753

52. Olival KJ, Hosseini PR, Zambrana-Torrelio C, *et al.* (2017) Host and viral traits predict zoonotic spillover from mammals. *Nature* **546**:646.

53. Anthony SJ, Johnson CK; PREDICT Consortium, *et al.* (2017) Global patterns in coronavirus diversity. *Virus Evolution* **3**(1):vex012. DOI:10.1093/ve/vex012

54. Mollentze N, Streicker DG. (2020) Viral zoonotic risk is homogenous among taxonomic orders of mammalian and avian reservoir hosts. *Proceedings of the National Academy of Sciences of the United States of America* **117**(17):9423–9430. DOI:10.1073/pnas.1919176117

55. Maldonado LL, Bertelli AM, Kamenetzky L. (2021) Molecular features similarities between SARS-CoV-2, SARS, MERS and key human genes could favor the viral infections and trigger collateral effects. *Scientific Reports* **11**:4108. https://doi.org/10.1038/s41598-021-83595-1

56. Cui J, Han N, Streicker D, *et al.* (2007) Evolutionary relationships between bat coronaviruses and their hosts. *Emerging Infectious Diseases* **13**(10):1526–1532. DOI:10.3201/eid1310.070448

57. Guo H, Hu BJ, Yang XL, *et al.* (2020) Evolutionary arms race between virus and host drives genetic diversity in bat severe acute respiratory syndrome-related coronavirus spike genes. *Journal of Virology* **94**(20):e00902-20. DOI:10.1128/JVI.00902-20

58. MacLean OA, Lytras S, Weaver S, *et al.* (2021) Natural selection in the evolution of SARS-CoV-2 in bats created a generalist virus and highly capable human pathogen. *PLOS Biology*, March 12. https://doi.org/10.1371/journal.pbio.3001115

59. Liu K, Tan S, Niu S, *et al.* (2021) Cross-species recognition of SARS-CoV-2 to bat ACE2. *Proceedings of the National Academy of Sciences* **118**(1):e2020216118. https://doi.org/10.1073/pnas.2020216118

60. El-Sayed A, Kamel M. (2021) Coronaviruses in humans and animals: the role of bats in viral evolution. *Environmental Science and Pollution Research* **28**(16):19589–19600. https://doi.org/10.1007/s11356-021-12553-1

61. Campos FS, Lourenco-de-Moraes R. (2020) Ecological fever: The evolutionary history of coronavirus in human-wildlife relationships. *Frontiers in Ecology and Evolution*, October 15. https://doi.org/10.3389/fevo.2020.575286

62. Zhu Z, Lian X, Su X, *et al.* (2020) From SARS and MERS to COVID-19: A brief summary and comparison of severe acute respiratory infections caused by three highly pathogenic human coronaviruses. *Respiratory Research* 21, 224. https://doi.org/10.1186/s12931-020-01479-w

63. Cui J, Li F, Shi ZL. (2019) Origin and evolution of pathogenic coronaviruses. *Nature Reviews Microbiology* **17**:181–192. https://doi.org/10.1038/s41579-018-0118-9

64. Subudhi S, Rapin N, Misra V. (2019) Immune system modulation and viral persistence in bats: Understanding viral spillover. *Viruses* **11**(2):192. DOI:10.3390/v11020192

65. Sohayati AR, Hassan L, Sharifah SH, *et al.* (2011) Evidence for Nipah virus recrudescence and serological patterns of captive Pteropus vampyrus. *Epidemiology and Infection* **139**(10):1570–1579. DOI:10.1017/S0950268811000550

66. Amman BR, Jones ME, Sealy TK, *et al.* (2015) Oral shedding of Marburg virus in experimentally infected Egyptian fruit bats (Rousettus aegyptiacus). *Journal of Wildlife Diseases* **51**(1):113–124. DOI:10.7589/2014-08-198

67. Schuh A, Amman B, Jones M, *et al.* (2017) Modelling filovirus maintenance in nature by experimental transmission of Marburg virus between Egyptian rousette bats. *Nature Communications* **8**:14446. https://doi.org/10.1038/ncomms14446

68. Subudhi S, Rapin N, Bollinger TK, *et al.* (2017) A persistently infecting coronavirus in hibernating Myotis lucifugus, the North American little brown bat. *Journal of General Virology* **98**(9):2297–2309. DOI:10.1099/jgv.0.000898

69. Jeong J, Smith C, Peel A, *et al.* (2017) Persistent infections support maintenance of a coronavirus in a population of Australian bats (Myotis

macropus). *Epidemiology and Infection* **145**(10):2053–2061. DOI:10.1017/ S0950268817000991

70. Banerjee A, Subudhi S, Rapin N, *et al.* (2020) Selection of viral variants during persistent infection of insectivorous bat cells with Middle East respiratory syndrome coronavirus. *Scientific Reports* **10**, 7257. https://doi.org/10.1038/ s41598-020-64264-1

71. Afelt A, Devaux C, Serra-Cobo J, Frutos R. (2018) *Bats, Bat-Borne Viruses, and Environmental Changes.* https://www.intechopen.com/books/bats/ bats-bat-borne-viruses-and-environmental-changes

72. Kading RC, Kingston T. (2020) Common ground: The foundation of interdisciplinary research on bat disease emergence. *PLOS Biology*, November 9. https://doi.org/10.1371/journal.pbio.3000947

73. Else H. (2020) How a torrent of COVID science changed research publishing — in seven charts. *Nature*, December 16. https://www.nature.com/articles/ d41586-020-03564-y

74. Wade N. (2021) The origin of COVID: Did people or nature open Pandora's box at Wuhan? *Bulletin of the Atomic Scientists*, May 5. https://thebulletin. org/2021/05/the-origin-of-covid-did-people-or-nature-open-pandoras-box- at-wuhan/

75. BBC. (2021) Li Wenliang: 'Wuhan whistleblower' remembered one year on. *BBC News.* https://www.bbc.com/news/world-asia-55963896

76. Moutinho S, Wadman M. (2021) Is Russia's COVID-19 vaccine safe? Brazil's veto of Sputnik V sparks lawsuit threat and confusion. *Science*, April 30. https://www.sciencemag.org/news/2021/04/russias-covid-19-vaccine-safe- brazils-veto-sputnik-v-sparks-lawsuit-threat-and

77. Woodward A. (2020) Trump barred a top health expert from speaking freely about the coronavirus. Its one of many ways the administration has muzzled scientists. *Insider*, February 28. https://www.businessinsider.com/ trump-gags-top-us-coronavirus-official-history-censoring-science-2020-2

78. Bieber F. (2020) Global nationalism in times of the COVID-19 pandemic. *Nationalities Papers* **50**(1):13–25. DOI:10.1017/nps.2020.35

79. Vinuales J, Moon S, Le Moli G, Burci G-L. (2021) A global pandemic treaty should aim for deep prevention. *Lancet* **397**(10287):1791–1792. https:// DOI:10.1016/S0140-6736(21)00948-X

80. Morse SS, Mazet JAK, Woolhouse M, Parrish CR. (2012) Prediction and prevention of the next pandemic zoonosis. *Lancet* **380**:1956–1965. https://doi. org/10.1016/S0140-6736(12)61684-5

10 Epilogue

"It's impossible to predict what will happen next in the pandemic."

Michael Osterholm,
Center for Infectious Disease Research and Policy,
Minneapolis Star Tribune, May 6, 2022

Contents

1. COVID-19 Pandemic Continues
   a. Endemic disease is likely
   b. Excess mortality
2. COVID-19 Vaccines
   a. Global availability
   b. Impact of SARS-CoV-2 variants
3. Collateral Damage
   a. Economic impact
   b. Other (non-COVID vaccines) vaccination programs
   c. Tuberculosis, HIV, and malaria control and mortality
4. COVID-19 Clinical Updates
   a. Immunocompetent adults
   b. Long-COVID = Persistent infection
   c. Immunocompromised patients
   d. Treatment effectiveness
5. SARS-CoV-2 Mutations
6. SARS-CoV-2 Origin: Revisited

The first nine chapters of this book focus on the first two years of the COVID-19 pandemic (2020–2021). The Epilogue highlights some of the major events and activities that occurred during the first half of 2022.

1. COVID-19 Pandemic Continues

The number of COVID-19 cases and deaths worldwide exceeded 500,000,000 and 6,000,000, respectively, by the end of June 2022,[1-2] and the actual number of cases and deaths is greater than reported. The number of cases continues to rapidly increase and is further underestimated by the recent availability of home testing, where the results are often not reported.[3] The WHO estimates the number of deaths is likely 30–50% higher since the pandemic started.[4] The number of daily deaths has started to level off in 2022 (Figure 10.84). This is due in large part to improvements in treating patients and the increasing availability of vaccines (Figure 10.85).[5]

Early on during the pandemic, there was hope that SARS-CoV-2 could be eradicated (i.e., the disappearance of SARS-CoV-2 worldwide)

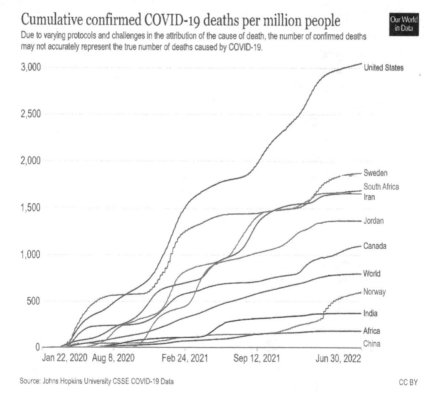

Cumulative confirmed COVID-19 deaths per million people

Due to varying protocols and challenges in the attribution of the cause of death, the number of confirmed deaths may not accurately represent the true number of deaths caused by COVID-19.

Source: Johns Hopkins University CSSE COVID-19 Data

CC BY

Figure 10.84. Cumulative COVID-19 deaths per million population from January 22, 2020 to June 30, 2022, in the world and the nine countries highlighted in Chapters 2 and 3.[2]

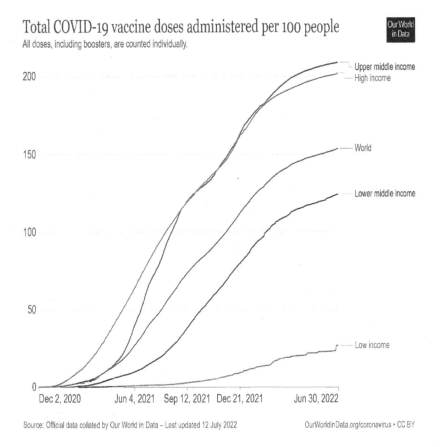

Total COVID-19 vaccine doses administered per 100 people

All doses, including boosters, are counted individually.

Source: Official data collated by Our World in Data – Last updated 12 July 2022   OurWorldInData.org/coronavirus • CC BY

Figure 10.85. COVID-19 vaccine doses administered per 100 people as of June 3, 2022.[5]

or eliminated (i.e., a very low incidence of disease worldwide), similar to what occurred with its close relative, SARS-CoV-1. However, at the end of June 2022, the COVID-19 pandemic is still ongoing, with new waves of SARS-CoV-2 in various locations across the world. This is even true of the five countries (China, Hong Kong, Singapore, Australia, and New Zealand) that had specific eradication or elimination goals. These countries achieved transient success in eliminating COVID-19 cases during 2020. However, in 2021, COVID-19 outbreaks reappeared.[6] For example, in October 2021, China experienced its largest and most widespread outbreak (over 500 cases and 19 of 31 provinces had one or more cases) of COVID-19.[7] This outbreak occurred despite China's very strict "zero-COVID" elimination policy that included quarantining infected people, their contacts, and the contacts of the contacts. In 2022, China had additional large outbreaks in Beijing and Shanghai.[8]

Factors that make eradication or elimination of SARS-CoV-2 unlikely include the limitations of the present COVID-19 vaccines and the continuing emergence of new variants. The currently available vaccines can prevent most cases of severe disease, but are less capable of preventing transmission of SARS-CoV-2 between people.[9–14] Additionally, the continuing limited availability of vaccines in some low-income countries (Figure 10.85),[2,15] the refusal of a substantial percentage of the world's population to receive COVID-19 vaccines,[16] and the inability of immunocompromised people to adequately respond to vaccines[17] lessen the potential impact that vaccines could have in ending the pandemic.

a. Endemic disease is likely

The ongoing occurrence of new SARS-CoV-2 variants also makes it more likely that endemic disease will occur once the COVID-19 pandemic ends.[18] A number of SARS-CoV-2 variant strains (e.g., Alpha, Beta, Gamma, Delta, Epsilon, Eta, Iota, Kappa, Mu, Zeta, Omicron, etc.) evolved since the pandemic began. The Delta variant was predominant across the globe for most of 2021, and research suggested that changes to the spike protein caused the Delta variant to be ~50% more transmissible than previous COVID-19 variants.[19–21] There was initial concern that the Delta variant was causing more severe illness than previous variants; however, most studies suggested that this was not the case.[20] The Omicron variant was initially identified in November 2021. During the past eight months, there has been further evolution of the Omicron variant with resultant subvariants (e.g., Omicron: B.1.1.529, BA.1, BA.1.1, BA.2, BA.3, BA.4, and BA.5).[21] Each of these Omicron variants have substantially higher transmission rates than the Delta variant, and the most recent Omicron variant, BA.5, is the most transmissible of all of them. Current data suggest Omicron variants cause less severe disease.[21] The Omicron variants are also better able to escape immunity induced by COVID-19 vaccines and/or immunity induced by infections with previous SARS-CoV-2 variants. The increased transmissibility and greater ability to escape the immune response has led to large surges in cases and significant stress on the healthcare systems in many countries (see "Impact of SARS-CoV-2 Variants" below).

The continuing emergence of new SARS-CoV-2 variants makes it very difficult to predict when the COVID-19 pandemic will end, but at some point, SARS-CoV-2 is very likely to become an endemic disease. While it is possible that endemic COVID will be similar to endemic influenza with a seasonal pattern in non-tropical countries; to date, there is little evidence that SARS-CoV-2 has a seasonal pattern. Indeed, some of the largest COVID-19 waves have occurred in temperate regions in the summer, including the most recent one due to BA.4 and BA.5.

b. Excess mortality

The term excess mortality quantifies the deaths due to the direct and indirect impact of the COVID-19 pandemic (Chapter 6 examines excess deaths through 2020 and this section updates this information through 2021). COVID-19 excess mortality is determined by examining the number of total deaths in 2019 versus 2020 and 2021. The WHO reported an excess mortality of ~14.9 million deaths (range 13.3 million to 16.6 million) for the period between January 1, 2020, and December 31, 2021.[22] This estimate includes the following: (1) reported deaths due to COVID-19, (2) an estimate of unreported deaths due to COVID-19, and (3) deaths associated with the wider impact of the pandemic on health systems (e.g., people delaying care for various health conditions) and society (e.g., disruption of essential services and supplies). The excess mortality exceeded the reported deaths at the end of 2021 by approximately 3-fold.[23]

2. COVID-19 Vaccines

a. Global availability

With the announcement in early 2020 that many pharmaceutical companies were trying to develop SARS-CoV-2 vaccines, there was hope that vaccines might be the solution to ending the pandemic. Four vaccines obtained emergency use approval in December 2020 (two mRNA vaccines developed by Pfizer-BioNTech and Moderna-NIH, and two viral vector vaccines developed by AstraZeneca-Oxford and the Gamaleya Institute, see Chapter 5). Since that time, additional COVID-19 vaccines also received Emergency Use Approval. Subsequently, most of these vaccines obtained full regulatory approval, and over 12 billion vaccine doses have been administered globally as of June 2022.[15]

The COVAX program was created in 2020 to try to ensure that low- and lower-middle-income countries would have equitable access to COVID-19 vaccines (Chapters 2 and 3). Since then, more than 70% of the vaccines shipped to low-income countries have come from the COVAX facility. However, insufficient quantities of vaccines were available to meet the global demand in 2021. This resulted in huge inequities in the distribution of vaccines between high- and upper-middle-income countries compared to low- and lower-middle-income countries (Figure 10.85).[5] Low-income countries had only vaccinated ~5% of their populations (at least one dose) by the end of 2021, despite having 52% of the world's population.[24] COVAX did not meet its goal of delivering 2.2 billion doses of vaccines to participating countries by the end of January 2022, nor its global target to vaccinate 70% of people by mid-2022. In response to these problems, COVAX changed its strategy to focus specifically on low-income countries.[25]

Some special populations were not included in the initial COVID-19 vaccine studies; therefore, recommendations were not initially available for them. For example, despite the increased risk of COVID-19 in pregnant women and their babies,[26,27] many countries did not recommend the vaccine or have not made any recommendations regarding their use (Figure 10.86),[28] and the majority of pregnant women are still not getting the vaccines.[29] Children also were not included in the initial COVID-19 vaccine trials. However, Pfizer and Moderna have now completed studies of their COVID vaccines in children greater than 6 months of age, and these vaccines are now approved for Emergency Use Authorization (EUA) by the Food and Drug Administration (FDA) and European Medicines Agency (EMA).[30]

b. Impact of SARS-CoV-2 variants

Defining a correlate of immune protection against SARS-CoV-2 disease continues to be an area of intense research. High serum levels of neutralizing antibodies correlate with protection against infection, severe disease, and death, but these antibodies decrease over months to a level where infection with SARS-CoV-2 can occur (Chapters 4, 5). Conversely, low or undetectable antibody levels, such as those associated with rituximab therapy (depletes B-lymphocytes by binding to the CD20 transmembrane surface protein), are

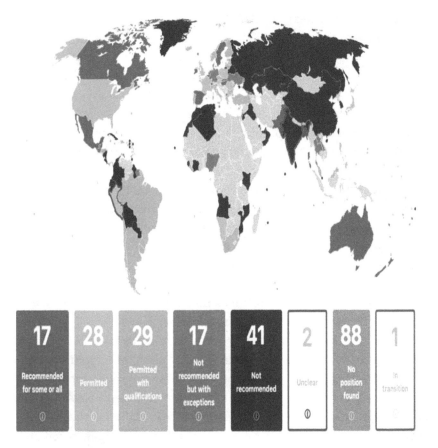

Figure 10.86. John Hopkins University COVID-19 Maternal Immunization Tracker (COMIT) showing the status of each country's recommendation for whether pregnant women should receive the vaccine.[28]

associated with increased COVID-19-related deaths, and persistent COVID-19 infection.[30A,30B] Alternatively, cell-mediated immunity also appears to be quite important in protecting against severe disease (see Immunocompetent Adults below). There still is no agreement about which cell-mediated immunity test(s) to use to determine if a person is protected against disease.[9,10]

Over the past 18 months, studies have examined the effectiveness of various COVID vaccines in preventing mild to moderate disease versus severe disease. The Phase 3 vaccine efficacy trials and subsequent effectiveness studies suggest that the mRNA vaccines have the highest effectiveness (>90%) against severe disease compared to viral-vector vaccines (66–92%)

and inactivated vaccines (50–70%).[11-14] All of the COVID vaccines are more effective at preventing severe disease than mild-moderate disease and less effective at preventing transmission of SARS-CoV-2. The ability of the vaccines to prevent infection and breakthrough mild-to-moderate disease decreases over time, but the ability to protect individuals against severe disease has remained relatively high. Even after the highly transmissible Delta variant became the predominant global strain, vaccination resulted in a 5-fold lower risk of symptomatic infection and a greater than 10-fold lower risk of hospitalization and death.[12]

The Omicron variant is even more contagious than the Delta variant but does not cause more severe disease. The Omicron variant does have a greater capacity to escape both natural and vaccine-induced immunity.[20,21,31] As of June 2022, Omicron has further mutated into the BA.4 and BA.5 variants, which appear to be more contagious than prior Omicron variants, and are currently the predominant SARS-CoV-2 global strains.

SARS-CoV-2 vaccines are focused on developing immunity to the spike protein. Notably, mutations that have developed globally in the Delta and Omicron variants in the S-protein are accruing at a 4-fold greater rate than those that develop in influenza H3N2.[32] Omicron's rapid mutational ability to evade immunity has led the FDA to recently announce that bivalent vaccines, containing the original vaccine strain and a BA.4 or BA.5 strain, should be used in the fall of 2022, analogous to multistrain influenza vaccines.[33] A potential longer-term answer is the ongoing research on the development of pan-coronavirus vaccines that can provide immunity against SARS-CoV-2 variants and other coronaviruses, analogous to current attempts to develop universal influenza vaccines.[34-36] A recent study using computer modeling has suggested that it may be possible to predict SARS-CoV-2 variants of concern that might occur within the next 4 months, thus offering the possibility that the need for new vaccines might be predictable.[37]

3. Collateral Damage

a. Economic impact

The impact of COVID-19 on the global economy in 2020 resulted in an overall 3.2% decrease in economic growth, with a greater impact on advanced economies (-4.6%) than emerging and developing economies

(–2.1%).[38] The International Monetary Fund (IMF) predicted that overall global growth would increase by 6% (5.6% in advanced economies and 6.4% in emerging and developing economies) in 2021. However, the IMF warned that the inequity in vaccine access between countries was becoming the principal fault line along which the global recovery splits into two blocs — those that can look forward to further normalization of economic activity (almost all advanced economies) and those that will still face resurgent infections and rising COVID-19 death tolls. In April 2022, the IMF revised its projections further downward, noting that the war in Ukraine was also having a marked impact of the global economy.[39]

b. Other (non-COVID vaccines) vaccination programs

The COVID-19 pandemic caused a major disruption in immunization services globally.[40] The percentage of children who received three doses of the DPT vaccine in 2021 fell to 81%, a 5% decline compared to 2019. This resulted in 25 million children being un or under-vaccinated in 2021. This decrease is 2 million more than in 2020 and 6 million more than in 2019. Similar decreases occurred for other routine recommended vaccines, including measles and human papillomavirus.[41] The decline was due to many pandemic-related factors, including increased numbers of children living in conflict and fragile settings, supply chain disruptions, resource diversion to emergency response efforts, and outbreak containment measures that limited routine immunization service access and availability. This has already led to an increase in outbreaks of vaccine-preventable diseases, including measles, which increased by 79% in the first few months of 2022.[42]

c. Tuberculosis, HIV, and malaria control and mortality

In 2020, global case detection of tuberculosis was reduced by at least 18% compared to 2019, with a projected global increase in tuberculosis mortality of 20% between 2020 and 2025.[43,44] Similarly, with HIV, it has been reported that global HIV testing was 41% less in 2020 compared with 2019, with an associated 1.06-fold increase in HIV mortality.[44] For malaria, the WHO has estimated that malaria cases in 2020 increased by 14,000,000 and deaths increased by 47,000 compared with 2019.[44] It will be extremely important to further analyze the impact of COVID-19 on these and other infectious diseases, so that we can minimize the future collateral damage of COVID-19 and other pandemics.[44–46]

4. COVID-19 Clinical Updates

a. Immunocompetent adults

Since the beginning of the COVID-19 pandemic in early 2020, SARS-CoV-2 global case fatality rates have declined from greater than 7% to less than 1% as of July 2022 (ourworldindata.com), reflecting vaccination, better treatments, new variants, and other factors. To facilitate better future disease prevention and management, efforts are ongoing to better understand the natural history of COVID-19. A human volunteer study in the United Kingdom (UK) inoculated 34 seronegative young adults with SARS-CoV-2.[47] Eighteen became infected and 89% of those infected experienced mild-to-moderate symptoms beginning 2–4 days after inoculation. SARS-CoV-2 viral loads peaked at 5 days and were largely gone by 10 days. IgG-neutralizing antibodies were detectable in 100% of those infected by 14 days. In the future, human volunteer studies could allow a better understanding of how COVID-19 infection is different from other coronavirus infections.

It is increasingly clear that prior coronavirus infections alter the natural history of COVID-19 infection. In a study of 52 household contacts of patients with COVID-19 infection, 26 contacts who remained SARS-CoV-2 PCR-negative were more likely to have pre-existing T cells specific to spike, nucleocapsid, membrane, envelope, and ORF1 SARS-CoV-2 epitopes that cross-reacted with human endemic coronaviruses (nonSARS-CoV-2 coronaviruses) than the 26 contacts who became PCR positive.[48] Similarly, prior SARS-CoV-2 infection was 46% protective against subsequent SARS-CoV-2 Omicron BA.2 infection, and this protection increased to 55% with two doses of the BNT162b vaccine (Pfizer) and >70% with three doses.[49] However, it has also been shown that all-cause mortality increases in a graded fashion, according to the number of COVID-19 infections an individual has, with or without vaccination against SARS-CoV-2. This increased mortality risk persists at least 6 months after the last infection.[50] Further investigation will be necessary to understand why some prior coronavirus infections can prevent subsequent SARS-CoV-2 infection, and others predispose to greater mortality.

It has also been shown that COVID-19 infection increases the near future risk of symptomatic manifestations of many other diseases. A cohort of 73,435 US Veterans with COVID-19 who survived at least 30 days after their COVID-19 diagnosis and were not hospitalized was compared with 4,990,835 Veterans who did not have COVID-19 and were not hospitalized.[51] Beyond the first 30 days after a COVID-19 diagnosis and in six months of follow-up, the COVID-19 group had an increased risk of respiratory failure, insufficiency and respiratory arrest (HR 3.37), cardiac dysrhythmias (HR 8.41), heart failure (HR 3.94), pulmonary embolism (HR 2.63), and neurocognitive disorders (HR 3.17).[51] In a much larger case-control study where 1,284,437 COVID-19 patients from eight countries were compared with an equal number of control patients with another respiratory infection, it was found that the increased risk duration of certain neuropsychiatric diseases varied significantly.[52] For example, the increased risk of mood and anxiety disorders returned to baseline within two months, whereas cognitive deficit (brain fog), dementia, psychotic disorders, ischemic stroke, intracranial hemorrhage, and seizure risk were still increased at the end of the 2-year follow-up period, and this risk changed as new SARS-CoV-2 variants emerged.[52] Much additional research will need to be done to understand how COVID-19 infection affects the pathogenesis of these other diseases.

b. Long-COVID = Persistent infection

Multiple studies have substantiated the importance of persistent symptoms after COVID-19 infection, so-called Long-COVID, recently renamed Post-acute Sequelae of COVID-19 (Chapter 4, Case #9).[53] More severe COVID-19 symptoms increase the likelihood of developing Long-COVID, with 55% of those with COVID-19 severe enough to require hospitalization having Long-COVID symptoms up to two years.[54] Conversely, in a prospective study of 33,281 laboratory-confirmed SARS-CoV-2 infections compared withe 62,957 never-infected controls as to the presence of Long-COVID symptoms 6, 12, and 18 months after infection, those with asymptomatic infection did not develop Long-COVID.[54A] Also, the risk of Long-COVID varies with the variant causing infection; those with the Delta variant were twice as likely to have Long-COVID as those with the Omicron variant (10.8% vs. 4.5%).[55]

While the precise cause of Long-COVID has not yet been determined, multiple 2022 publications have demonstrated persistent SARS-CoV-2 infection in the gastrointestinal (GI) tract. A study looking at longitudinal shedding of SARS-CoV-2 RNA in respiratory and fecal samples found that oropharyngeal shedding of viral RNA was gone by 4 months; however, fecal RNA shedding was still present in 12.7% of patients at 4 months and 3.8% at 7 months, and fecal shedding correlated with GI and other systemic symptoms.[56] In a study of 44 patients with underlying inflammatory bowel disease approximately 7 months after mild COVID-19, 73% were found to have RNA evidence of SARS-CoV-2 in their GI mucosa, unrelated to immunosuppression or degree of gut inflammation; 66% of those with persistent RNA had Long-COVID symptoms versus 0% of those without detectable RNA.[57] An investigation of 37 patients with Long-COVID found that 60% had spike protein circulating in their blood up to 12 months after infection, suggesting active SARS-CoV-2 replication is occurring somewhere in the body.[58] Not only does there appear to be greater, long-term SARS-CoV-2 replication in the GI tract than in the respiratory tract, one small study comparing SARS-CoV-2 isolates from the respiratory tract versus the GI tract found greater genetic diversity in the GI tract variants.[59]

These studies collectively indicate that persistent GI SARS-CoV-2 infection likely plays an important role in Long-COVID. Further work needs to be done to better understand what is unique about the GI tract in facilitating persistent infection and in-host SARS-CoV-2 evolution, especially related to whether such individuals have a localized GI immune deficit or systemic immune deficit that makes this viral persistence possible, and whether persistent SARS-CoV-2 infection occurs elsewhere besides the GI tract.

c. Immunocompromised patients

Substantial evidence now exists that COVID-19 can cause long-term infection in immunocompromised patients that is associated with much higher mortality (Chapter 4, Case #7).[60,61] Such patients have been shown to have persistent SARS-CoV-2 replication that is greater than the general population, can go on for more than one year, and does not resolve without aggressive treatment of their COVID-19 or improvement in their underlying immunity (Chapter 4, SARS-CoV-2 mutation).[62] This persistent SARS-CoV-2 replication is associated with continuous in-host evolution that is increasingly thought to be the source of new variants of concern (Chapter 4, SARS-CoV-2 mutation and SARS-CoV-2 mutations below).[63–67]

Three more publications looking at prolonged, in-host SARS-CoV-2 mutations in immunocompromised hosts will further demonstrate this point.[65–67] One study found that each time a patient received convalescent plasma, new mutations appeared, especially in the spike protein (Chapter 4, Pathogenesis).[65] In another study, in Germany, when six immunocompromised hosts were treated with bamlanivimab (which binds to the spike protein ACE2-binding site), viral clearance did not occur, and 5/6 patients developed the E484K mutation soon after treatment.[66] The background prevalence of the E484K mutation in nonimmunocompromised hosts was 3/1270, strongly suggesting the mutation occurred due to the immunologic pressure of the treatment.[66] One additional immunocompromised patient with cholangiocarcinoma also developed a spike protein mutation (Q493R) after receiving bamlanivimab and etesivimab.[67] Rapid development of mutations in immunocompromised hosts could be the reason for their increased mortality.

It is likely that the immune deficits that predispose to persistent infection, in-host SARS-CoV-2 evolution, and higher mortality can be caused by both B-cell and T-cell lymphocyte deficits.[1,2,48,60–67,67A,67B] As an example of a B-cell lymphocyte deficit, patients with rheumatoid arthritis treated with rituximab had only a 22% response rate to either Pfizer's, Moderna's or AstraZeneca's vaccines vs 98% of control patients.[67A,67C] An example of a T-cell defect that can predispose to poor outcomes with COVID-19 is shown by HIV patients with low CD4 lymphocyte counts, that cannot clear the virus until treated adequately with antiretroviral therapy.[67D,67E]

d. Treatment effectiveness

Clinicians all over the world have tried many drugs that might improve COVID-19 patient outcomes, including treatments already approved for other diseases (drugs, blood anticoagulants, convalescent plasma) and many new pharmaceutical agents (Chapter 4, Case #4). After 2.5 years of the pandemic, we now have 6 different classes of drugs that reduce hospitalizations and mortality; steroids (intravenous, oral, and inhaled), IL-6 inhibitors, spike protein binding inhibitors, anticoagulants, and two new oral drugs (molnupiravir, paxlovid) (Table 10.30; updated from Chapter 4,

Table 10.30.   Revised COVID-19 treatment recommendations (compare with Table 4.6).

COVID-19 Treatment	Study	Comment[91,92]
Effective		
Steroids	RCT	>30% mortality reduction, intubated patients
Budesonide (inhaled)	RCT	One outpatient study suggests decreased hospitalization, mortality
Anticoagulation	RCT	Mortality benefit in non-ICU patients, but not in ICU patients
IL-6 inhibitors	RCT	Mortality benefit
Monoclonal Ab	RCT	Decreases hospitalization and mortality; resistance may develop
Molnupiravir (oral)	RCT	Outpatient treatment, decreases hospitalization and mortality
Ritonavir/PF-07321332 (oral)	RCT	Outpatient treatment, decreases hospitalization and mortality
Partially effective		
Remdesivir	RCT	No mortality benefit, decreased hospitalization 5 days
Ineffective		
Convalescent Plasma	RCT	No benefit, unless high titer
Hydroxychloroquine	RCT	No benefit, not recommended
Ivermectin	RCT	No benefit, not recommended
Lopinavir-ritonavir	RCT	No benefit, not recommended

Table 4.9), but so far, only monoclonal antibodies that block spike protein binding have been shown to decrease viral transmission.[68–79]

Two new oral agents — Molnupiravir (RNA-polymerase fidelity antagonist) and Paxlovid (ritonavir/PF-07321332, a 2-drug combination, protease inhibitor) — were approved under the US EUA in November 2021, and December 2021, respectively; both reduce hospitalizations and mortality (Table 10.30).[77–79] If priced low enough for use in developing countries, they could have a major impact on improving outcomes and decreasing transmission.[80,81] In particular, Molnupiravir has already been shown to decrease transmission in a ferret animal model.[77] Mathematical modeling suggests the two agents might work even better used together.[82] An interesting phenomenon for both drugs has been a rebound of symptoms, occurring in 2.31% of patients within 7 days after treatment and 5.87% of patients within 30 days after treatment with Paxlovid.[83] For Molnupiravir, rebound occurred in 3.75% of patients at 7 days and 8.21% at 30 days.[83] This suggests the possibility that virus replication is only temporarily suppressed by these drugs, in some patients.[83]

Since the immunologic pressure of convalescent plasma and monoclonal antibodies have both been shown to provoke adaptive SARS-CoV-2 mutations (Chapter 4, Case #4), it is reasonable to wonder whether drugs such as Paxlovid and Molnupiravir may have the same effect. For example, HIV, with its similar mutation rate to SARS-CoV-2 (Chapter 4, Pathogenesis), rapidly developed resistance mutations (in less than one to two years) when treated with one or two drugs but not with three drugs.[84,85] Similarly, influenza A became 92% resistant to amantadine in one year after Chinese farmers used amantadine to prevent influenza in chickens.[86] Molnupiravir is a nucleoside analog that causes RNA polymerase transcription errors that may be lethal to the virus, in a somewhat analogous fashion to azidothymidine, the first drug used to treat HIV infection.[87] The concern related to SARS-CoV-2, is that, in addition to creating lethal mutants, it may also lead to a much greater frequency of SARS-CoV-2 variants.[88,89] A possible solution would be multidrug therapy, which would minimize the appearance of mutations, analogous to 3-drug therapy for HIV infection, and this is especially important, if they are considered for long-term use with Long-COVID or immunocompromised hosts, where persistent viral replication would likely increase the risk of drug resistance.

5. SARS-CoV-2 Mutations

SARS-CoV-2 has an approximately 30,000 nucleotide genome, with an estimated yearly mutation rate of 0.7×10^{-3} base substitutions/nucleotide site/year for the original pandemic strain, and greater than 2.0×10^{-3} for many of the variants of concern, nearly identical to the mutation rates of HIV and influenza A, 1,000 times greater than most bacteria, and 10,000,000 times greater than human genome mutation (Chapter 4, Figure 4.58).[89A] Statistically, every virus replication will result in a change in at least one nucleotide in the genome. Many will be nonsense mutations, some will be lethal to the virus, but some will lead to new ways the virus can interact with or adapt to its host. Each group of SARS-CoV-2 virus variants within a single host is considered a quasispecies, and it will keep changing as long as the virus is replicating.[88] During peak COVID-19 infection within each infected human, there are likely millions of variants within the current quasispecies (Chapter 9, Figure 9.81).[90]

Importantly, the genomic location of SARS-CoV-2 mutations is not random, with less than 20 nucleotide mutation hot spots identified out of 30,000 possible nucleotides, occurring predominantly in structural proteins, with spike protein mutations occurring at the highest frequency (Table 10.31).[91–93] Non-random, genomic mutations are consistent with recent evolutionary findings in plants, where genomic mutation hot spots (mutation bias) occur predominantly in areas encoding environmentally interactive proteins, with significantly fewer mutations occuring in essential (metabolic and reproductive) genes, suggesting hot spots have evolved to facilitate adaptation to new host environments.[94]

As discussed above, it is increasingly likely that immunocompromised hosts may be the source of the SARS-CoV-2 variants of interest and variants of concern.[63–67] This likely occurs through a combination of adaptive and convergent evolution, with the possibility that even simultaneous, multi-mutational jumps could be involved.[30,46,95–97] One study found a link between a single immunocompromised host's SARS-CoV-2 variant (B.1.616) and an outbreak, a possible "smoking gun", that suggested immunocompromised hosts may be the source of Variants of Interest and Variants of Concern.[93] The largest group of immunocompromised hosts in the world is thought to be those with inadequately treated HIV infection in Africa (2/3s of all global HIV infections).[46,98] Until successful strategies for global SARS-CoV-2 control can be developed, we should continue to see new Variants of Concern come from different parts of the world, likely from immunocompromised hosts, at regular intervals.[98]

6. SARS-CoV-2 Origin: Revisited

Coming full circle, we close out with this fundamental question: Do we know the origin of SARS-CoV-2? The answer is still no, but we are much closer. It is increasingly likely that the pandemic began in the Huanan Seafood Wholesale Market in Wuhan, and involved at least two zoonotic transmissions, the first around November 18, 2019, involving lineage B viruses, and the second within a few weeks involving lineage A viruses.[99,100]

No hard evidence exists as to what zoonotic intermediate host was the source of these viruses, but the progenitor virus most likely came from horseshoe bats (*Rhinolophus*), associated with a highly complex reticulate evolution.[99–101] Computer modeling of viral bat to human spillover events in Southeast Asia suggests that a median of 66,000 SARS-related coronavirus spillover events occur annually, largely associated with hotspots of SARS-CoV-2 viral diversity in southern China, Myanmar, Lao PDR, and northern Vietnam.[102] Such spillover events may relate to the consumption of exotic foods in China and other Asian countries, with a recent study identifying 102 mammalian-infecting viruses (including coronaviruses) in a survey of 1,941 such animals sampled across China.[103] These findings collectively suggest that we need to definitively identify the intermediate host(s) of SARS-CoV-2, ascertain the chain of transmission that brought it to humans, and finally determine how best to block future transmission in wet markets or any other sources of these animal hosts that will put humans at risk.

References

1. Richie H, Ortiz-Opsina E, Bellekian D, *et al*. (nd) Cumulative confirmed COVID-19 cases per million people. Our World in Data. https://ourworldindata.org/covid-cases. Accessed: June 30, 2022.

2. Richie H, Ortiz-Ospina E, Bellekian D, *et al*. (nd) Cumulative confirmed COVID-19 deaths per million people. Our World in Data. Published online at OurWorldinData.org. https://ourworldindata.org/covid-deaths. Accessed: June 30, 2022.

3. Blauer B, Neuzo J. (2022) Home testing confounds COVID-19 testing data. John Hopkins Coronavirus Resource Center. https://coronavirus.jhu.edu/pandemic-data-initiative/data-outlook/home-tests-confound-covid-19-testing-data. Accessed June 28, 2022.

4. WHO. (nd) The true death toll of COVID-19. Estimating global excess mortality. World Health Organization. https://www.who.int/data/stories/the-true-death-toll-of-covid-19-estimating-global-excess-mortality. Accessed: November 3, 2021.

5. Richie H, Ortiz-Opsina E, Bellekian, *et al*. (nd) COVID-19 vaccine doses administered per 100 people as of November 11, 2021. Our World in Data. https://ourworldindata.org/covid-vaccinations#how-many-covid-19-vacci-nation-doses-have-been-administered. Accessed June 30, 2022.

6. De Foo C, Grépin KA, Cook AR, *et al.* (2021) Navigating from SARS-CoV-2 elimination to endemicity in Australia, Hong Kong, New Zealand, and Singapore. *The Lancet* **398**:1547–1551. DOI:10.1016/S0140-6736(21)02186

7. Yeung J. (2021) China doubles down on zero-Covid-19 as it battles most widespread outbreak since Wuhan. CNN, November 4. https://www.cnn.com/2021/11/04/china/china-delta-covid-outbreak-strategy-intl-hnk/index.html

8. Yuan S. (2022) Zero COVID in China: What next? *The Lancet* **399**:1856–1857. http://dx.doi.org/10.1016/s0140-6736%2822%2900873-x

9. Nature. (2021) COVID vaccine immunity is waning — how much does that matter. *Nature* **597**:606–607. https://media.nature.com/original/magazine-assets/d41586-021-02532-4/d41586-021-02532-4.pdf

10. Abbasi J. (2021) The flawed science of antibody testing for SARS-CoV-2 immunity. *JAMA* **326**(18):1781–1782. DOI:10.1001/jama.2021.18919

11. Scobiie HM, Johnson AG, Surhar AB, *et al.* (2021) Monitoring incidence of covid-19 cases, hospitalizations, and deaths, by vaccination status — 13 jurisdictions, April 4 – July 17, 2021. *Morbidity and Mortality Weekly Report* **70**(37):1284–1290. DOI:10.15585/mmwr.mm7037e1

12. Singanayagam A, Hakki S, Dunning J, *et al.* (2021) Community transmission and viral load kinetics of the SARS-CoV-2 delta (B.1.617.2) variant in vaccinated and unvaccinated individuals in the UK: A prospective, longitudinal, cohort study. *Lancet Infectious Diseases* **22**(2):183–195. https://doi.org/10.1016/S1473-3099(21)00648-4

13. Zheng C, Shao W, Chen X, *et al.* (2022) Real-world effectiveness of COVID-19 vaccines: A literature review and meta-analysis. *International Journal of Infectious Diseases* **114**:252–260. https://doi.org/10.1016/j.ijid.2021.11.009

14. CDC. (nd) Interim clinical considerations for use of COVID-19 vaccines currently approved or authorized in the United States. Centers for Disease Control and Prevention. https://www.cdc.gov/vaccines/covid-19/clinical-considerations/covid-19-vaccines-us.html

15. Richie H, Ortiz-Ospina E, Bellekian D, *et al.* (nd) Coronavirus (COVID-19) Vaccinations. Our World in Data. https://ourworldindata.org/covid-vaccinations

16. Lazarus JV, Wyka K, White TM, *et al.* (2022) Revisiting COVID-19 vaccine hesitancy around the world using data from 23 countries in 2021. *Nature Communications* **13**:3801. https://doi.org/10.1038/s41467-022-31441-x

17. Lee ARYB, Wong SY, Chai LYA, *et al.* (2022) Efficacy of covid-19 vaccines in immunocompromised patients: Systematic review and meta-analysis. *BMJ* **376**:e068632. DOI:10.1136/bmj-2021-068632

18. del Rio C, Malani PN. (2022) COVID-19 in 2022 — the beginning of the end or the end of the beginning? *JAMA* **327**(24):2389–2390. DOI:10.1001/jama.2022.9655

19. Mallapaty S. (2022) COVID-19: How Omicron overtook Delta in three charts. *Nature News*, March 4. https://www.nature.com/articles/d41586-022-00632-3

20. Taylor CA, Patel K, Pham H, *et al.* (2021) Severity of disease among adults hospitalized with laboratory-confirmed COVID — confirmed COVID-19 before and during the period of SARS-CoV-2 B.1.617.2 (Delta) predominance — COVID-NET, 14 States, January–August 2021. *Morbidity and Mortality Weekly Report* **70**(43):1513–1519. https://www.cdc.gov/mmwr/volumes/70/wr/mm7043e1.htm?s_cid=mm7043e1_w

21. CDC. (2022) What you need to know about variants. Centers for Disease Control and Prevention. https://www.cdc.gov/coronavirus/2019-ncov/variants/variant.html

22. WHO. (2022) 14.9 million excess deaths associated with the COVID-19 pandemic in 2020 and 2021. World Health Organization, May 5. https://www.who.int/news/item/05-05-2022-14.9-million-excess-deaths-were-associated-with-the-covid-19-pandemic-in-2020-and-2021

23. Richie H, Ortiz-Ospina E, Bellekian D, *et al.* (nd) What is the cumulative number of confirmed COVID-19 deaths? Our World in Data. https://ourworldindata.org/covid-deaths

24. Usher AD. (2021) A beautiful idea: How COVAX has fallen short. *Lancet* **397**:2322–2325. DOI:10.1016/s0140-6736(21)01367-2

25. Usher AD. (2021) Vaccine shortages prompt changes to COVAX strategy. *Lancet* **398**:1474. DOI:10.1016/s0140-6736(21)02309-6

26. Desisto CL, Wallace B, Simeone RM, *et al.* (2021) Risk for stillbirth among women with and without COVID-19 at delivery- United States, March 2020–September 2021. *Morbidity and Mortality Weekly Report* **70**(47):1640–1645. https://www.cdc.gov/mmwr/volumes/70/wr/mm7047e1.htm

27. CDC. (2021) CDC health advisory COVID-19 vaccination for pregnant people to prevent serious illness, deaths, and adverse pregnancy outcomes from COVID-19. *Morbidity and Mortality Weekly Report*, September 29.

28. Rosen J. (2021) Global policies on COVID-19 vaccination in pregnancy vary widely by country according to new online tracker. Hub, Johns

Hopkins University, June 28. https://hub.jhu.edu/2021/06/28/tracker-map-of-vaccine-policies-for-pregnant-women/. Accessed: June 29, 2022.

29. Naqvi S, Saleem S, Naqvi F, *et al.* (2022) Knowledge, attitudes, and practices of pregnant women regarding COVID-19 vaccination in pregnancy in 7 low- and middle-income countries: An observational trial from the Global Network for Women and Children's Health Research. *BJOG: An International Journal of Obstetrics & Gynaecology,* May 21. https://doi.org/10.1111/1471-0528.17226

30. FDA. (2022) Coronavirus (COVID-19) update: FDA authorizes Moderna and Pfizer-BioNTech COVID-19 vaccines for children down to 6 months of age, June 17, 2022. The US Food and Drugs Administration. https://www.fda.gov/news-events/press-announcements/coronavirus-covid-19-upda te-fda-authorizes-moderna-and-pfizer-biontech-covid-19-vaccines-chil-dren#:~:text=For%20the%20Moderna%20COVID%2D19,through%20 17%20years%20of%20age

30A. MacKenna B, Kennedy NA, Mehrkar A, *et al.* (2022 Jul) Risk of severe COVID-19 outcomes associated with immune-mediated inflammatory diseases and immune-modifying therapies: a nationwide cohort study in the OpenSAFELY platform. *Lancet Rheumatol.* **4**(7):e490–e506. doi: 10.1016/ S2665-9913(22)00098-4.

30B. Jorge Calderón-Parra, Elena Múñez-Rubio, Ana Fernández-Cruz, *et al.* Incidence, Clinical Presentation, Relapses and Outcome of Severe Acute Respiratory Syndrome Coronavirus 2 (SARS-CoV-2) Infection in Patients Treated With Anti-CD20 Monoclonal Antibodies, *Clinical Infectious Diseases*, Volume 74, Issue 10, 15 May 2022, Pages 1786–1794, https://doi.org/10.1093/cid/ciab700

31. Callaway E. (2022) What Omicron's BA.4 and BA.5 variants mean for the pandemic. *Nature*, June 23. https://www.nature.com/articles/d41586-022-01730-y

32. Kistler KE, Huddleston J, Bedford T. (2021) Rapid and parallel adaptive mutations in spike S1 drive clade success in SARS-CoV-2. *bioRxiv*, Sep 14. DOI:10.1101/2021.09.11.459844

33. FDA. (2022) Coronavirus (COVID-19) update: FDA recommends inclusion of Omicron BA.4/5 component for COVID-19 vaccine booster doses. The US Food and Drugs Administration, June 30. https://www.fda.gov/news-events/press-announcements/coronavirus-covid-19-update-fda-recommends-inclusion-omicron-ba45-component-covid-19-vaccine-booster

34. Lowe D. (2022) Are pan-coronavirus vaccines possible? *Science*, April 21. https://www.science.org/content/blog-post/are-pan-coronavirus-vaccines-possible

35. Morens DM, Taubenberger JK, Fauci AS. (2021) Universal coronavirus vaccines — an urgent need. *New England Journal of Medicine* **386**: 297–299. DOI:10.1056/NEJMp2118468

36. NIH. (2021) NIH launches clinical trial of universal influenza vaccine candidate. National Institutes of Health, June 1. https://www.nih.gov/news-events/news-releases/nih-launches-clinical-trial-universal-influenza-vaccine-candidate

37. Maher MC, Bartha I, Weaver S, *et al.* (2022) Predicting the mutational drivers of future SARS-CoV-2 variants of concern. *Science Translational Medicine* **14**(633):eabk3445. DOI:10.1126/scitranslmed.abk3445

38. IMF. (2021) Fault lines widen in the global recovery. *World Economic Outlook*, International Monetary Fund, July. https://www.imf.org/en/Publications/WEO/Issues/2021/07/27/world-economic-outlook-update-july-2021

39. IMF. (2022) War sets back the global economy. *World Economic Outlook*, International Monetary Fund, April. https://www.imf.org/en/Publications/WEO/Issues/2022/04/19/world-economic-outlook-april-2022

40. SeyedAlinaghi S, Karimi A, Mojdeganlou H, *et al.* (2022) Impact of COVID-19 pandemic on routine vaccination coverage of children and adolescents: A systematic review. *Health Science Reports* **5**(2):e00516. DOI:10.1002/hsr2.516

41. UNICEF. (2022) COVID-19 pandemic leads to major backsliding on childhood vaccinations, new WHO, UNICEF data shows. UNICEF, July. https://www.unicef.org/press-releases/covid-19-pandemic-leads

42. UNICEF. (2022) Measles cases are spiking globally. UNICEF, May. https://www.unicef.org/stories/measles-cases-spiking-globally#:~:text=04%20May%202022,and%20other%20vaccine%2Dpreventable%20diseases

43. Dheda K, Perumal T, Moultrie H, *et al.* (2022) The intersecting pandemics of tuberculosis and COVID-19: Population-level and patient-level impact, clinical presentation, and corrective interventions. *Lancet Respiratory Medicine* **10**(6):603-622. DOI:10.1016/S2213-2600(22)00092-3

44. Chanda-Kapata P, Ntoumi F, Kapata N, *et al.* (2022) Tuberculosis, HIV/AIDS and malaria health services in sub-Saharan Africa — a situation analysis of the disruptions and impact of the COVID-19 pandemic. *International Journal of Infectious Disease*. https://doi.org/10.1016/j.ijid.2022.03.033

45. Pai M, Kasaeva T, Swaminathan S. (2022) COVID-19's devastating effect on tuberculosis care — a path to recovery. *New England Journal of Medicine* **386**:1490–1493. DOI:10.1056/NEJMp2118145

46. Corey L, Corbett-Detig R, Beyrer C. (2022) Expanding Efforts and Support to Respond to the HIV and COVID-19 Intersecting Pandemics. *JAMA* **327**(13):1227–1228. DOI:10.1001/jama.2022.3517

47. Killingley B, Mann AJ, Kalinova M, *et al.* (2022) Safety, tolerability and viral kinetics during SARS-CoV-2 human challenge in young adults. *Nature Medicine* **28**(5):1031–1041. DOI:10.1038/s41591-022-01780-9

48. Kundu R, Narean JS, Wang L, *et al.* (2022) Cross-reactive memory T cells associate with protection against SARS-CoV-2 infection in COVID-19 contacts. *Nature Communications* **13**(1):80. https://doi.org/10.1038/s41467-021-27674-x

49. Altarawneh HN, Chemaitelly H, Ayoub HH, *et al.* (2022) Effects of previous infection and vaccination on symptomatic omicron infections. *New England Journal of Medicine* **387**:21–34. DOI:10.1056/NEJMoa2203965

50. Al-Aly Z, Bowe B, Xie Y. (2022) Outcomes of SARS-CoV-2 reinfection. *Nature Portfolio*, June 17. https://doi.org/10.21203/rs.3.rs-1749502/v1

51. Al-Aly Z, Xie Y, Bowe B. (2021) High-dimensional characterization of post-acute sequelae of COVID-19. *Nature* **594**:259–264. https://doi.org/10.1038/s41586-021-03553-9

52. Taquet M, Sillett R, Zhu L, *et al.* (2022) Neurological and psychiatric risk trajectories after SARS-CoV-2 infection: An analysis of 2-year retrospective cohort studies including 1,284,437 patients. *Lancet Psychiatry*, August 17. https://doi.org/10.1016/S2215-0366(22)00260-7

53. Lopez-Leon S, Wegman-Ostrosky T, Perelman C, *et al.* (2021) More than 50 Long-term effects of COVID-19: A systematic review and meta-analysis. *medRxiv*. DOI:10.1101/2021.01.27.21250617

54. Huang L, Li X, Gu X, *et al.* (2022) Health outcomes in people 2 years after surviving hospitalisation with COVID-19: A longitudinal cohort study. *Lancet Respiratory Medicine*. DOI:10.1016/S2213-2600(22)00126-6

54A. Hastie, C.E., Lowe, D.J., McAuley, A. *et al.* (2022) Outcomes among confirmed cases and a matched comparison group in the Long-COVID in Scotland study. *Nat Commun* **13**, 5663. https://doi.org/10.1038/s41467-022-33415-5

55. Antonelli M, Pujol JC, Spector TD, Ourselin S, Steves CJ. (2022) Risk of long COVID associated with Delta versus Omicron variants of SARS-CoV-2. *Lancet* **399**(10343):2263–2264. DOI:10.1016/S0140-6736(22)00941-2

56. Natarajan A, Zlitni S, Brooks EF, *et al.* (2022) Gastrointestinal symptoms and fecal shedding of SARS-CoV-2 RNA suggest prolonged gastrointestinal infection. *The New York Medical Journal* **3**(6):371–387.e9. DOI:10.1016/j. medj.2022.04.001

57. Zollner A, Koch R, Jukic A, *et al.* (2022) Postacute COVID-19 is characterized by gut viral antigen persistence in inflammatory bowel diseases. *Gastroenterology* **163**(2):495–506.e8. DOI:10.1053/j.gastro.2022.04.037

58. Swank Z, Senussi Y, Alter G, Walt DR. (2022) Persistent circulating SARS-CoV-2 spike is associated with post-acute COVID-19 sequelae. *medRxiv*, June 16. https://doi.org/10.1101/2022.06.14.22276401

59. Wang Y, Wang D, Zhang L, *et al.* (2022) Intra-host variation and evolutionary dynamics of SARS-CoV-2 populations in COVID-19 patients. *Genome Medicine* **13**:30. https://doi.org/10.1186/s13073-021-00847-5

60. Pinato DJ, Tabernero J, Bower M, *et al.* (2021) Prevalence and impact of COVID-19 sequelae on treatment and survival of patients with cancer who recovered from SARS-CoV-2 infection: Evidence from the OnCovid retrospective, multicentre registry study. *Lancet Oncology.* https://doi.org/10.1016/S1470-2045(21)00573-8

61. Belsky JA, Tullius BP, Lamb MG, *et al.* (2021) COVID-19 in immunocompromised patients: A systematic review of cancer, hematopoietic cell and solid organ transplant patients. *Journal of Infection* **82**(3):329–338. DOI:10.1016/j.jinf.2021.01.022

62. Kim DY, Lin MY, Jennings C, *et al.*; CDC Prevention Epicenter Program. (2022) Duration of replication-competent SARS-CoV-2 shedding among patients with severe or critical coronavirus disease 2019 (COVID-19). *Clinical Infectious Diseases.* DOI:10.1093/cid/ciac405

63. Corey L, Beyrer C, Cohen MS, *et al.* (2021) SARS-CoV-2 variants in patients with immunosuppression. *New England Journal of Medicine* **85**:562–566. DOI:10.1056/NEJMsb2104756

64. Harari S, Tahor M. (2022) Evolutionary insight into the emergence of SARS-CoV-2 variants of concern. *Nature Medicine* **28**:1357–1358. https://doi.org/10.1038/s41591-022-01892-2

65. Weigang S, Fuchs J, Zimmer G, *et al.* (2021) Within-host evolution of SARS-CoV-2 in an immunosuppressed COVID-19 patient as a source of immune escape variants. *Nature Communications* **12**:6405. https://doi.org/10.1038/s41467-021-26602-3

66. Jensen B, Luebke N, Feldt T, *et al.* (2021) Emergence of the E484K mutation in SARS-CoV-2-infected immunocompromised patients treated with

bamlanivimab in Germany. *Lancet Regional Health.* https://doi.org/10.1016/j.lanepe.2021.100164

67. Focosi D, Novazzi F, Genoni A, *et al.* (2021) Emergence of SARS-COV-2 spike protein escape mutation Q493R after treatment for COVID-19. *Emerging Infectious Diseases.* https://doi.org/10.3201/eid2710.211538

67A. Jyssum I, Kared H, Tran TT, *et al.* (2022 Mar) Humoral and cellular immune responses to two and three doses of SARS-CoV-2 vaccines in rituximab-treated patients with rheumatoid arthritis: a prospective, cohort study. *Lancet Rheumatol.* **4**(3):e177–e187. doi: 10.1016/S2665-9913(21)00394-5.

67B. Dzinamarira T, Murewanhema G, Chitungo I, *et al.* (2022 May 16) Risk of mortality in HIV-infected COVID-19 patients: A systematic review and meta-analysis. *J Infect Public Health.* **15**(6):654–661. doi: 10.1016/j.jiph.2022.05.006.

67C. MacKenna B, Kennedy NA, Mehrkar A, et al. (June 8, 2022) Risk of severe COVID-19 outcomes associated with immune-mediated inflammatory diseases and immune-modifying therapies: a nationwide cohort study in the OpenSAFELY platform. *Lancet Rheumatol.* https://doi.org/10.1016/S265-9913(22)00098-4

67D. Cele S, Karim F, Lustig G, *et al.* (2022) SARS-CoV-2 prolonged infection during advanced HIV disease evolves extensive immune escape. *Cell Host & Microbe* **30**:154–62. https://doi.org/10.1016/j.chom.2022.01.005

67E. Maponga TG, Jeffries M, Tegally H, et al. (2022 Jul 6) Persistent SARS-CoV-2 infection with accumulation of mutations in a patient with poorly controlled HIV infection. *Clin Infect Dis.* ciac548. doi: 10.1093/cid/ciac548.

68. Yu L-M, Bafadhel M, Dorward J, *et al.* (2021) Inhaled budesonide for COVID-19 in people at high risk of complications in the community in the UK (PRINCIPLE): A randomized, controlled, open-label, adaptive platform trial. *Lancet.* https://doi.org/10.1016/S0140-6736(21)01744-X

69. Guimaraes PO, Quirk D, Furtado RH, *et al.* (2021) Tofacitinib in patents hospitalized with COVID-19 pneumonia. *New England Journal of Medicine* **385**:406–415. DOI:10.1056/NEJMoa2101643

70. WHO Rapid Evidence Appraisal for COVID-19 Therapies (REACT) Working Group. (2021) Association between administration of IL-6 antagonists and mortality among Patients hospitalized for COVID-19. A meta-analysis. *JAMA* **326**(6):499–518. DOI:10.1001/jama.2021.11330

71. REMAP-CAP, ACTIV-4a, and ATTACC Investigators. (2021) Therapeutic anticoagulation with heparin in noncritically ill patients with COVID-19. *New England Journal of Medicine* **385**:790–802. DOI:10.1056/NEJMoa2105911

72. Cooper MH, Christensen PA, Salazar E, *et al.* (2021) Real-world assessment of 2,879 COVID-19 patients treated with monoclonal antibody therapy: A propensity score-matched cohort study. *Open Forum Infectious Diseases* **8**(11):ofab512. https://doi.org/10.1093/ofid/ofab512

73. Dougan M, Nirula A, Azizad M, *et al.* (2021) Bamlanivimab plus etese-vimab in mild or moderate COVID-19. *New England Journal of Medicine* **385**:1382–1392. DOI:10.1056/NEJMoa2102685

74. Gupta A, Gonzalez-Rojas Y, Juarez E, *et al.* (2021) Early treatment for COVID-19 with SARS-CoV-2 neutralizing antibody Sotrovimab. *New England Journal of Medicine* **385**:1941–1950. DOI:10.1056/NEJMoa2107934

75. O'Brien MP, Forleo-Neto E, Musser BJ, *et al.* (2021) Subcutaneous REGEN-COV antibody combination to prevent COVID-19. *New England Journal of Medicine* **385**(13):1184–1195.

76. Cohen MS, Nirula A, Mulligan MJ, *et al.* (2021) Effect of bamlanivimab vs placebo on incidence of COVID-19 among residents and staff of skilled nursing and assisted living facilities: A randomized clinical trial. *JAMA* **326**(1):46–55

77. Aripaka P. (2021) Britain approves Merck's COVID-19 pill in world first. *Reuters,* November5.https://www.reuters.com/business/healthcare-pharmaceuticals/britain-approves-mercks-oral-covid-19-pill-2021-11-04/

78. Merck. (nd) Merck and Ridgeback's Molnupiravir, an oral COVID-19 antiviral medicine, receives first authorization in the world. Merck & Co. https://www.merck.com/news/merck-and-ridgebacks-molnupiravir-an-oral-covid-19-antiviral-medicine-receives-first-authorization-in-the-world/

79. Pfizer. (2021) Pfizer's novel COVID-19 oral antiviral treatment candidate reduced risk of hospitalization or death by 89% in interim analysis of phase 2/3 EPIC-HR study. Pfizer, November 5. https://www.pfizer.com/news/press-release/press-release-detail/pfizers-novel-covid-19-oral-antiviral-treatment-candidate

80. Guarascio F, Erman M. (2021) Merck COVID-19 pill sparks calls for access for lower income countries. Reuters, October 17. https://www.reuters.com/business/healthcare-pharmaceuticals/merck-covid-19-pill-sparks-calls-access-lower-income-countries-2021-10-17/

81. Cox RM, Wolf JD, Plemper RK. (2021) Therapeutically administered ribonucleoside analogue MK-4482/EIDD-2801 blocks SARS-CoV-2 transmission in ferrets. *Nature Microbiology* **6**:11–18. https://doi.org/10.1038/s41564-020-00835-2

82. Czuppon P, Débarre F, Gonçalves A, *et al.* (2021) Success of prophylactic antiviral therapy for SARS-CoV-2: Predicted critical efficacies and impact of

different drug-specific mechanisms of action. *PLOS Computational Biology* **17**(3):e1008752. https://doi.org/10.1371/journal.pcbi.1008752

83. Wang L, Berger NA, Davis PB, *et al.* (2022) COVID-19 rebound after Pax-lovid and Molnupiravir during January-June 2022. *medRxiv*, June 22. https//doi.org/10.1101/2022.06.21.22276724

84. Ho DD. (1995) Time to hit HIV, early and hard. *New England Journal of Medicine* **333**:450–451. DOI:10.1056/NEJMs199508173330710

85. Collier AC, Coombs RW, Schoenfeld DA, *et al.* (1996) Treatment of human immunodeficiency virus infection with saquinavir, zidovudine, and zalcit-abine. *New England Journal of Medicine* **334**:1011–1018. DOI:10.1056/NEJM19960413341602

86. Hayden FG. (2006) Antiviral resistance in influenza viruses — implications for management and pandemic response. *New England Journal of Medicine* **354**:785–788. DOI:10.1056/NEJMp068030

87. Kabinger F, Stiller C, Schmitzová J, *et al.* (2021) Mechanism of molnupira-vir-induced SARS-CoV-2 mutagenesis. *Nature Structural & Molecular Biology* **28**:740–746. https://doi.org/10.1038/s41594-021-00651-0

88. Haseltine WA. (2021) Supercharging new viral variants: The dangers of molnupiravir (Part 1). *Forbes*, December 8. https://www.forbes.com/sites/williamhaseltine/2021/11/01/supercharging-new-viral-variants-the-dan-gers-of-molnupiravir-part-1/?sh=76d543576b15

89. Nelson CW, Otto SP. (2021) Mutagenic antivirals: The evolutionary risk oflowdoses.https://virological.org/t/mutagenic-antivirals-the-evolutionary-risk-of-low-doses/768

89A. Tay JH, Porter AF, Wirth W, Duchene S. (2022 Feb 3) The Emergence of SARS-CoV-2 Variants of Concern Is Driven by Acceleration of the Substitu-tion Rate. *Mol Biol Evol.* **39**(2):msac013. doi: 10.1093/molbev/msac013

90. Domingo E, Sheldon J, Perales C. (2012) Viral quasispecies evolution. *Microbiology and Molecular Biology Reviews* **76**(2):159–216. DOI:10.1128/MMBR.05023-11

91. Laamarti M, Alouane T, Kartti S, *et al.* (2020) Large scale genomic analy-sis of 3067 SARS-CoV-2 genomes reveals a clonal geo-distribution and a rich genetic variations of hotspots mutations. *PLOS One* **15**(11):e0240345. DOI:10.1371/journal.pone.0240345

92. Pachetti M, Marini B, Benedetti F, *et al.* (2020) Emerging SARS-CoV-2 mutation hot spots include a novel RNA-dependent-RNA polymerase var-iant. *Journal of Translational Medicine* **18**:179. https://doi.org/10.1186/s12967-020-02344-6

93. Wilkinson SAJ, Richter A, Casey A, *et al.* (2022) Recurrent SARS-CoV-2 mutations in immunodeficient patients. *medRxiv*, March 2. https//doi.org/10.1101/2022.03.02.22271697

94. Monroe JG, Thanvi S, Carbonell-Bejerano P, *et al.* (2020) Mutation bias shapes gene evolution in Arabidopsis thaliana. *bioRxiv*, June 18. https://doi.org/10.1101/2020.06.17.156752

95. Martin DP, Weaver S, Tegally H, *et al.* (2021) The emergence and ongoing convergent evolution of the N501Y lineages coincides with a major global shift in the SARS-CoV-2 selective landscape. *medRxiv*, July 25. DOI:10.1101/2021.02.23.21252268

96. Rochman ND, Wolf YI, Faure G, *et al.* (2021) Ongoing global and regional adaptive evolution of SARS-CoV-2. *Proceedings of the National Academy of Sciences* **118**(29):e2104241118. https://doi.org/10.1073/pnas.2104241118

97. Van Dorp L, Acman M, Richard D, *et al.* (2020) Emergence of genomic diversity and recurrent mutations in SARS-CoV-2. *Infection Genetics Evolution* **83**:10435. https//doi.org/10.1016/j.meegid.2020.104351

98. WHO. (2021) HIV/AIDS. Key facts. World Health Organization, November 30. https://www.who.int/news-room/fact-sheets/detail/hiv-aids#:~:text=There%20were%20an%20estimated%2037.7,2.0%20million%5D%20people%20acquired%20HIV

99. Worobey M, Levy JI, Serrano LM, *et al.* (2022) The Huanan Seafood Wholesale Market in Wuhan was the early epicenter of the COVID-19 pandemic. *Science*, July 26. DOI:10.1126/science.abp8715

100. Pekar JE, Magee A, Parker E, *et al.* (2022) The molecular epidemiology of multiple zoonotic origins of SARS-CoV-2. *Science*, July 26. DOI:10.1126/science.abp8337

101. Lytras S, Hughes J, Martin D, *et al.* Exploring the natural origins of SARS-CoV-2 in the light of recombination. Genome *Biology and Evolution*, **14**(2):evac018. DOI:10.1093/gbe/evac018

102. Sánchez CA, Li H, Phelps KL, *et al.* (2022) A strategy to assess spillover risk of bat SARS-related coronaviruses in Southeast Asia. *Nature Communications* **13**:4380. https://doi.org/10.1038/s41467-022-31860-w

103. He W-T, Hou X, Zhao J, *et al.* (2022) Virome characterization of game animals in China reveals a spectrum of emerging pathogens Cell, March 31. https://doi.org/10.1016/j.cell.2022.02.014

11 The Human Side

Disasters provoke human response. The Coronavirus Pandemic was no exception.

Once COVID-19 infected a community, certain activities occurred, no matter where you lived...

We waited in lines....

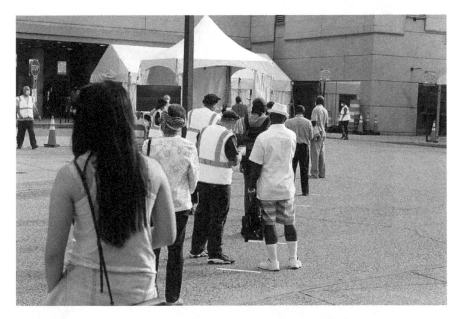

Figure 11.87. COVID-19 testing. Checking-In for COVID-19 Testing at Baltimore Convention Center at West Conway and South Sharpe Street in Baltimore MD, US on Friday morning, June 19, 2020.

Photo credit: Elvert Barnes Photography
https://commons.wikimedia.org/wiki/File:02.CheckIn.CV19Test.BaltimoreMD.19June2020_(50023384657).jpg

Stores sold out....

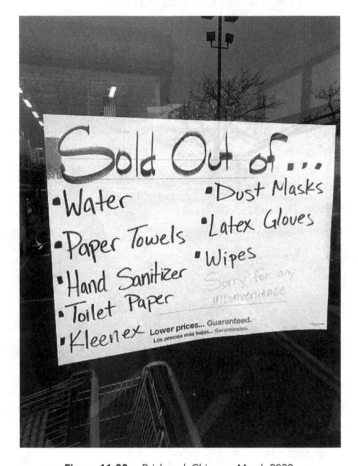

Figure 11.88.   Brickyard, Chicago, March 2020.
Photo credit: Awkwafaba
https://commons.wikimedia.org/wiki/File:Sold_out_during_COVID-19_outbreak_at_home_
improvement_box_store_in_Brickyard.jpg

Emergency rooms overflowed with COVID-19 patients.

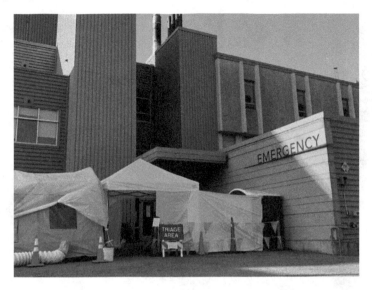

Figure 11.89.   COVID triage outside an hospital's emergency room, March 2020.
Photo credit: James Brooks
https://commons.wikimedia.org/wiki/File:Bartlett_Regional_Hospital_COVID_triage.jpg

Then ICUs.

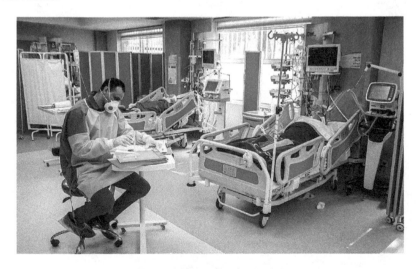

Figure 11.90.   Pandemic ICU.
Source: Fars News Agency — Mohsen Atayi/CC BY 4.0
https://commons.wikimedia.org/wiki/File:Pandemic_photomontage_COVID-19.png

Then entire hospitals.

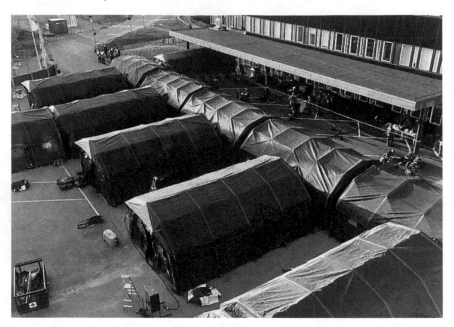

Figure 11.91.   Field hospital in Gothenburg, Sweden, March 2020.
Photo credit: Helen Sjoland
https://commons.wikimedia.org/wiki/File:%C3%96stra_Sjukhuset_COVID-19_F%
C3%A4ltsjukhus.jpg

We experienced ventilator, dialysis machine, drugs, and oxygen shortages.

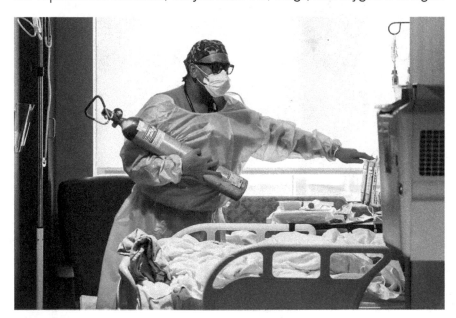

Figure 11.92.   Oxygen tank being replaced for a COVID patient by a US Navy Critical Care Nurse in Lafayete, Louisiana, August 26, 2021.
Photo credit: Mass Communication Specialist 2nd Class Michael H. Lehman.
https://commons.wikimedia.org/wiki/File:NEPLO_Surges_Medical_Teams_Back_Into_COV-ID_Hotspot210826-N-PC620-0047.jpg

And patients died....
Time of Death: 7:19pm
By: Dr. Craig Spencer, NYC ED physician, With permission.

We stop the drips.
Turn off the ventilator.
And wait.
You think of their family. At home. Sobbing.
Someone starts saying a prayer.
You can't help but cry.
This isn't what we do.
You stand by. You wait.
This isn't what we do.
You stand by. You wait.
Time of death: 7:19pm.

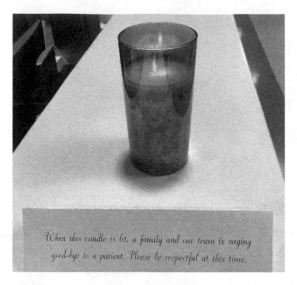

Figure 11.93.   Respect for the dying. Grand Strand Medical Center, Myrtle Beach, South Carolina, US, fall 2020.
Photo courtesy of R. Sherertz.

Sometimes in overwhelming numbers.

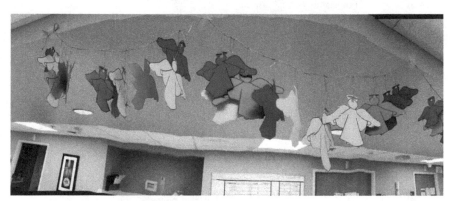

Figure 11.94.   One angel for every patient that died. Grand Strand Medical Center, Myrtle Beach, South Carolina, US, fall 2020.
Photo courtesy of R. Sherertz.

Requiring unprecedented body storage methods.

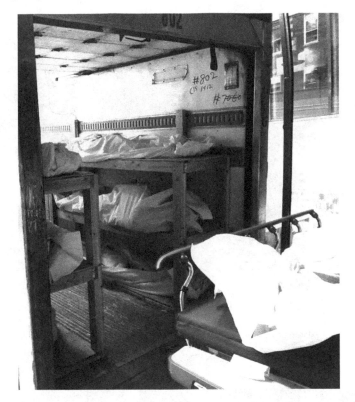

Figure 11.95.   Refrigerated truck holding the COVID-19-deceased in Hackensack, NJ, April 27.
Photo credit: Lawrence Purce
https://commons.wikimedia.org/w/index.php?search=COVID-19-deceased+in+Hackensack%2C+NJ%2C++April+27.&title=Special:MediaSearch&go=Go&type=image

Some parts of the world allowed funerals to be attended.

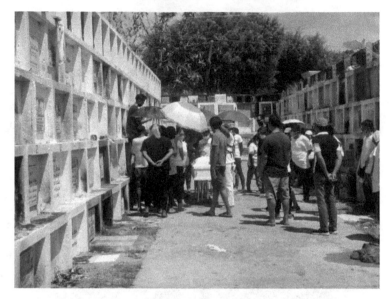

Figure 11.96.   Baliuag, Bulacan, Philippines, March 2020.
Photo credit: Judgefloro
https://commons.wikimedia.org/wiki/File:8136Coronavirus_pandemic_in_Baliuag,_Bulacan_68.jpg

Some did not.

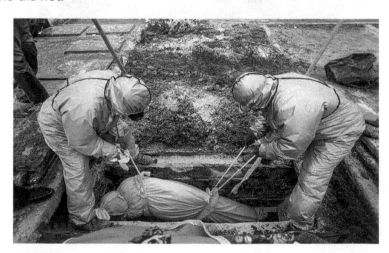

Figure 11.97.   Temporary graves in Hamadan, Iran, during the COVID-19 pandemic, March 2020.
Photo credit: Behzad Alipour
https://commons.wikimedia.org/wiki/File:Temporary_graves_in_Iran_during_COVID-19_pandemic_1.jpg

Sometimes, mass COVID-19 cemeteries became necessary.

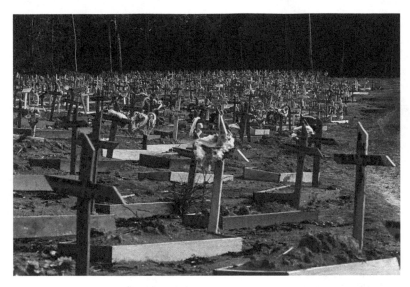

Figure 11.98. COVID-19 cemetery, Manaus Brazil. Foto Marcio James/Semcom PM Manaus Cemitério, November 16, 2020.
https://commons.wikimedia.org/wiki/File:Secretaria_de_Sa%C3%BAde_da_PM_de_Manaus_(50608864473).jpg

In heavily infected countries, drastic measures were taken: Stay-at-home orders were issued.

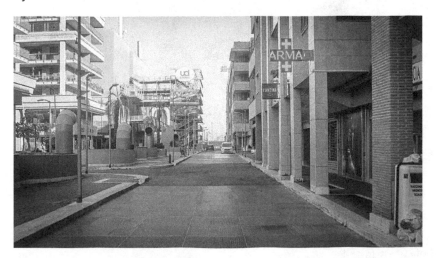

Figure 11.99. COVID-19 lockdown, Fiumicino (Rome), Italy.
Photo credit: Nicola
https://commons.wikimedia.org/wiki/File:Italy_Lockdown_-_IMG_6490_(49727982548).jpg

Airplane travel was greatly decreased.

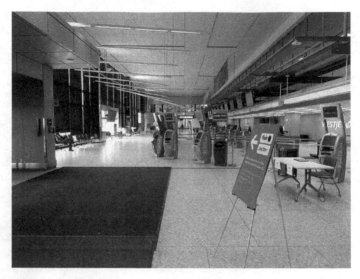

Figure 11.100. Edmonton International Airport departures area, empty of passengers because of travel and entry restrictions during COVID-19, April 2020.
Photo credit: Khoshhat
https://commons.wikimedia.org/wiki/File:Edmonton_International_Airport_departures_area_Covid-19_impact.jpg

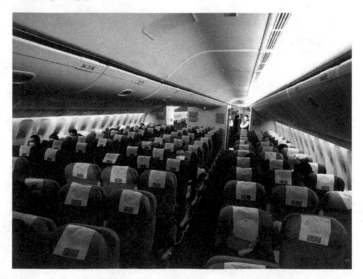

Figure 11.101. Near empty flight from PEK to LAX in March 2020.
Photo credit: Mx. Granger
https://commons.wikimedia.org/wiki/File:A_nearly_empty_flight_from_PEK_to_LAX_amid_the_COVID-19_pandemic_1.jpg

Mask orders were issued. Embraced by some. Not by others.

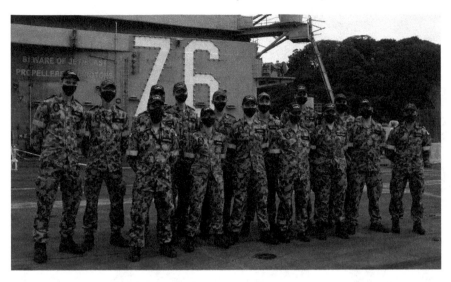

Figure 11.102.   Mask wearing by Royal Australian Navy. October 31, 2021.
Photo credit: Mass Communication Specialist Seaman George Cardenas
https://commons.wikimedia.org/wiki/File:Sailors_from_HMAS_Brisbane_tour_USS_Ronald_
Reagan_while_wearing_face_masks_in_November_2021.jpg

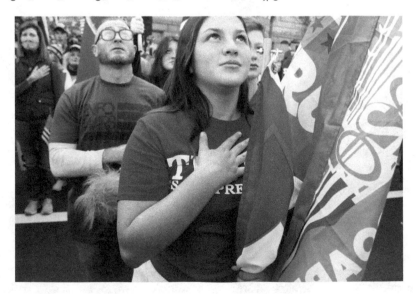

Figure 11.103.   Lack of mask wearing at a Trump rally, November 2020.
https://commons.wikimedia.org/wiki/File:41.Rally.MAGA.PennAve.WDC.14Novem-
ber2020_(50802949458).jpg

Some schools were closed.

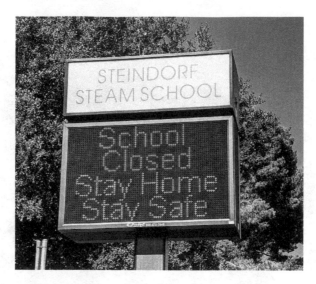

Figure 11.104.   School closure.
Photo credit: Travis Wise, May 15, 2020
https://commons.wikimedia.org/wiki/File:Steindorf_STEAM_School,_San_Jose,_California,_May_15,_2020.jpg

Some stayed open.

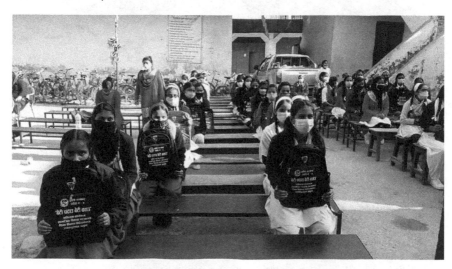

Figure 11.105.   Photo credit: Krishna590, February 2021.
https://commons.wikimedia.org/wiki/File:Student_condition_in_covid.jpg

Protests to the many societal interventions happened globally.

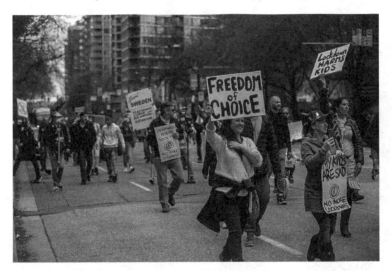

Figure 11.106.   Protest march, Vancouver, British Columbia, April 2020.
Photo credit: GoToVan
https://commons.wikimedia.org/wiki/File:COVID-19_Vancouver%27s_largest_protest,_
April_26th_2020_(49823131178).jpg

But … Humanity is resilient and found solutions.
Socializing while social distancing.

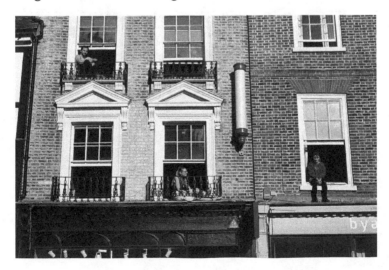

Figure 11.107.   Social distancing, April 2020.
Photo credit: Gyles Glover
https://commons.wikimedia.org/wiki/File:Social_distance_on_Kings_Parade.jpg

Music with social distancing.

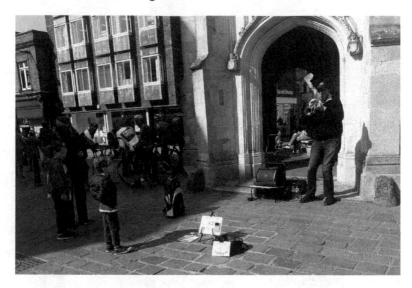

Figure 11.108.   Busking at the Cross in Chichester, England, April 2021.
Photo credit: Djm-leighpark
https://commons.wikimedia.org/wiki/File:Busking_at_the_Cross_in_Chichester,_England_
following_lockdown_step_2_easing_Wednesday_14_April_2021.jpg

And Love… it happens with or without pandemic interventions.

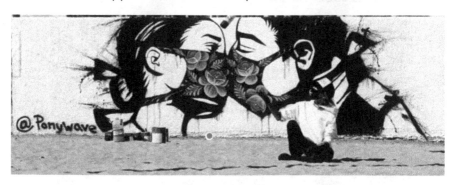

Figure 11.109.   Love during the pandemic.
Photo credit: Top Pony Wave, with permission.
https://www.greylockglass.com/2020/05/05/street-art-is-having-a-moment-is-it-a-pivotal-
one

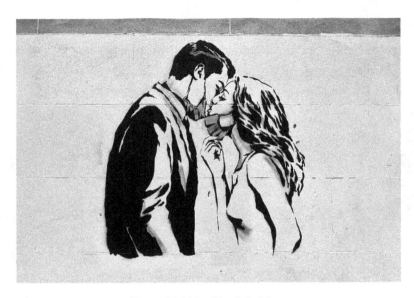

Figure 11.110. The Rebel Bear.
Photo credit: Daniel Naczk, April 2020
https://commons.wikimedia.org/wiki/File:Glasgow._Bank_Street._Graffiti._jpg.jpg

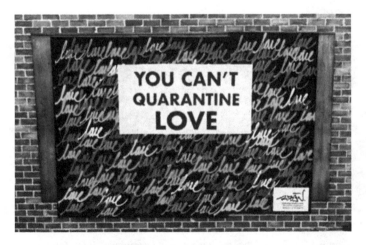

Figure 11.111. Photo credit: Ruben Rojas, with permission.
https://www.nytimes.com/2020/05/01/arts/design/street-murals-art-los-angeles-virus.html

And Hope and Faith persisted.

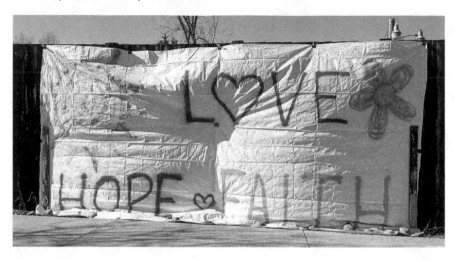

Figure 11.112.   Love, Hope, Faith during the pandemic.
Photo credit: Xnatedawgx, May 2020.
https://commons.wikimedia.org/wiki/File:Love,_Hope_%26_Faith_sign_during_the_pandemic._2020-05-04.jpg

We thanked our healthcare workers and first responders.

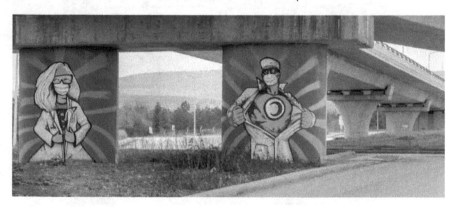

Figure 11.113.   Ankara healthcare workers murals, Murat Karabulut.
https://commons.wikimedia.org/wiki/File:Ankara_healthcare_workers_murals_(1).jpg

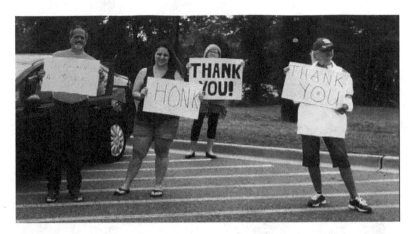

Figure 11.114. Grand Strand Medical Center, Myrtle Beach, South Carolina, US, with permission.

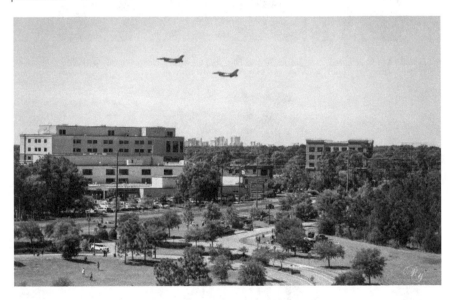

Figure 11.115. The South Carolina Air National Guard performing a flyover with F-16 fighter jets celebrating healthcare providers, Grand Strand Medical Center, Myrtle Beach, South Carolina, US.
Photo credit: Paul Yurkin, with permission.

We remained optimistic that SARS-CoV-2 could be defeated.

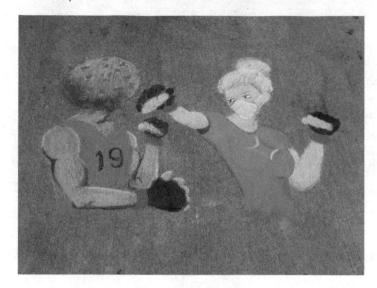

Figure 11.116.   Sidewalk art, Grand Strand Medical Center, Myrtle Beach, South Carolina, US.

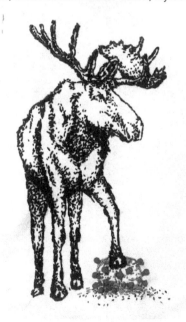

Figure 11.117.   Artist: Betsy Sherertz, Oslo, Norway. Needlework: Elizabeth Sherertz, Murrells Inlet, South Carolina, US, with permission.

Finally, in December 2020, definitive hope arrived, in the form of COVID-19 vaccines.

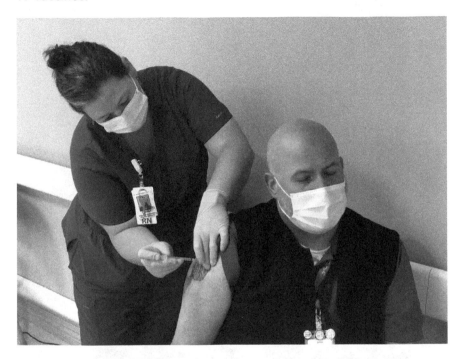

Figure 11.118.   Grand Strand Medical Center, Myrtle Beach, South Carolina, US, with permission.

And a new optimism was felt.

Go Be Free
By: Jax Sherertz, Age: 9, with permission.

Covid is a horrible thing,
Making our notifications go "Ring Ring Ring!"
Stay inside,
Stay away from others, and put those masks on!
Everyday we sit in our house nearly locking ourselves inside,
But the truth is, we don't have to hide!
Now we have vaccines for this horrible virus, and things are opening up and all you need is a mask! Or sometimes also a negative test.
So make a reservation and let the world do the rest.
You can go to Disneyland, or Disney World which is even better!
Or you can see a movie like The Croods 2 or Raya and The Last Dragon, which in my opinion, rules!
So here I say, Go, Be, Free!!!

We must remember what happened, learn from our mistakes and do better in the future.

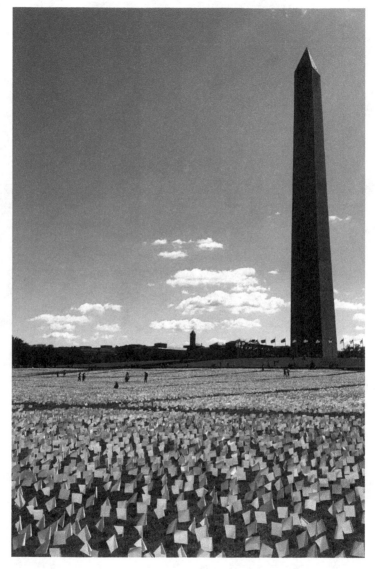

Figure 11.119. September 26, 2021, 687,764 white flags, one for each US COVID-19 death through that date.
Photo credit: L. Kaplowitz, with permission.

Acknowledgments

We are greatly indebted to Drs. Alejandro Cravioto, Kari Johansen, Lisa Kaplowitz, Douglas Lyles, Jim Peacock, and Dick Wenzel for reviewing various chapters in this book, and especially to Chuck Diggins and Dr. Larry Givner for reviewing the entire book.

We would further like to thank the many people who shared or helped us create images that could be used in this book: Jeffrey Aronson (Figure 1.4), Rebecca Abramson (Figures 3.37, 3.39, 3.43, 3.44, 3.45, 3.46, 3.47), Elvert Barnes (Figures 11.87 and 11.103), Awkwafaba (Figure 11.88), James Brooks (Figure 11.89), Mohsen Atayi (Figure 11.90), Helen Sjoland (Figure 11.91), Michael Lehman (Figure 11.92), Robert Sherertz (Figures 11.93, 11.94), Lawrence Purce (Figure 11.95), Judgefloro (Figure 11.96), Behzad Alipour (Figure 11.97), Marcio James (Figure 11.98), Nicola (Figure 11.99), Khoshhat (Figure 11.100), Mx. Granger (Figure 11.101), George Cardenas (Figure 11.102), Travis Wise (Figure 11.104), Krishna590 (Figure 11.105), GoToVan (Figure 11.106), Gyles Glover (Figure 11.107), Djm-leighpark (Figure 11.108), Pony Wave (Figure 11.109), Daniel Naczk (Figure 11.107), Ruben Rojas (Figure 11.111), Xnatedawgx (Figure 11.112), Murat Karabulut (Figure 11.113), Paul Yurkin (Figure 11.115), Betsy Sherertz/Beth Sherertz (Figure 11.117), Lisa Kaplowitz (Figure 11.119), Grand Strand Medical Center (Figures 11.114, 11.116, 11.118), and Ruth Karron (Figure 11.118).

We also are thankful to our families for their patience and understanding while we spent many hours during the past few years researching and writing this book.

Index

access to COVID-19 tools (ACT)-Accelerator programs, 195, 213, 214

acquired immunodeficiency syndrome (AIDS) patients, 153, 154, 446

Adult Respiratory Distress Syndrome (ARDS), 166

Advisory Committee on Immunization Practices (ACIP), xxii, 262

Aedes aegypti, 326, 341, 342, 345

Aedes albopictus, 343

Africa, 13, 31, 32, 48, 49, 62, 97–100, 105, 106,108, 229, 231, 234, 292, 296, 301, 323, 328, 331, 333, 338, 340, 343–350, 355, 361, 414, 446

African Task Force for Coronavirus, 32

agricultural society, 299

airborne transmission, 123, 124, 324, 350, 352–354, 363

allergic rhinitis, 156, 356

"America First" policy, 207

American Society of Testing and Materials (ASTM), 124

Americas regions, 23, 45–48, 86–97

anaphylaxis, vaccine-related, 206

angiotensin-converting enzyme 2 (ACE2) receptor, Figure 4.56, 4.57, 4, 120, 159–162, 164, 168, 170

angiotensin 2 receptor blockers (ARB), 160

Antarctica, 23, 54

antibody tests, 131–133

anticoagulation, 139, 140, 144–146, 167, 173, 353

antigen tests, 131, 132

anti-inflammatory drugs, 151

anti-inflammatory effect, 146, 159

antiphospholipid syndrome, 171

antituberculous treatment, 350

Aristotle's Theory of Spontaneous Generation, 302

Asia region, 41
    containment and mitigating policy, 15, 41, 64, 70, 82, 107, 254, 409
    population movement restrictions, 71

asymptomatic infection, 11, 149, 165, 322, 333, 363, 441

Atlas, Scott Dr.; Stanford School of Medicine, 91

Australia, 43, 108, 253, 296, 302, 433

Azar, Alex; Health and Human Services Secretary under President Trump, 89

azithromycin (antibiotic), 135

bacille Calmette-Guerin (BCG) vaccine, 258, 350

bacterial pneumonia, 161, 166, 351

bamlanivimab, monoclonal antibody targeting SARS-CoV-2 spike protein, 144

basic reproduction number, R_0, 9–11,
     319, 321, 325, 331, 332
bat coronavirus strain, 290
bats, Table 9.29, Figure 9.83, 5, 6, 13,
     169, 287, 289–293, 295, 296, 298,
     304, 322, 325, 328, 336, 351, 359,
     362–364, 417–420, 447
Beijing China Xinfadi Agricultural
     Market, 72
Bhattacharya, Jay Dr.; Stanford School
     of Medicine, 82
Biden, Joe; US President, 414
Bill & Melinda Gates Foundation, 201
Biomedical Advanced Research
     Development Authority (BARDA),
     207
blood clotting system, 155
Bolsonaro, Jair; President of Brazil, 107
Bordetella Pertussis (Pertussis), 298,
     333, 334
Borrelia burgdorferi (Lyme disease), 322
brake strategy, 83
Brazil, 13, 44, 86, 107, 147, 168, 169,
     202, 203, 231, 232, 257, 259, 263,
     268, 302, 411, 421, 467
breath, shortness of, 121, 126, 139,
     149, 150, 156, 157
Brix, Deborah Dr.; Coronavirus
     Response Coordinator under
     President Trump, 90
broad-spectrum antiviral activity, 28
bubonic plague, 336, 337

Campbell, William Dr.; Nobel
     Laureate, 303
Canada, 23, 45, 47, 48, 61, 86, 96,
     97, 106, 231, 261
     deaths per capita in, 45, 48, 96
     economic impact, 96

healthcare system, 96
     mitigation policy in, 97
     testing and tracking system, 96
     travel restrictions, 96
Caplan, Arthur Dr.; New York
     University School of Medicine, 267
cardiac fibroblasts, 164
cardiomyocyte infection, 164
cardiovascular disease, 133, 219, 222
case fatality rates (CFRs), COVID-19,
     6, 11, 29, 45, 105, 106, 121, 147,
     209, 210, 259
CD4 lymphocytes, 154, 162, 168
CD8 lymphocytes, 162, 168
Centers for Disease Control (CDC)
     Africa CDC, 32
     China CDC, 410
     European CDC (European Centre
          for Disease Prevention and
          Control), 232
     US CDC, 29, 31, 32, 84, 89, 91, 92,
          98, 125, 132, 149, 150, 210,
          252, 261, 263, 264, 271, 288,
          294, 327, 410, 416
C. difficile colitis, 323
central nervous system (CNS), 155
cerebrospinal fluid, 153
cerebrovascular disease, 133
chest CT (computerized tomography),
     Figures 4.49, 4.52, 4.54,
     Table 4.7, 126, 127, 129, 135, 140
chickenpox infection (Varicella zoster
     virus), 333
children, xxii, 16, 29, 78, 120,
     148–153, 215, 218, 224, 232,
     233, 250–254, 267, 270–272, 329,
     333–335, 338, 344, 351, 416, 436,
     325, 439
     asymptomatic infection, 149

COVID risk-free environment, 416
signs and symptoms in, 150
vaccination programs, 251, 439
China, 1, 2, 5, 6, 23, 24, 26–30, 32,
33, 34, 40–45, 49, 61, 71–75, 106,
107, 136, 152, 154, 157, 169, 201,
204, 217, 231, 233, 251, 257, 268,
288, 290–294, 318, 337, 338, 343,
352, 353, 410, 421, 433, 434, 447
COVID-19 cases in, 29, 30, 44, 45,
103, 149, 234
economic impact, 63, 74, 217
essential activities, 71
essential workers, 71
income support and debt relief, 74
lockdowns, 45, 63, 76, 78, 91, 108,
225, 254, 272, 409
outbreaks, 72
quarantines, 45, 76
SARS-CoV-2 elimination approach,
70, 71
shuts down public transportation, 27
social media platform, 73
Wuhan epidemic curve, Figure 2.8,
26
cholera (Vibrio cholerae), 336
cholesterol, 139
chronic lung disease, 133
chronic lymphocytic leukemia, 171
cinchona bark, 345
Clark, Helen; Prime Minister New
Zealand, 40
clinical manifestations, COVID-19,
Table 4.4, 120, 122, 151, 154, 157,
165, 172, 347
arterial thrombosis, 412
asymptomatic, 67, 72, 120, 121,
130, 147, 149, 152, 165, 166,
170, 322, 326, 328, 332–334,
340, 343, 345, 348, 349, 351,
352, 353, 363
autopsy, 162
central nervous system (CNS), 155
chest CT, CTA scans, Figures 4.49,
4.52, 4.54, Table 4.7, 127, 129,
135, 140
chest X-ray, Figures 4.49, 4.54,
Table 4.7, 126, 127, 129, 135,
139, 140, 153
common symptoms, 121
diagnostic testing, PCR vs antigen
vs antibody, Figures 4.50, 4.51,
Table 4.8, 130–132
embolic and thrombotic events,
120, 134
emergency department findings,
Table 4.5, 121, 128
encephalitis, 155, 156, 196, 417
encephalopathy, 155
fatal outcome, 120, 139, 140
gastroenteritis, 297, 327
Guillain-Barre, 155
immunocompromised patients,
121, 153, 442
laboratory abnormalities, Table 4.6,
Figures 4.53, 4.55, 126, 128,
137, 141
long COVID/long haulers, 156, 157,
441, 442
meningitis, 153, 155, 298, 325, 333
Multisystem Inflammatory
Syndrome in Children
(MIS-C), Tables 4.10, 4.11,
4.12, 148–151
myocardial infarction, 138,140, 159
myocarditis, 163
persistent infection, 120, 140, 142,
171, 413, 431, 441–443

pneumonia, 5, 6, 26, 29, 119, 126,
    127, 129, 130, 134–136, 138,
    145, 153–156, 161, 166, 318,
    322, 336, 351, 417
pregnancy, 120, 152, 153
pulmonary embolus, 122,135
reinfection, 120, 139, 140, 142,
    158, 167, 412, 413
risk factors for hospital admission,
    133
seizure, 155, 441
stroke, 122, 154, 155, 157, 412,
    441
symptoms, xix, xxiii, 11, 67, 80,
    119–121, 123, 125, 145,
    149–152, 155, 157, 158, 167,
    169, 206, 353, 363, 412,
    440–442, 444
time course of appearance of viral
    antigens, viral antibodies,
    Figure 4.50, 130
transmission risk, 120–125, 350
treatment, Tables 4.9, 10.30, 143,
    444
venous thrombosis, 120, 122, 136,
    139, 412
clinical updates, 2022, 440–445
immunocompetent adults, 413,
    437, 440
immunocompromised patients,
    413, 431, 442
persistent infection, 413, 431,
    441–443
treatment effectiveness, 443
Clostridium difficile (colitis), 297, 323
Clostridium tetani (tetanus), 298, 321
coagulopathy, 159, 166, 167
Coalition for Epidemic Preparedness
    Innovation (CEPI), 39, 201, 214

Cohen, Glenn Dr., Harvard Law
    School, 265
collateral damage, Chapter 6, 249,
    250, 438, 440
birth rate, decreased, 250
drug shortages, 251, 255
economic impact, 74, 82, 96, 266,
    409, 431, 438
elective surgeries, 249, 251, 252
equipment shortages, 249, 255,
    258
ethical issues, 140, 148, 222, 225,
    228, 238, 250, 258, 264–267,
    272, 273
excess deaths, Figure 6.68, 255,
    256, 435
immigrants, 250, 261
influenza, 249, 253, 254, 262, 267,
    268
malaria control, 439
misinformation, 101, 249, 257
outpatient visits, 251
prisoners, 250, 260
psychological impact, 254
racial disparities, 219, 250, 259,
    260
routine vaccinations, decreased,
    252
RSV infections, 253
school closure impacts, 270
sexually transmitted diseases
    (STDs), 335
tuberculosis and hiv control, 439
vaccination programs, 217, 223,
    431, 439
vaccines, exclusion of pregnant
    females, 262
vaccines, use for political
    advantage, 232

colonization (colonialism), 288,
302–304, 323, 361
community-acquired pneumonia, 130,
135, 136
community, psychological impact, 254
contact tracing, 6, 63, 68, 71, 73, 80,
82, 89, 93, 102, 348, 350, 354, 355,
361
containment and mitigating steps,
63, 64
China vs. India, 71
elimination vs mitigation, 70, 71
government policies, 64, 75, 82, 100
Iran vs. Jordan, 62, 101
quick approach, 70, 71
South Africa vs. African Region, 98
Sweden vs. Norway, 78
US vs. Canada, 86
control measures, 43, 101, 108, 354,
355, 409
convalescent plasma, 126, 139, 143,
145, 146, 148, 168, 170, 171, 353,
443–445
coronary artery calcium (CAC), 164
coronary artery disease, 139, 154,
160, 164
coronaviruses, Table 1.1, xix, 9, 11,
15, 23, 31, 35, 37, 39, 40, 43–45,
48, 61, 70, 74, 75, 78, 96, 100, 102,
104, 108, 130, 133, 165, 167
animal species infected, 289
betacoronavirus, 6
ecology of, Figure 7.69, 289
evolution, Figure 9.81, 13, 14,
169–172, 289, 292, 294,
295, 351, 403, 411, 413, 416,
418–420, 434, 442, 443, 446,
447

human coronaviruses, 1, 5, 7, 8
human population, 171, 295, 296,
363
replication, Figure 1.2, 1, 3, 4, 130,
142, 169–171, 342, 350, 442,
445
structure, Figure 1.1, 3
coronavirus strain (SARS-CoV-2), 1
Coronavirus Task Force, 89–91
Corynebacterium diphtheriae
(diphtheria), 298, 333, 334
COVID-19 cemetery, 467
COVID-19 pandemic; see also
individual entries, xix, xxi, 9, 11, 15,
23, 31, 35, 37, 39, 40, 43, 44, 45,
48, 61, 70, 74, 75, 78, 96, 100, 102,
104, 130, 133, 167, 196, 207, 211,
213, 219, 221, 224, 250, 251, 253,
254, 258, 267, 270, 271, 404–406,
408, 409, 414, 416, 431, 432–435,
439, 440, 466
admissions, risk factors, 133
adult manifestations of, 122
birth rate impact, 250
Canada, 23, 45, 47, 48, 61, 86, 96,
97, 106, 231, 261
case fatality by focus countries
during 2020, 433
cases per million people,
Figures 2.13, 2.15, 2.17, 2.20,
2.24, 43, 45, 46, 47, 50, 53
deaths per million people,
Figures 2.14, 2.16, 2.18, 2.21,
2.25, 43–48, 50, 52, 53, 79,
84, 86, 87, 89, 90, 96, 99, 100,
103–106, 432
endemic disease, 211, 212, 434,
435

excess mortality, 255, 431, 435
fatality rates, 11, 121, 259, 335, 353, 440
flattening the curve, Figure 1.5, 15, 70
mask wearing, 38, 45, 63, 70, 76–78, 80, 90, 92–95, 105, 121, 123–125, 210, 218, 350, 352, 354, 357, 409, 423, 469
mitigation strategies, 15, 70, 76, 82, 85, 86, 97, 107, 108, 270, 403, 409
respiratory diseases, 5, 16, 31, 253, 254
risk factors controversy, 133
Solidarity Response Fund, 39
tests per 1000 people, 80
vaccination program, 208, 211, 216, 223, 226, 228, 230
waves, 16, 76, 87, 97, 106, 108, 337, 409, 433, 435
WHO declaration of pandemic, 24
Wuhan epidemic curve, 319
COVID-19 testing, 147, 320, 459
COVID-19 Tools Accelerator programs, 37
COVID-19 treatment, 143, 147, 444
  anticoagulation, 139, 140, 144–146, 167, 173, 353, 444
  convalescent plasma, 126, 139, 145, 146, 148, 168, 170, 171, 353, 443, 445
  effectiveness, 71, 120, 124, 125, 142, 168, 173, 212, 223, 225, 229, 431, 437, 443
  hydroxychloroquine, 143, 146, 147, 251, 257, 258, 444
  interleukin-6 (IL-6) inhibitors, 443, 444
  impact on mortality, 147
  ivermectin, 143, 146, 303, 444
  lopinavir-ritonavir, 143, 146, 444
  molnupiravir, 443–445
  monoclonal antibodies against spike protein, 353, 444
  remdesivir, 28, 99, 126, 139, 143, 146, 148, 170, 258, 444
  ritonavir/PF-07321332, 444
  steroids, 135, 142, 143, 146, 155, 156, 166, 173, 353, 443, 444
COVID-19 Vaccine Access (COVAX) Program and Facility, 214–216, 219, 227, 228, 238, 269, 436
COVID-19 vaccines, xix, xx, 40, 195, 196, 198–201, 204, 207, 209, 210, 212, 214–226, 229–234, 237, 238, 263, 264, 266, 268, 269, 272, 273, 408, 410, 413, 414, 477
  characteristics of, Tables 5.13, 5.14, Figure 5.61, 199–201, 204
  clinical evaluation of, Table 5.15, 201–203
  delivery and distribution, Figures 5.63, 5.65, Table 5.17, 205, 212, 218, 220, 225
  development of, Figure 5.60, Table 5.13, 40, 196, 201, 207, 263, 272, 335, 349
  effectiveness of, 223, 225, 229, 258, 437
  effect of prior COVID-19, 250, 271
  ethical issues, 258, 261
  foreign policy agenda, 268
  global availability, 435
  high risk groups for early vaccine administration, 265
  impact of variants, 169

inequity, Figures 5.67, 10.85, 234, 237, 403, 406, 413, 433, 439

life-threatening allergic reaction, 206

mandatory, xxi, 76, 268, 338

maternal immunization, 437

mRNA vaccines, Figure 5.62, 195, 204, 205, 207–9, 435, 437

nationalism for, 38, 216

pillars of ACT, Acceleratory" to "Accelerator Program", insert "Table 5.16, 39, 214

prediction of GDP growth by country, 84

pregnant women, Figure 10.86, 153, 250, 262, 263, 264, 436, 437

prioritization criteria, Table 5.17, Figure 5.64, 221, 222, 267

Prioritization Roadmap of, 220

prioritizing groups, 195, 219

SARS-CoV-2 variants, 13, 14, 195, 210, 212, 411, 412, 431, 434, 435, 436, 438, 441, 445, 446

side effects, 203, 206, 207, 338

spike protein vaccines, 434

vaccine administration by focus countries, 264

vaccine hesitancy, Tables 5.18, 5.19, 195, 196, 224, 228–237, 354

vaccine hesitancy, United States vs international media coverage, Figure 5.66, 236

vaccine passports, 250, 264–266

vaccine prioritization by country, 221

vaccination programs, 208, 211, 216, 223, 226, 228, 230

viral vector vaccines, 435

C-reactive protein (CRP), 128, 129

Crimean War, 300

cumulative COVID-19 cases, 31, 43, 46, 47, 50–53

cyclophosphamide, 170, 171

cystic fibrosis, 222

cytokine storm, 120, 144, 154, 165, 166, 167, 343

cytomegalovirus, 153, 154

deaths per capita, xx, 45, 48, 52, 79, 84, 86, 90, 96, 97, 99, 100, 103–106

decreased mortality, 142

deep venous thrombosis (DVT), 136, 139

Delta variant, 14

Dengue virus (*Flavivirus Dengue virus*), 297, 336, 343, 360

dexamethasone, 126, 136, 139, 143, 146, 148, 155

diabetes, 133, 134, 139, 159, 160, 173, 202, 219, 222, 356

diagnostic testing, antigens, antibodies, PCR for RNA, 130

dichlorodiphenyltrichloroethane (DDT), 346

diphtheria (*Corynebacterium diphtheriae*), 196, 224, 252, 325, 333–335

diphtheria, tetanus toxoids and pertussis-containing (DTP) vaccine, 136, 138, 139, 144, 224

disease pathogenesis, 362, 419, 423

droplet nuclei, 124

drug shortages, 251, 255

Eastern Mediterranean region, 23, 51, 100

Ebola, 28, 100, 144, 171, 172, 196,
    201, 231, 295, 297, 304, 318, 325,
    328, 354, 404, 406, 417, 419
    hemorrhagic fever, 154, 297, 328,
        340
    treatment of, 144, 151
    virus outbreak, 28, 343
Ebola virus, 28, 171, 201, 297, 328
echo studies, COVID-19, 163
economic impact of pandemic, 74,
    82, 96, 266, 431, 438
eculizumab, monoclonal antibody
    against complement protein C5,
    121, 126, 171
education system, 270
    educators, 270
    digital learning, 270, 271
    elementary school, 271
    impact on learning, 271
    mitigation policies, 15, 41, 70, 76,
        82, 85, 86, 97, 107, 108, 254,
        270, 272
    school closures impact, 270–272
    student education, 271
    virtual learning, 270
EK SARS-CoV-2 mutation 484K, 443
elderly populations, vaccine, 221
elective surgeries, 251, 252
embolic and thrombotic events, 134
    deep venous thrombosis, 136, 139,
        412
    myocardial infarctions, 138
    pulmonary emboli, 120, 129, 136,
        138, 139, 155
    strokes, 120, 136, 138, 139, 155,
        156
Emergency Use Authorization (EUA),
    92, 99, 132, 196, 198, 263

emerging infectious disease,
    definition of, 288, 304
emerging infectious diseases (EIDs),
    288, 296, 297, 303, 304, 359, 417,
    418, 422
    accelerating occurrence, 299
    agricultural society, Neolithic
        Period, 299
    bats, 418
    city size, 359
    colonization (colonialism), 323, 361
    famine, 287, 301, 303
    Germ Theory, 297, 303, 304, 337,
        338, 340, 347–350, 361, 362,
        364
    global trends, 317, 357, 359
    historically important infectious
        diseases, 1940–2020,
        Table 7.20, Figures 7.70, 8.74,
        880, 297, 299, 330, 360
    historically important infectious
        diseases, pre-1940, Table 7.21,
        Figures 7.70, 8.73, 8.74,
        880, 298, 299, 330, 339,
        360
    slavery, 301, 303, 304
    war, xxiii, xxvx, 287, 300, 322, 326,
        352, 439
encephalopathy, 155
endemic disease, 211, 212, 431, 434
England, 77, 92, 107, 143, 147, 149,
    207, 216, 217, 223, 300, 339, 472
    COVID-19 vaccine, 223
    healthcare system, 251
epidemic, causes, Table 8.23, 318,
    324–335
    chickenpox (*Varicellovirus human
        herpesvirus 3*), 333

diphtheria (*Corynebacterium diphtheriae*), 298, 333–335
dysentery (*Shigella*), 298
ebola (*Ebola virus*), 28, 201, 297, 328
epidemic typhus (*R.prowazekii*), 300
influenza A and B (*Orthomyxovirus A, B*), 212, 330
Marburg (*Marburg virus*), 297, 328
measles (*M.morbillivirus*), 333, 334
meningitis (*N.meningitidis*), 153, 298, 333
Middle East Respiratory Syndrome (MERS) (*Betacoronavirus MERS-CoV*), 2, 6, 8, 13, 16, 28, 29, 146, 168, 201, 287, 289–297, 304, 325, 328, 329, 354–356, 359, 417, 418, 420
mumps (*Paramyxovirus rubulavirus*), 196, 298, 325, 333, 334
Norovirus (*Norovirus norwalk*), 325, 327
pertussis (*Bordetella pertussis*), 298, 333, 334
polio (*Enterovirus poliovirus*), 252, 297, 298, 325, 327
rubella (*Rubivirus rubellae*), 325, 333
Severe Acute Respiratory Syndrome (SARS) (*Betacoronavirus SARS-CoV*), 5, 6, 417
scarlet fever (*Streptococcus. pyogenes*), 298, 333, 334, 335
syphilis (*Treponema pallidum*), 336
tuberculosis (*Mycobacterium tuberculosis*), 336
Zika (*Flavivirus zika*), 263, 325, 326, 341–345

epidemics, 1,7, 33, 34, 317, 320, 324–328, 330, 334, 336, 340, 348, 349, 354, 405, 406, 418, 421
    airborne transmission, 123, 124, 324, 350, 352–354, 363
    body fluid transmission, 324
    definition of, 288
    droplet transmission, 324
    epidemic curve, 319
    vector-borne, 324, 326
epidemic typhus (*Rickettsia prowazekii*), 298, 300, 325, 326
epidemiology, 220, 303, 317
erythrocyte sedimentation rate (ESR), 128, 129, 150
etesevimab, monoclonal antibody against SARS-CoV-2 spike protein, 144
ethical issues, 120, 140, 147, 148, 249, 258, 267
    drug trials, 249, 258
    education system, 270
    equipment shortages, 249, 255, 258
    immigrants, 250, 261
    prisoners, 260
    racial disparities, 219, 250, 259, 260
    vaccines, 250, 253, 254, 258, 261–263, 265–269, 272, 273
Europe, 28, 30, 45, 46, 61, 76–79, 92, 105, 107, 124, 149, 198, 216, 228–232, 234, 251, 270, 296, 301, 322, 328, 332, 333, 337, 338, 340, 344, 346, 349, 353, 361
    COVID-19 cases, 28, 42–48, 77, 107, 149, 234
    outpatient clinic visits, 251

public response, 77
travel restrictions, 32, 76, 96
vaccine hesitancy, xix, 195, 196,
    224, 228–237, 354
wearing masks, 77, 90, 92–94,
    125
European Commission, 30, 38, 40,
    226, 227
European Council, 421
European masks, N95 equivolent, EN
    Type IIR and FFP P2, 124
European Investment Bank, 40
European Medicines Agency (EMA),
    201, 436
European Union, 76
    color-coded system, 76
    travel policies, 76
excess mortality, 255, 435

famine, 301
fatality rate, 2, 6, 8, 10, 11, 16, 29, 52,
    105, 195, 209, 353
fatal outcome, COVID-19 reinfection,
    139
    treatment effectiveness, 443
fecal-oral transmitted, Tables 8.22,
    8.23, 8.24, 321, 323, 327, 331
Federal Reserve Board, 410
Federal Trade Commission, 410
field hospital in Gothenburg, 462
Finlay, Carlos Dr.; Physician
    co-discover of the importance of
    mosquitoes in Yellow Fever, 345
first pandemic wave, 52, 87, 89
flattening the curve, Figure 1.5, 15,
    70
Flavivirus West Nile virus (West Nile
    encephalitis), 297, 322
food allergies, 156

foreign policy agenda, 268
front-line health and social workers,
    219

Galen's Miasma Theory, 302
Gamaleya COVID-19 vaccine, 201,
    208, 209, 269
Gamaleya Research Institute in Russia,
    198
gastrointestinal (GI) tract, persistent
    SARS-CoV-2 infection, 442
gastrointestinal infection mortality
    (Shigella), 327
generalized pain (COVID-19), 157
gene sequencing data, 27
genetic factors, 134, 413
genetic mutations, 12, 14, 209
genetic recombination, 12
geriatric male, 121, 139, 154
Germ Theory, 337, 338, 340,
    347–350, 361, 362, 364
gestational age, 152
Global Alliance for Vaccines and
    Immunization (Gavi), 214–217
Global Alliance Partners, 39, 99
global health security, 404
Global Immunization Division, 252
Global Influenza Plan, 7
global non-exclusive voluntary
    licensing, 37
global pandemic treaty, 421
Global Preparedness Monitoring
    Board 2019 Annual Report on
    Global Preparedness for Health
    Emergencies, 88
global spread of COVID-19,
    Figure 2.6 (12/31/19-3/10/20),
    Figure 2.7 (3/10/20), Figure 2.10
    (1/22/20-12/30/20), Figures 2.11,

2.12 (2/23/20-12/30/20), 24, 25, 36, 42, 361

Africa regions, Figure 2.9 (2/16/20-5/22/20), 31

Canada, 23, 45, 47, 48, 61, 86, 96, 97, 106, 231, 261

Canada vs United States, Figures 2.17, 2.18 (1/1/20-12/30/20), 47

China, 1, 2, 5, 6, 23, 24, 26–30, 32, 33, 34, 40,45, 49, 61, 63, 71–75, 106, 107, 136, 152, 154, 157, 169, 201, 204, 217, 231, 233, 251, 257, 268, 288, 290–294, 318, 337, 338, 343, 352, 353, 410, 421, 433, 434, 447

China vs India, Figures 2.13, 2.14 (1/4/20-12/30/20), 43,44

COVID-19 outbreaks, 72

COVID testing globally, Figure 2.19 (1/1/20-12/28/20), 49

impact on economy, 63

India, xxiv, xxxi, 14, 23, 43–45, 61, 71, 73–75, 106, 147, 201, 231, 233, 251, 255, 259, 268, 269, 338, 344, 348, 355, 411, 414

Iran, 6, 23, 34, 51–53, 62, 100–104,

Iran vs Jordan, Figures 2.22, 2.23 (1/29/20-1/5/21), Figures 2.24, 2.25 (1/22/20-12/30/20), 51–53

Jordan, 6, 23, 51– 53, 62, 100–104, 106, 225

mortality, focus countries, Figure 3.48 (3/14/20-12/31/20), 106

Norway, 23, 45, 46, 61, 75, 78–86, 96, 101, 103, 104, 106, 201, 259, 261, 476

Norway vs Sweden, Figures 2.15, 2.16 (1/22/20-12/30/20), 46

South Africa, 23, 48–50, 62, 98, 99, 106, 168, 169, 202, 203, 210, 211, 234, 253, 414

South Africa vs other African countries, Figures 2.20, 2.21 (1/22/20-12/27/20), 50

Sweden, 23, 45, 46, 61, 78–83, 85, 86, 106, 107, 233, 261

United States, xxiii, xxiv, 23, 38, 45, 74, 123, 150, 198, 212, 250, 322, 330, 471

waves, 1, 16, 76, 87, 97, 106, 108, 168, 337, 409, 433, 435

WHO declaration of pandemic, 24

WHO regions, Figures 2.11, 2.12, (3/8/20-12/30/20), 42

global vaccination, 338, 423

global warming, 322, 349, 357, 358, 364, 418

glucocorticoids, 171

"God Committees", 255

Google mobility trends, 70

Gorgas, William, Dr.; Physician co-discover of the importance of mosquitoes in Yellow Fever, 345

Gostin, Lawrence; Professor, Georgetown University Law School, 265

Government Response Stringency Index, Figures 3.27, 3.28, 3.29, 3.30, 3.31, 3.32, 3.33, 3.34, 64–69

citizens, debt/contract relief for, 69

contact tracing policy, 68
containment and mitigation policy,
    64
face covering policy, 68
Government Stringency Index
government support of an
    individual's income, 69
government support of debt or
    contract relief, 69
public transport closure policy, 67
stay at home policy, 65
testing people stringency, 67
workplace closure policy, 66
Grand Strand Medical Center, 464,
    475–477
Great Barrington Declaration, focused
    protection, 82, 91, 92
Great Pox (smallpox), 328
gross domestic product (GDP), 96
Guangdong Province of China, 5
Guillain-Barre, 155
Gupta, Sunetra Dr.; Oxford University,
    82

Hansen's disease, 324
Health and Social Care Inspectorate,
    80
healthcare sectors, 64
healthcare systems, xix, 1, 15, 48, 64,
    434
healthcare workers (HCWs), 123, 221
    personal protective equipment, 93,
        121, 124, 318
heart disease, 120, 159, 161, 162, 202
heart failure, 134, 154, 159, 160, 356,
    441
herd immunity, 10, 11, 76, 78, 80, 82,
    91, 92, 107, 205, 210, 320, 340,
    342, 362

high-income countries, 38, 105,
    106, 196, 207, 213, 215–217, 221,
    224, 226, 227, 229, 231, 234, 237,
    264–266, 270, 408, 410, 413, 414
Hispanic ethnicity, 134, 149
historic infectious diseases mortality,
    330
HIV infection, 153, 171, 348, 350,
    445, 446
Hong Kong, 6, 43, 71, 108, 231, 433
Huanan Seafood Wholesale Market,
    26, 73, 446
human contact, transmission, 77, 326
human coronaviruses, 5, 8
Human COVID Genetic Effort, 413
human genetic factors, 413
human immune system, 170
human immunodeficiency virus
    (Lentivirus HIV-1), 336
humanity, xxx, xxxii, 153, 154, 292,
    299, 333, 336, 359, 364, 422
humanity, images, Chapter 11, 459
    COVID-19 ICU care, 461
    COVID-19 overwhelming hospitals,
        461, 462
    COVID-19 triage, 461
    COVID-19 testing lines, 459
    dying-related images, 464
    empty airports, airplanes, 468
    equipment shortages, O2, 463
    funerals, 466
    healthcare worker appreciation,
        474, 475
    honoring the dead, 478
    hope, 474
    love, 474
    mask wearing or not, 469, 472, 473
    mass graves, 467
    optimism, 476, 477

protest marches, 471
refrigerator truck for bodies, 465
school closings or not, 470
sidewalk art, 476
social distancing, 471, 472
societal lockdown, 467
stores sold out, 460
vaccination, 477
human settlements, Neolithic period,
    300
human tissue tropisms, 419, 420
human-to-human transmission, 5, 6
hydrophobia, 322
hydroxychloroquine, 144, 146, 147,
    251, 257, 258
hypertension, 133, 134, 139, 154,
    156, 157, 159–161, 202, 356
hypogammaglobulinemia, 171

ignorance, 288, 302, 303, 337, 338,
    340, 347, 349, 350, 364
IHR committee see International
    Health Regulation (IHR) committee,
    27
immigrants, 261
Immigration and Customs
    Enforcement (ICE) group, 261
immune response, 142, 158, 159, 166,
    168, 204, 205, 212, 290, 411, 434
immunity, 10, 11, 13, 76, 78, 80, 82,
    91, 92, 107, 108, 120, 133, 142,
    154, 162, 165, 166, 168, 205, 210,
    254, 320, 322, 333, 337, 338, 340,
    342–345, 348, 351, 354, 361, 362,
    364, 434, 437, 438, 442
immunocompetent adults, 413, 437,
    440
immunocompromised patients, 121,
    153, 413, 442

immunoglobulin, 149, 155
immunomodulatory agents, 151
incubation period, 319, 320, 347–349,
    351–353, 357
Independent Oversight and Advisory
    Committee (IOAC), 404
Independent Panel for Pandemic
    Preparedness and Response, 40,
    108, 405, 407, 409, 410
India, xxiv, xxxi, 14, 23, 43, 44, 45, 61,
    71, 73–75, 106, 147, 201, 231, 233,
    251, 255, 259, 268, 269, 338, 344,
    348, 355, 411, 414
    countrywide lockdown, 44
    COVID-19 cases, 44, 45
    economic impact, 74
    global public health, 14
    Individual Indian states, 73
    informal economy, 73
    migrant laborers, 74
    rural communities, 74
    strict lockdown, 71, 74
ineffective treatment, 143, 146, 444
inequity, 413
infectious disease, definition of, 288
infectious diseases, xxi, xxii, 125, 165,
    166, 201, 296–303, 321, 324, 328,
    330, 333–336, 354–357, 359, 360,
    363, 403, 418, 420–422
    treatment, xix, xxii, 37, 99, 120,
        137, 138, 140, 144, 146, 147,
        151, 153, 161, 166, 167, 171,
        202, 257, 258, 323, 324,
        326, 328–330, 333, 337, 340,
        342–345, 347, 348, 350, 352,
        353, 403, 422, 423, 442–445,
        497, 498
infectivity fatality rates (IFR), 11, 121,
    147, 353

inflammation blocking mechanism,
  160
inflammatory CNS syndromes, 155
inflammatory parameters, 129, 151
influenza (*Influenza virus*), 2, 7, 8, 9,
  12, 13,16, 108, 123, 124, 146, 157,
  162, 165, 171, 172, 173,186, 297,
  212, 226, 228, 238, 249, 253, 254,
  262, 267, 268, 295, 325, 326, 329,
  330. 332, 333, 335, 336, 351, 352,
  354, 356, 357, 360, 361, 362, 364,
  430, 435, 445
  H1N1 virus, 8, 12
informal economy, India, 73
intellectual property, 37, 408, 414
intensive care units (ICUs), 1, 28, 324
International Health Regulation (IHR)
  committee, 27, 28
International Money Fund (IMF), 84,
  103
International Vaccine Access Center
  (IVAC), 252
in vitro and in vivo activity, remdesivir,
  28
Iran, 6, 23, 34, 51–53, 62, 100–104,
  106, 225, 466
  economic effect, 102
  isolation policies, 102
  methanol alcohol, 101
  Obama administration, 102
  public health activities, 101
  SARS-CoV-2 testing, 100, 102
  social distancing, 101
  Trump administration, 102
  WHO public health experts, 101
Israel, 224–228, 264
  COVID-19 vaccine, 226, 264
  ethical issues, 225, 228, 264

Italy, 30, 34, 45, 76, 85, 147, 233,
  250, 259, 271, 346
ivermectin, 143, 146, 303, 444

Japan, 27, 28, 71, 108, 201
Jenner, Edward Dr.; discoverer of
  smallpox vaccine, 303
Jenner, William, 338
Johnson & Johnson (Janssen)
  vaccines, 207
Joint Allocation Taskforce (JAT), 219
Jordan, 23, 51–53, 62, 100–104, 106,
  225
  deaths per capita, 52, 100,
    103–106
  economy, 52, 101–104

Kawasaki disease, 150, 151, 152
kidney disease, 157, 161
Koch, Robert Dr.; physician discoverer
  of *M.tuberculosis*, 303
Korea, quick approach, 71
Kulldorff, Martin Dr., Harvard
  University biostatistician, 81

laboratory abnormalities, 126, 128,
  137, 141
laboratory data, 9, 319
lactate dehydrogenase (LDH), 126,
  128
Lancet COVID-19 Commission, 40
left ventricular systolic dysfunction,
  164
Legionella pneumophila (pneumonia),
  297, 322
Legionnaire's disease, 322
leprosy (*Mycobacterium leprae*), 298,
  321, 323, 324

lessons learned, 70, 147, 148, 231
  China vs. India, 71
  Iran vs. Jordan, 101
  South Africa vs African Region, 98
  Sweden vs Norway, 78
  United States vs Canada, 86
life-threatening allergic reaction,
  vaccines, 206
Lister, Joseph Dr.; physician
  discoverer of antisepsis, 303
Li Wenliang, Dr.; physician sounding
  alarm about COVID-19, 73
lockdowns, 63, 71, 76, 78, 91, 108,
  254, 272, 409
long COVID/long haulers, 156
lopinavir-ritonavir, HIV medication
  used to treat COVID-19 early in
  pandemic, 146
low-income countries, 35, 106, 434,
  436
lung disease, 120, 133, 161, 166
Lyme disease (*Borrelia burgdorferi*),
  321, 322
lymph node (lymphadenitis), 336
lymphocyte immune responses, 151
lymphocytopenia, 126, 128, 135, 148

malaria (*Plasmodium falciparum*), 336,
  344
Marburg hemorrhagic fever (*Marburg
  virus*), 328
Marburg virus, 297, 328
masks, xxv, xxvi, xxxii, xxxiii, 38, 45,
  63, 70, 76–78, 80, 90, 92–95, 105,
  121, 123–125, 210, 218, 350, 352,
  354, 357, 409, 423, 469
meadows, Mark; White House Chief
  or Staff under President Trump, 90

measles (*Measles morbillivirus*), 333
medical supplies availability, 90
meningococcal infection (*Neisseria
  meningitidis*), 333
Merck Pharmaceutical Company, 201
messenger RNA (mRNA), 4
Messonnier, Nancy Dr. head of US
  CDC Respiratory Branch, 31
methicillin-resistant *Staphylococcus
  aureus* (MRSA), 321
methylprednisolone, 143, 146, 149
microorganisms, xxi, 297, 299, 302,
  303, 364
Middle East Respiratory Syndrome
  (MERS), 28, 29, 146, 168, 201, 325,
  328, 329, 354–356, 359
middle-income countries, 105, 206, 217,
  218, 221, 224, 228, 265, 266, 272
migrant laborers, 74
misinformation, 101, 257
mitigation policies, 15, 70, 76, 82, 85,
  86, 97, 107, 108, 270, 403, 409
Moderna-NIH, 198, 200, 435
monoclonal antibodies, 144, 146,
  148, 168, 353, 444, 445
mortality, xix, 8, 9, 12, 13, 16, 39, 84,
  85, 86, 92, 100, 108, 120, 121, 129,
  133, 134, 142–148, 151, 153, 154,
  164, 165, 173, 212, 213, 255, 256,
  259, 260, 294, 300–302, 321–335,
  337–340, 344–349, 351–354, 361,
  363, 364, 431, 435, 439, 440,
  442–444
mosquito-borne infection, 340, 345
mRNA vaccines, 195, 204, 207, 208,
  209, 435, 437
Muller, Paul Hermann, chemist
  discoverer of DDT, 346

multidrug-resistant (MDR) organism, 350

Multisystem Inflammatory Syndrome in Children (MIS-C), 120, 148–152, 158
   case definition for, 150, 318
   clinical and pathologic findings, 151
   Kawasaki disease, 150–152
   Toxic Shock Syndrome, 151

mumps (*Mumps virus*), 298, 333, 334

mutation rate vs species genome size, Figure 4.58, 172

Mycobacterium leprae (leprosy), 298, 324

Mycobacterium tuberculosis (tuberculosis), 298, 324, 329, 336, 349

myocardial infarctions, 138

nasopharynx, 124, 132

National Health Commission in China, 318

nationalism, 213, 421

National Labor Relations Board, 410

Neisseria meningitidis (epidemic meningitis), 298, 333

New England Journal of Medicine (NEJM) editorial, 92

New Zealand, 40, 43, 71, 107, 433

nomenclature methods for naming SARS-CoV-2, variants, 14

non-COVID-19 drug indications, 251

non-COVID-19 mortality, 255

non-COVID Emergency Department visits, 251

nonwhite race, 133

Norovirus infection (*Norovirus norwalk*), 327

Northwest Evaluation Association, 271

Norway, 61, 78–83, 85, 86, 106, 201, 259, 261
   GDP growth in 2020-2023, 83
   lockdown, cost-benefit analysis, 82
   stringent policy, 83

Novovax recombinant nanoparticle vaccine, 211

O_2 requirements, 128

Obama administration, 102

obesity, 108, 126, 129, 133, 134, 159, 160, 173, 202, 219

Okonjo-Iweala, Ngozi Dr. Chair Gavi Board, 40

older age, 133

Omicron variants, 434, 438, 441

Operation Warp Speed, 207, 227, 232

Our World in Data Statistics and Research COVID-19 Pandemic website, 43

outbreaks, 24, 26–30, 32, 33, 35, 40, 41, 48, 72, 73, 75, 89, 96, 100, 105, 262, 263, 317–325, 327, 334–336, 338, 342, 343, 351, 354–356, 433, 439, 446
   definition of, 322
   environmental source, 323
   incubation period, 319, 320, 347–349, 351–353
   infectious diseases, 321, 324, 328, 330, 333–336, 354–357, 359, 360, 363
   investigation, 12, 62, 152, 162, 318, 353, 356, 403, 421, 422, 440, 442

person-to-person transmission, 8, 9, 319, 321, 322, 325, 332, 349
point-source outbreaks, Figure 8.71, 319
propagated outbreaks, Figure 8.72, 319, 320
vector-borne, 296, 324, 326, 361
outbreak, self-limited, causes, Table 8.22, 320–324
C.difficile colitis, 321
legionellosis, 321
leprosy, 298, 321, 323, 324
Lyme disease, 321
MRSA infection, 323, 324
rabies, 196, 321, 322
tetanus, 196, 224, 321, 322
typhoid fever, 298, 300, 321, 323, 324
West Nile encephalitis, 321
outpatient clinic visits, 251
Oxford-AstraZeneca vaccine, 198
Oxford Coronavirus Government Response Tracker (OxCGRT), 64

Pan American Health Organization (PAHO), 231
pandemic management
early interventions, 422
global vaccination, 423
investigation, 422
R&D, 423
pandemics, xix, xx, 2, 5, 7, 11–13, 16, 37, 70, 93, 108, 262, 272, 291, 295, 302, 303, 317, 320, 331, 335–338, 340, 342, 344, 346, 348, 349, 351, 352, 354, 357, 359–362, 364, 403–406, 408, 409, 414, 418, 421, 422, 440

1918 influenza A, 362, 363
airborne transmission, 124, 324, 350, 352–354, 363
air travel trends, Figure 8.76, 358, 364
asymptomatic infection, 149, 165, 205, 322, 333, 363, 441
bat species diversity, Figure 8.79, 360
body fluid transmission, 324
definition of, 322
droplet transmission, 324
environmental source, 323
factors predisposing to, Table 8.25, 362
fatality rate, 10, 16, 353
fatigue, 77, 93, 94, 97, 122, 156, 157, 158, 203, 206
Germ Theory, 337, 338, 340, 347–350, 361, 362, 364
global warming, Figure 8.77, 322, 349, 357, 358, 418
herd immunity, 10, 11, 76, 78, 80, 82, 91, 92, 107, 205, 210, 320, 340, 342, 362
land use trends, Figure 8.78, 357, 359, 363
mortality, xix, 120, 121, 129, 133, 134, 142–148, 151, 153, 154, 164, 165, 173, 212, 213, 255, 256, 259, 260, 294, 300–302, 322, 324–330, 333–335, 337–340, 344–349, 351–354, 361–364
person-to-person transmission, 8, 319, 321, 322, 325, 332, 349
population size vs infectious disease trends, 329

public health measures, 232, 361

R_0, Figures 1.3, 1.4, Table 8.24,
8-11, 331

SARS-CoV-2 vs influenza A, 172

ship traffic trends, 357

superspreaders, xxi, 123, 317, 348,
354, 355, 357

transmission, Table 1.2, Table 8.24,
8, 9, 331, 332

transmission route, 362

vector-borne, 336

waves, 1, 16, 76, 87, 97, 106, 108,
168, 337, 409, 433, 435

pandemics, causes, 335

cholera (*Vibrio cholerae*), 336

COVID-19 (*Betacoronavirus
SARS-CoV-2*), 6

dengue (*Dengue virus*), 336

dengue, global distribution,
Figure 8.75, 341

HIV (*Lentivirus human
immunodeficiency virus*), 336

influenza (*Orthomyxovirus A*), 352

malaria (*Plasmodium falciparum*),
344

plague (*Yersinia pestis*), 336

Plasmodium falciparum, 336

smallpox mortality over three
centuries, 339

smallpox (*Variola virus*), 336

syphilis (*Treponema pallidum*), 336

tuberculosis (*Mycobacterium
tuberculosis*), 336

SARS-CoV-2, 352–354

SARS-CoV-2 vs 1918 Influenza A",
Table 8.26, 362, 363

yellow fever (*Flavivirus yellow fever
virus*), 335

yellow fever, global distribution,
Figure 8.75, 341

pangolins tissue, 291

Pasteur, Louis Dr. developed rabies
vaccine, 303

pathogenesis, xxi, 146, 158, 159, 161,
167, 356, 362, 413, 419, 423, 443,
445

ACE2 receptor, 120, 159–162, 164,
168

coagulopathy, 159, 167

heart disease, 159

immune response, 159

lung disease, 159

PCR vs. antigen vs. antibodies,
diagnostic testing, Figures 4.50,
4.51, Table 4.48, 130–132

Pence, Mike; Vice President under
President Trump, 89

penicillin, 153, 328, 346, 347

pericardial effusions, 163

peri-coronary adipose tissue
attenuation, CT scan, 164

persistent infection, SARS-CoV-2, 120,
140, 142, 171, 442, 443

personal protective equipment (PPE),
1, 30, 93, 121, 124, 318

person-to-person transmission, 8, 9,
319, 321, 322, 325, 332, 349

pertussis (*Bordetella pertussis*), 196,
224, 262, 333–335

Pfizer-BioNTech vaccines, 204

physical therapy evaluation, 121

plague (*Yersinia pestis*), 336

Plasmodium falciparum (malaria), 336,
344

pneumococcal pneumonia, 145

polio (*Enterovirus poliovirus*)
epidemic, causes, 224

poliovirus infection, 327

politics, minimizing its impact, 409,
410, 411

polymerase chain reaction (PCR), 8, 131

polymorphonuclear (PMN) leukocytes, 162

population fatality rate (PFR), 10

population movement restrictions, 71

possibly effective treatments, 143

pre-competitive drug discovery, 38

pregnant women, 250, 262–264, 436, 437

Pregnant Women & Vaccines against Emerging Epidemic Threats (PREVENT) group, 263

preventing pandemics, Table 9.27, 9.28, 404–407

previous pandemics, 9, 37, 93, 212, 336

propagated outbreaks, 319

prophylactic anticoagulation, 144

public gatherings, 63, 65, 81

public health responses, 95, 107, 168, 409, 410

   contact tracing, 348, 350, 354, 355, 361

   containment, 61, 64, 70, 82, 84, 86, 100, 107, 354,

   elimination, 433, 434

   lockdown, 62, 63, 70–74, 76, 210, 225, 253, 254, 270, 272

   mandating interventions, 268

   mask wearing, 254, 423, 469

   mitigation, 1,15, 23, 41, 43, 45, 82–84, 86, 254

   public health movement, 350

   quarantines, 45, 76

   quick approach, 70, 71

   risk assessment, 27, 28

social distancing, 15, 70, 90, 92–94, 101, 254, 270, 210, 352, 354, 471, 472, 409

surveillance systems, 323

Public Health Emergency of International Concern (PHEIC), 27, 404

public humiliation, 91

public transportation, 27, 63

pulmonary embolism (PE), 138, 139, 441

quarantines, 45, 76

quick approach, 70, 71

rabies (*Rabies virus*), 196, 298, 321, 322, 417

RAND Europe analysis found, 216

randomized clinical trials (RCTs), 142

Rapid European COVID-19 Emergency Response research (RECOVER) Social Sciences team, 232

reassortment process, 12

Redfield, Robert Dr.; Head of the US CDC under President Trump, 89

Reed, Walter Dr., codiscoverer of mosquitos importance in yellow fever transmission, 345

reinfection vs. persistent infection, 120, 140

remdesivir, 28, 126, 148, 170, 258, 353, 444

renin-angiotensin system, 159

respiratory allergies, 356

respiratory diseases, 5, 16, 31, 253, 254

respiratory failure, 29, 159, 161, 166, 441

respiratory tract, 5, 7, 8, 16, 120, 124,
   130, 159, 169–171, 173, 324, 325,
   329, 332, 356, 362, 442
Rickettsia prowazekii (epidemic
   typhus), 298, 326
rituximab, monoclonal antibody
   against CD-20 cell surface receptor,
   436
RNA human pathogens, 417
R$_0$, basic reproduction number, 9,
   321, 325, 332
   mathematical modelling, 320
   herd immunity, 210
routine vaccination decrease, 252
Royal African Company, 301
RSV infections, 253
Rubella virus (rubella), 298, 333
Ryan, Michael Dr. WHO Health
   Emergencies Program, 30

SAGE see Strategic Advisory Group
   of Experts on Immunization (SAGE),
   xxii, 220
SAGE Vaccine Hesitancy working
   group, 229
Salmonella typhi (typhoid fever), 298,
   323, 354
sarilumab, monoclonal antibody
   against interleukin IL-6, 144
SARS-COV-2; see also individual
   entries, xix, 1–4, 6, 7, 10, 13, 14,
   16, 23, 24, 27, 28, 30, 32, 33,
   35, 37, 38, 40, 41, 43, 48, 49,
   54, 61–63, 71, 73, 76, 89, 92, 98,
   99, 100, 102, 105, 108, 119–121,
   123–126, 130–132, 135, 139, 140,
   142, 144–146, 148–153, 155, 156,
   158–163, 165–173, 195, 196, 201,
   205, 209–212, 223, 227, 234, 250,
   251, 255, 258, 260, 261, 263,
   267, 268, 272, 287–297, 303, 304,
   336, 352, 354, 356, 359–363, 403,
   411–413, 416–418, 420, 431–436,
   438, 440–476
   animal host, bats, 362
   animal host, intermediate, 362
   animal host, natural, 362
   evolution of, 292
   flattening the curve, 15, 70
   genomic data, 292, 419
   infection-induced immunity, 10
   intermediate host, 6, 289, 291, 447
   mitigation, 92, 210
   mortality, factors affecting,
      Tables 4.9, 10.30, 8, 142–145,
      439, 444, 445
   mutations, 167, 169, 171, 172, 209,
      297, 438
   origin of, 13, 446
   pangolins tissue, 291
   post-acute sequelae of, 412, 441
   reinfection, 120, 140, 412, 413
   replication cycle of, 4
   source of, 288, 443, 446
   spike protein, 142, 144, 145, 159,
      169, 171, 172, 201, 204, 434,
      438
   spread, WHO region, 24, 41
   structure of, 3
   superspreaders, 123
   survival on surfaces, 125
   variant of concern, 13
SARS-CoV-2 variants, 13, 14, 144,
   209, 210, 431, 434, 435, 436, 438,
   441, 445, 446
   Alpha, 434

Beta, 434

Delta, 434

Gamma, 434

Omicron, 434

scarlet fever, 298, 325, 333, 334

second pandemic wave, 99, 100

  African region, 100

  Americas region, 86

Securities and Exchange Commission, 410

self-limited outbreaks, 321

Semmelweis, Ignac Dr. discovered the importance of handwashing, 303

sepsis and septic shock, 166

Severe Acute Respiratory Syndrome (SARS), 5, 73, 146, 288, 328

Shanghai Laboratory, 27

Shaw, Jana Dr. SUNY Upstate Medical University, 265

Shigella dysenteriae (dysentery), 298, 327

Shigella outbreaks, 327

shortness of breath, COVID-19, 122

sickle cell trait, 345

side effects, drugs 203, 206, 207, 338

Singapore, 6, 43, 71, 354, 433

Sirleaf, Ellen Johnson former Liberian President, 40

slavery, 301, 303, 304

sleep disturbance, 157

smallpox (Variola virus), 336

smell, loss of, 121, 122, 156, 161

Snow, John Dr.; discoverer of the epidemiology of cholera, 303

social distancing, 63, 68, 70, 90, 92–95, 101, 210, 254, 270, 352, 354, 471, 472

Solidarity Call to Action, 37, 38, 213

Solidarity program, 213

South Africa, 13, 23, 48–50, 62, 98, 99, 106, 168, 169, 202, 203, 210, 211, 234, 253, 331, 414

  AstraZeneca vaccine, 211, 234

  cases and deaths, 48–52, 96–98, 106

  intensive care capabilities, 98

South Korea, 27, 30, 43, 71, 108

Staphylococcus aureus, 297, 321, 324

state authority handoff, 90

stay-at-home orders, 63, 467

steroids, 99, 135, 142, 143, 155, 156, 166, 173, 353, 443

Strategic Advisory Group of Experts on Immunization (SAGE), xxii, 220, 221, 228–230

Streptococcus pyogenes (scarlet fever), 298, 333, 334, 354

strokes, 257

suicide rates, 255

superspreaders, xxi, 123, 348, 354, 355, 357

supplemental oxygen, 135, 143

Supply Chain Task Force, 38

surface spike protein, 159

surfaces, SARS-CoV-2 survival, 125

symptoms, 121

surface transmission, 125

Sweden, 23, 45, 46, 61, 78–83, 85, 86, 106, 107, 233, 261, 462

  coronavirus deaths per capita, 79

  daily deaths per capita, 79

  GDP growth in 2020–2023, 83

  limiting public gatherings, 63, 81

  lockdowns, concept of, 78

  pandemic strategy, 81

  public health strategy, 80

  testing and contact tracing, 71, 80

syphilis (Treponema pallidum), 336

technical working groups, 32

Tedros Adhanom Ghebreyesus WHO Director General, 23, 27–30, 32, 38–41, 57, 61, 62, 105, 195, 229, 404–406, 410, 421

Tegnell, Anders Dr., Swedish Public Health Advisor, 78, 80

temporary graves in Hamadan, 466

testing per capita, 504

tetanus (*Clostridium tetani*), 196, 224, 298, 302, 321, 322

tetanus antitoxin, 322

therapeutic anticoagulation, 144, 145, 167

third wave, xxxiii, 48, 87, 234

thromboembolism, 145

tick-borne infection, 322

tocilizumab, 143, 144, 146

Toxic Shock Syndrome, 151

Trade-Related Aspects of Intellectual Property Rights (TRIPS), Figure 9.82, 414, 415

trade restrictions, 32

transmissibility, 12, 14, 212, 351, 434

transmission risk
    healthcare workers, 123
    personal protective equipment, xxiv, 1, 121–124
    superspreaders, xxi, 123, 348, 354, 355, 357
    surfaces, SARS-CoV-2 survival, 125
    symptoms vs no symptoms, 121

transmission risk, 350

transmitted symptomatic COVID-19 disease, 72

travel restriction, 32, 76, 96, 252, 423

treatment effectiveness
    decreased mortality, 142
    ethics, 147, 267
    ineffective, 143, 146, 444
    mortality, impact on, 147
    possibly effective, 143

treatment effectiveness, 142, 443

Treponema pallidum (syphilis), 328

Trump administration, 89, 90–93, 97, 102, 207, 216, 410, 422
    Coronavirus Task Force, 89–91
    first pandemic wave, 87, 89
    press conferences, 91
    public health and medical issues, 91
    public humiliation, 91
    science-based approach, 89
    social distancing, 15, 63, 68, 70, 90, 92–95, 101, 254, 270, 352, 354, 409, 471, 472
    state authority handoff, 90
    vaccine development, 82, 93, 403, 422, 423
    wearing masks, 77, 90, 92–94, 125, 354, 357

tuberculoid leprosy, 324

tuberculosis (*Mycobacterium tuberculosis*), 336

typhoid fever (*Salmonella typhi*), 196, 321, 323

Typhoid Mary, 323

unemployment rates, 2

UNICEF, vaccine delivery, 205, 217

United Nations Children's Fund (UNICEF), 214

United States (US), xxi, xxii, xxiii, xxiv, 14, 16, 31, 38, 44, 48, 49, 52, 74, 77, 79, 84, 86–89, 91–93, 96, 97, 102, 106, 107, 123, 125, 147, 149,

153, 157, 198, 201, 205, 207, 216,
217, 221, 227, 228, 232, 235, 236,
253–255, 257, 259–261, 264–268,
271, 272, 322, 330, 338, 353, 410,
412, 414, 421, 441, 444, 459, 463,
464, 475–478
  CDC (US) recommendations, 92
  per capita mortality rate, 92
  personal protective equipment, 1,
    30, 93, 121, 318
  political issues, 89
  SARS-CoV-2 testing, 43, 89, 92, 98,
    102
University of Washington, 90, 253
USAID Emerging Pandemic Threat
  initiative, 418
USAID's (United States Agency for
  International Development), 38
US COVID-19 vaccination program,
  228
US Department of Veterans Affairs
  healthcare database, 157
US Food and Drug Administration
  (FDA), 92, 201, 436
US National Institute of Health, 412

vaccination efforts, 172, 252, 338,
  423
vaccination program, 208, 211, 216,
  226, 228, 230
vaccines, xix, xx, xxi, xxxiii, 2, 13,
  37–40, 92, 99, 100, 105, 126, 159,
  168, 169, 172, 195–202, 204–220,
  222–235, 237, 238, 250, 253, 254,
  258, 261–263, 265–269, 272, 273,
  295, 328, 334, 335, 352, 353, 361,
  364, 405, 406, 408, 410, 411, 413,
  414, 432–439, 443, 477

vaccine development timeline, Figure
  5.59, 197, 422
vaccine hesitancy, xix, 195, 196, 224,
  228–237, 354
  determinants of vaccine hesitancy,
    229, 230
  governments, recommendations,
    232
  one region impacts other regions,
    233
  overcoming hesitancy, 196, 235,
    236
  regions and countries, xix, 23, 32,
    41, 196, 230
  working group, 229
vaccine passports, 250, 264
vaccine tracker websites, 198
Vahlne, Anders Dr., Karolinska
  Institutet, 80
Values Framework, 220
variant of concern (VoC), 13, 14, 144,
  209, 210, 431, 434, 435, 436, 438,
  441, 445, 446
Varicella zoster virus (chickenpox),
  298, 333
Variola virus (smallpox), 298, 336, 338
vascular system, 135
vector-borne, 321, 324, 326, 361
ventilators, xxvi, xxviii, xxxi, xxxii, 39,
  90, 122, 124, 128, 143–145, 147,
  164, 166, 258, 259
ventricular dilatation, 164
Vibrio cholerae (cholera), 336, 348
viral genomic data, 419
viral RNA transcription, 144
viral shedding, 353, 363
viral spike protein, 4
viral transmission, 12, 418, 444

viral vector vaccines, 435
Virological.org, 27
vitamin B12 deficiency, 156
vitamin D deficiency, 156
VoC *see* variant of concern (VoC), 13

water treatment, 323
wearing masks, 63, 77, 90, 92–94,
    125, 354, 357
WeChat, 73
Wellcome Trust, 39, 61, 201
West African Health Organization, 32
wet markets, 5, 6, 291–293, 304
WHA *see* World Health Assembly
    (WHA), 40, 405
Whitmer, Gretchen, Michigan
    Governor, 95
work and school closures, 63
World Bank, 39, 52, 101, 108, 214,
    330
World Health Assembly (WHA), 40,
    405
World Health Organization (WHO),
    1, 2, 6–8, 24, 26–35, 37–41, 51,
    52, 54, 62, 77, 80, 93, 94, 98, 99,
    101, 102, 105, 108, 143, 195,
    196, 212, 213, 215, 218, 219, 220,
    228, 231–234, 252, 253, 257, 258,
    261–266, 288, 292, 293, 324, 329,

330, 338, 340, 343, 345–347, 350,
    404, 405, 407, 409, 410, 421, 422,
    432, 435, 439
COVID-19 Tools Accelerator
    programs, 37
global health program, 39
Global Influenza Plan, 7
Health Emergencies Program, 30,
    404
Joint Allocation Taskforce, 219
pandemic fatigue, 77, 93, 94, 97
Solidarity Call to Action, 37, 213
Solidarity program, 195, 213
Strategic Advisory Group of Experts
    on Immunization, xxii, 220
technical reports, 41, 61, 62
Values Framework, 220
World Trade Organization (WTO), 414
Wuhan, 1, 2, 6, 26–29, 71–73, 75,
    136, 152, 288, 290–292, 421

yellow fever (*Yellow fever virus*), 336
Yersinia pestis (plague), 298, 336

zero-COVID elimination policy, 433
Zika virus infection (*Flavivirus Zika*),
    326
Zika virus outbreak, 28, 263
zoonotic disease emergence, 296

Figures and Tables

Figure Number	Title	Page
1.1	Structure of SARS-CoV-2	3
1.2	Replication cycle of SARS-CoV-2	4
1.3	The effect of R_0 (basic reproduction number) on how many cases occur in the next generation of a propagated outbreak.	10
1.4	The relation between the basic reproduction number of a virus, R0, and the proportion of the population that needs to be immunized to achieve herd immunity.	11
1.5	Flattening the curve.	15
2.6	Confirmed cases of COVID-19, by WHO region and epidemiological week, from Dec 31, 2019 to March 10, 2020.	24
2.7	Countries, territories or areas with reported confirmed cases of COVID-19, 25 as of March 10, 2020.	25
2.8	Epidemic curves of the estimated number of infections and observed number of new cases, along with the weekly mean lag time between the date of diagnosis, cumulative hospitalization rate and government reactions, measures, and major events in Wuhan from December 14, 2019 to February 23, 2020.3	26
2.9	Cumulative total COVID-19 cases reported by region in Africa from February 16 to May 22, 2020.	31
2.10	Total cumulative worldwide cases and deaths of COVID-19 from January 22 to December 30, 2020.	36
2.11	Total confirmed COVID-19 cases from February 23, 2020 to December 30. 2020.	42
2.12	Total cumulative deaths from COVID-19 by WHO region from March 8, 2020 to December 30, 2020.	42

2.13   Cumulative confirmed COVID-19 cases per million population.   43
        Comparison of China, India, Asia, and the World from January
        2020 to December 30, 2020.

2.14   Daily new confirmed COVID-19 deaths per million population.   44
        Comparison of China, India, Asia, and the World from January
        2020 to December 30, 2020.

2.15   Cumulative confirmed COVID-19 cases per million population.   46
        Comparison of Norway, Sweden, Europe, and the World from
        January 22, 2020 to December 30, 2020.

2.16   Cumulative confirmed COVID-19 deaths per million population.   46
        Comparison of Norway, Sweden, Europe, and the World from
        January 22, 2020 to December 30, 2020.

2.17   Cumulative confirmed COVID-19 cases per million population   47
        in the US, Canada, and the World from January 1, 2020 to
        December 30, 2020.

2.18   Cumulative confirmed COVID-19 deaths per million population   47
        in the US, Canada, and the World from January 1, 2020 to
        December 30, 2020.

2.19   Total COVID-19 tests done per 1,000 population from January 1,   49
        2020 to December 28, 2020.

2.20   Cumulative confirmed COVID-19 cases per million population.   50
        Comparison of South Africa, all other African countries, and the
        World from January 22, 2020 to December 27, 2020.

2.21   Cumulative confirmed COVID-19 deaths per million population.   50
        Comparison of South Africa, all other African countries and the
        World from January 22 2020 to December 27, 2020.

2.22   Cumulative confirmed COVID-19 cases in the WHO Middle East   51
        region
        from January 29, 2020 to January 5, 2021.

2.23   Cumulative confirmed COVID-19 deaths in the WHO Middle   52
        East region
        from January 29, 2020 to January 5, 2021.

2.24   Cumulative confirmed COVID-19 cases per million population.   53
        Comparison of Jordan and Iran from January 22, 2020 to
        December 30, 2020.

2.25   Cumulative confirmed COVID-19 deaths per million population. 53
        Comparison of Jordan and Iran from January 22, 2020 to
        December 30, 2020.

3.26   The overall Stringency Index of Government Polices for COVID-19, 65
        as of December 29, 2020.4 The Index is based on nine metrics
        that include school closures, workplace closures, cancellations
        of public events, restrictions of public gatherings, closure of
        public transport, stay at home requirements, public information
        campaigns, restrictions on internal movements, and international
        travel controls.

3.27   Stay at home component metric of the Stringency Index for 66
        COVID-19 from January 21, 2019 to December 31, 2020.

3.28   Stringency of workplace closure policy metric of the Stringency 66
        Index from January 21, 2019 to December 31, 2020.

3.29   Stringency of public transport closure policy metric of the Strin- 67
        gency Index from January 21, 2019 to December 31, 2020.

3.30   Stringency of testing people for evidence of COVID-19 infection 67
        metric of the Stringency Index from COVID-19 from January 21,
        2019 to December 29, 2020.

3.31   Stringency of contact tracing policy metric for the Stringency Index 68
        from January 21, 2019 to December 29, 2020.

3.32   Stringency of face covering policy metric of the Stringency Index 68
        from January 21, 2019 to December 29, 2020.

3.33   Government support of an individual's income metric of the 69
        Stringency Index from January 21, 2019 to December 31, 2020.

3.34   Government support of debt or contract relief for citizens Strin- 69
        gency Index from January 21, 2019 to December 31, 2020.

3.35   Reported outbreaks of COVID-19 in China in 2020. 72

3.36   Impact of the COVID-19 pandemic on China's economy when 74
        comparing the pre-pandemic period in 2019 and during the
        pandemic in 2020.

3.37   Impact of the COVID-19 pandemic on India's GDP from October 75
        2019 to June 2020.

3.38   Cumulative confirmed COVID-19 deaths per million population 79
        from January 22, 2020 to December 31, 2020 in the World and
        the nine countries highlighted in Chapter 3.

3.39   Norway's and Sweden's predicted GDP growth in 2020–2023. 83

3.40   International Money Fund (IMF)-predicted GDP growth in 2021   84
         for each country.

3.41   Early policy stringency and cumulative mortality† from COVID-19   85
         — 37 European countries, January 23 to June 30, 2020.

3.42   Cumulative confirmed map of COVID-19 deaths per million   87
         population, as of December 31, 2020.

3.43   This map shows areas of concern around the US on December 16,   88
         2020. Red counties are "sustained hotspots" with high sustained
         caseloads and a higher risk of health care capacity issues.

3.44   The percentages of Americans who have worn masks from April   94
         to September 2020.

3.45   Americans' social distancing habits from March to September 2020.   95

3.46   Iran's reported GDP from 2015 to 2020 and predicted GDP from   103
         2021 to 2025.

3.47   The GDP in Jordan from 1986 to 2019, with projections up until   104
         2026.

3.48   The case fatality rate in the World, Africa, Canada, China, India,   106
         Jordan, Norway, South Africa, Sweden, and the US, March 14 to
         December 31, 2020.

4.49   Case #2. X-ray, CT scan.   127

4.50   Time course for the detection of SARS-CoV-2 RNA (grey line),   130
         viral antigens (red line), and antibodies (blue lines).

4.51   Diagnostic testing available for SARS-CoV-2 infection: (a) PCR,   131
         (b) Antigens, (c) Antibodies.

4.52   Case #3. Chest CT angiogram   135

4.53   Case #3. COVID-consistent laboratory abnormalities with   137
         improvement after treatment (6-day period).

4.54   Case #4. (a) Admission Chest X-ray showing bilateral infiltrates,   140
         (b) Admission Chest CT showing bilateral ground glass infiltrates.

4.55   Case #4. COVID-consistent laboratory abnormalities (8-day period).   141

4.56   Hypothesis: Increased ACE-2 receptor density on bronchial   160
         mucosa (curving pink surface) leads to worse inflammation with
         COVID-19 infection.

4.57   Hypothesis: Chronic SARS-CoV-2 infection occurs and is tissue   170
         specific.

4.58   Relationship between mutation rate and species genome size.

5.59   Timeline for development of various vaccines.   197

5.60   The relative percentage of various vaccine platforms for the   198
        COVID-19 vaccine that are in clinical trials at the end of 2020.

5.61   Diagram of the three platforms used to make various COVID-19   204
        vaccines.

5.62   Diagram of the operation of an mRNA vaccine.   205

5.63   Countries that began vaccinating its population with a COVID-19   218
        vaccine prior to January 1, 2021.

5.64   Vaccination prioritization policies of various countries.   222

5.65   COVID-19 vaccines administrated per 100 people by the end of   225
        February 2020 in the countries highlighted in Chapter 3, except
        for Jordan and Iran (who had not yet received any vaccines at
        that time).

5.66   Percentage of negative media coverage in the US versus   236
        international media coverage.

5.67   Share of people vaccinated with at least one dose of COVID-19   237
        vaccines, as of June 30, 2021.

6.68   COVID-19 deaths compared with all-cause mortality in the US.   256

7.69   Ecology of coronaviruses causing severe disease in humans.   289

7.70   Historically important infectious diseases. Their rate of   299
        occurrence is accelerating. 100 million years ago (MYA) to
        2020 CE. YA = years ago.

8.71   Point-source outbreak.   319

8.72   Propagated outbreak.   320

8.73   A comparison of mortality per 100,000 population for 12 historic   330
        infectious diseases seen in the last 260 years.

8.74   Patterns of smallpox mortality in London, England, over three   339
        centuries.

8.75   Similar global distribution of yellow fever (top, 1960–2005) and   341
        dengue (bottom, 1960-2005).

8.76   Increasing global air travel in the last 80 years (1936–2016), trillions   358
        of passenger-kilometres per year.

8.77   Global warming from 1850 to 2020.   358

8.78   Estimated increases in land use for cropland and grazing. 100AD 359
        to 2016.

8.79   Estimated increase in the local number of bat species due to shifts 360
        in their geographical ranges driven by climate change between
        the 1901–1930 and 1990–2019 periods.

8.80   The appearance of historically important emerging infectious 360
        diseases in relationship to the global population.

9.81   Viral quasi-species are an important mechanism for the evolution 411
        of new coronavirus species.

9.82   A map outlines which countries support or oppose the move of 415
        waiving COVID-19 medical patents. Last updated: May 28, 2021.

9.83   Viral quasi-species are an important mechanism for the evolution 419
        of new coronavirus species, likely in bats as well.

10.84   Cumulative COVID-19 deaths per million population from January 432
        22, 2020 to June 30, 2022, in the world and the nine countries
        highlighted in Chapters 2 and 3.

10.85   COVID-19 vaccine doses administered per 100 people as of 433
        June 3, 2022.

10.86   John Hopkins University COVID-19 Maternal Immunization Tracker 437
        (COMIT) showing the status of each country's recommendation
        for whether pregnant women should receive the vaccine.

11.87   COVID-19 testing.   459
11.88   Stores sold out.   460
11.89   Emergency rooms overflowed with COVID-19 patients.   461
11.90   ICUs overflowed.   461
11.91   Hospitals overflowed.   462
11.92   We experienced ventilator, dialysis machine, drugs, and oxygen 463
        shortages.
11.93   Respect for the dying.   464
11.94   One angel for every patient that died   464
11.95   Requiring unprecedented body storage methods.   465
11.96   Some parts of the world allowed funerals to be attended.   466
11.97   Some funerals could not be attended.   466
11.98   Mass COVID-19 cemeteries.   467

11.99   COVID-19 lockdown.   467

11.100   Empty airports   468

11.101   Near empty airplanes   468

11.102   Some wore masks.   469

11.103   Some did not wear masks.   469

11.104   Some schools were closed   470

11.105   Some schools stayed open.   470

11.106   Social protests happened globally.   471

11.107   Some socialized in spite of social distancing.   471

11.108   Music in spite of social distancing.   472

11.109   Love in the pandemic with masks.   472

11.110   Love in the pandemic without masks.   473

11.111   You can't quarantine love.   473

11.112   Love, Hope, Faith during the pandemic.   474

11.113   Celebrating healthcare workers 1.   474

11.114   Celebrating healthcare workers 2.   475

11.115   Celebrating healthcare workers 3.   475

11.116   Optimism during the pandemic 1.   476

11.117   Optimism during the pandemic 2.   476

11.118   Vaccines brought hope.   477

11.119   We must remember those we lost.   488

Table Number	Name	Page
1.1	Severe Acute Respiratory Disease (SARS) Outbreaks Due To Coronaviruses First Detected in Humans during the 21st Century	2
1.2	Transmission and Mortality Rates of Previous Pandemics	9
3.3	Interventions that can help enable effective containment and mitigation of COVID-19.	63
4.4	Adult manifestations of COVID-19.	122
4.5	Emergency Department vital signs, O2 requirements.	128
4.6	Laboratory abnormalities in COVID-19 patients admitted to the hospital.	128
4.7	Chest imaging abnormalities in COVID-19 adult patients admitted to the hospital.	129
4.8	Sensitivity and/or specificity of PCR for SARS-CoV-2 versus antibody tests for diagnosing COVID-19 infection.	132
4.9	COVID-19 treatments tried globally through midyear 2021.	143
4.10	Signs and symptoms in pediatric (<18 years old) and adult (18–64 years old) patients with laboratory-confirmed COVID-19 (United States, February 12 to April 2, 2020).*	150
4.11	Case definition for Multisystem Inflammatory Syndrome in Children (MIS-C).	150
4.12	Clinical and pathologic findings that can help distinguish Kawasaki disease from MIS-C.	151
5.13	Characteristics of COVID-19 vaccines with published Phase 3 trial data being used by the end of 2020.	199
5.14	Additional COVID-19 vaccines characteristics.	200
5.15	Demographics and characteristics of the Phase 3 studies of the Pfizer, Moderna, AstraZeneca, and Gamaleya vaccines.	202
5.16	Pillars of the ACT-Accelerator.	214
5.17	WHO's values framework for allocation and prioritization of COVID-19 vaccination.	220
5.18	Vaccine Hesitancy Determinants.	230
5.19	Survey of the willingness of those living in various countries in different regions to be vaccinated with a COVID-19 vaccine.	231
7.20	Historically important emerging infectious diseases: 1940 to 2020.	297

7.21   Historically important emerging infectious diseases: Pre-1940.   298

8.22   Infectious diseases that cause self-limited outbreaks.   321

8.23   Infectious diseases that cause epidemics.   325

8.24   Infectious diseases that cause pandemics.   331

8.25   Summary of factors predisposing to pandemics.   362

8.26   Pandemic SARS-CoV-2 versus pandemic 1918 Influenza A.   363

9.27   Twelve different commissions and panels have examined outbreaks, epidemics, and pandemics, and the International Health Regulations (2005) during the past decade.   406

9.28   A timetable for immediate action. Who needs to do what, and when created by the Independent Panel for Pandemic Preparedness and Response for the WHO Executive Board.   407

9.29   Well known RNA human pathogens with bat reservoirs.   417

10.30   Revised COVID-19 treatment recommendations (compare with Table 4.6).   444